PAIN IN OSTEOARTHRITIS

PAIN IN OSTEOARTHRITIS

Edited by

David T. Felson MD, MPH
Department of Clinical Epidemiology
Boston University School of Medicine

Hans-Georg Schaible MD
Friedrich Schiller University of Jena

WILEY-BLACKWELL

A JOHN WILEY & SONS, INC., PUBLICATION

Published by John Wiley & Sons, Inc., Hoboken, New Jersey
Published simultaneously in Canada

Wiley-Blackwell is an imprint of John Wiley & Sons, formed by the merger of Wiley's global Scientific, Technical, and Medical business with Blackwell Publishing.

For general information on our other products and services or for technical support, please contact our Customer Care Department within the United States at (800) 762-2974, outside the United States at (317) 572-3993 or fax (317) 572-4002.

Wiley also publishes its books in a variety of electronic formats. Some content that appears in print may not be available in electronic formats. For more information about Wiley products, visit our web site at www.wiley.com.

Library of Congress Cataloging-in-Publication Data:

Pain in osteoarthritis / [edited by] David T. Felson, Hans-Georg Schaible.
    p. ; cm.
  Includes bibliographical references.
  ISBN 978-0-470-40388-4 (cloth)
1. Osteoarthritis–Complications. 2. Pain. I. Felson, David T. II. Schaible, H. -G.
[DNLM: 1. Osteoarthritis–physiopathology. 2. Pain–therapy. WE 348 P144 2008]
RC931.O67P35 2008
616.7′223–dc22

                                           2008049891

Printed in the United States of America

10 9 8 7 6 5 4 3 2 1

CONTENTS

PREFACE

In patients with osteoarthritis, pain is the key determinant of the decision to seek care, and the central symptom of their illness affecting their quality of life and ability to carry out their daily tasks. Pain and its relief are also the main focus of treatment, especially given the absence of structure modifying therapy for osteoarthritis. Given the centrality of pain to both the therapeutic contract between the clinician and the patient and as the patient's overriding symptom, it is surprising that previous books on osteoarthritis have not focused more prominently on this aspect of disease.

Perhaps one reason for the avoidance of a focus on pain might be the belief that pain originates in a diseased joint and that understanding the causes of disease and correcting the pathology would naturally result in alleviating the pain. For example, in rheumatoid arthritis the success in targeting the underlying inflammatory process has genuinely stabilized disease or even placed it in remission with attendant pain reduction. Why should osteoarthritis be any different?

By the time a person has clinical osteoarthritis, his/her joint has probably experienced longstanding cartilage wear, bony remodeling, perhaps modest synovial inflammation, and a weakness in bridging muscles. The structure of the joint may well have been remodeled. Many of the changes visible on MRI in patients even with early symptoms are impressive and suggest that pathology is extensive and has existed for some time prior to the development of symptoms. Our ability to reverse this pathology and create a healthier painless joint may be limited. Our attempts at pharmacologically protecting cartilage to prevent from further wearing away have not been successful, and it is arguable whether protecting 'cartilage in the face of extensive pathology involving structures outside, of cartilage is likely to be effective. Thus, new ideas in terms of treating the joint and alleviating pain in patients with osteoarthritis are needed.

In persons without disease, pain is a sensory experience that tells the body to avoid particular activities and motivates the person to avoid exposing the body to painful stimuli. During acute and chronic joint disease, the peripheral and central nociceptive system is often in a state of sensitization, forcing the patient to restrict movements of the afflicted joint and to avoid loading of the joint. In the long term, this, protective reaction may change and turn into a maladaptive state in which protective mechanisms may not operate in their normal way. Evidence, much of it summarized in this book, suggests that the mechanisms of pain in osteoarthritis may extend beyond the normal protective functioning of pain. It is thus likely that nervous system changes and pathological pain processes may, for many patients with osteoarthritis, be the source of their most severe, troublesome pain, pain that is the most disabling and causes the most problems with their daily functioning. Providing an understanding of this dysfunctional pain is a major goal of this book.

Understanding the pain of osteoarthritis involves a new multidisciplinary approach that combines insights from neuroscience with expertise in joint anatomy and physiology. It requires an understanding of how the peripheral nervous system works to transmit pain impulses to the central nervous system and when those messages become pathologically augmented. It also requires an understanding of how excess focal loading across a joint might cause damage to joint structures stimulating nociceptive fibers. Both the neuron and articular pathologies combine to provide a comprehensive picture of what causes pain in osteoarthritis.

In this book, the initial chapters describe the pathophysiology of the articular nervous system pathology of this system in states like osteoarthritis. In the second part, we cover the pain experience in osteoarthritis and clinical factors that contribute to that experience. Lastly, we provide for the clinician caring for patients with osteoarthritis a new paradigm about how to approach treatment, orienting treatment toward the different types of pathophysiology that pain may represent. On the one hand, pain may arise from the inflammatory changes that occur in joints with osteoarthritis. On the other hand, it may arise because of pathologic modifications of the peripheral nervous system, which enhance pain experience. Lastly, pain may arise from abnormal mechanical loading that targeted treatment may correct. We hope that this book provides clinicians who are caring for osteoarthritis patients with an appreciation, for the complexity of their pain and some creative approaches to diagnosing and treating their symptoms.

DAVID T. FELSON
HANS-GEORG SCHAIBLE

ACKNOWLEDGMENTS

For DTF: I appreciate the forebearance and support of my wife, Elaine, and daughter, Rachel, and my father who taught me to welcome and be excited by new approaches to difficult problems.

For H-GS: I thank my family for great support and patience, and I appreciate the enthusiasm and input of all my colleagues who share with me the interest and work on neurobiological mechanisms of pain.

I thank Mrs. Sabine Oppermann for her help with the book.

CONTRIBUTORS

Kim Louise Benneil, PhD, Director, Centre for Health, Exercise & Sports Medicine, School of Physiotherapy, The University of Melbourne, 202 Berkeley Street, Melbourne, Victoria 3010, Australia

David R. Blake, MD, FRCP, The Royal National Hospital for Rheumatic Diseases, Bath BA1 1RL, United Kingdom and School for Health, University of Bath, Claverton Down BA2 7AY, United Kingdom

Douglas Bourne, MSc, Faculty of Kinesiology, University of Calgary, 2500 University Drive, NW, Calgary AB T2N IN4, Canada

Kenneth D. Brandt, MD, Clinical Professor of Medicine, Kansas University Medical Center, 5755 Windsor Drive, Fairway, Kansas 66205, USA

Philip G. Conaghan, MBBS, PhD, FRACP, FRCP, Section of Musculoskeletal Disease, Leeds Institute of Molecular Medicine, University of Leeds, Leeds LS9 7TF, United Kingdom

Paul Creamer, MD, FRCP, Consultant Rheumatologist, Southmead Hospital, Bristol BS10 5NB, United Kingdom

David T. Felson, MD, MPH, Boston University School of Medicine, 650 Albany Street, Suite 200, Boston, Massachusetts 02118, USA

Blair D. Grubb, BSc, PhD, Department of Cell Physiology and Pharmacology, University of Leicester, PO Box 138, Leicester LEI 9HN, United Kingdom

Richard C. Haigh, MRCP, Department of Rheumatology, Royal Devon & Exeter Hospital (Wonford), Exeter EX2 5DW, United Kingdom

James L. Henry, PhD, Michael G. DeGroote Institute for Pain Research and Care, McMaster University, Health Sciences Centre 1J11, 1200 Main Street West, Hamilton, Ontario L8N 3Z5, Canada

Monica Herrera, MD, Department of Pharmacology, College of Medicine, University of Arizona, 1656 East Mabel, Room 118, Tucson, Arizona 85724, USA

Walter Herzog, PhD, Faculties of Kinesiology, Engineering, and Medicine, University of Calgary, 2500 University Drive NW, Calgary AB T2N 1N4, Canada

Rana Shane Hinman, PhD, Centre for Health, Exercise and Sports Medicine, School of Physiotherapy, The University of Melbourne, 202 Berkeley Street, Melbourne, Victoria 3010, Australia

Michael Anthony Hunt, MPT, PhD, Centre for Health, Exercise & Sports Medicine, School of Physiotherapy, The University of Melbourne, 202 Berkeley Street, Melbourne, Victoria 3010, Australia

Julia J. Inglis, Research Associate, Kennedy Institute of Rheumatology, Imperial College London, London W6 8LH, United Kingdom

Juan Miguel Jimenez-Andrade, PhD, Department of Pharmacology, College of Medicine, University of Arizona, 1656 East Mabel, Room 118, Tucson, Arizona 85724, USA

Bruce L. Kidd, Professor of Clinical Rheumatology, Barts & The London School of Medicine & Dentistry, London E1 2AD, United Kingdom

Jenny Lewis, PhD, MSc DiPCOT, The Royal National Hospital for Rheumatic Diseases, Bath BA1 1RL, United Kingdom

Patrick W. Mantyh, PhD, Department of Pharmacology, College of Medicine, University of Arizona, 1656 East Mabel, Tucson, Arizona 85724 and Research Service VA Medical Center, Minneapolis, Minnesota 55417, USA

Paul I. Mapp, MD, Academic Department of Rheumatology, University of Nottingham, City Hospital, Clinical Sciences Building, Nottingham NG5 1PB, United Kingdom

Candida S. McCabe, PhD, RGN, The Royal National Hospital for Rheumatic Diseases, Bath BA1 1RL, United Kingdom and School for Health, University of Bath, Claverton Down BA2 7AY, United Kingdom

Jason J. McDougall, AHFMR Senior Scholar, Arthritis Society Investigator, Department of Physiology and Pharmacology, University of Calgary, 3330 Hospital Drive NW, Calgary, Alberta T2N 4N1, Canada

Tuhina Neogi, MD, FRCPC, Boston University School of Medicine, 650 Albany Street, Suite 200, Boston, Massachusetts 02118, USA

Gunnar Ordeberg, MD, PhD, Department, of Orthopaedics, University Hospital, SE-751 85 Uppsala, Sweden

Hans-George Schaible, MD, Friedrich-Schiller University of Jena, Institute of Physiology, University Hospital of Jena, Teichgraben 8, D-07740 Jena, Germany

Joachim Scholz, MD, Department of Anesthesia and Critical Care, Massachusetts General Hospital, Neural Plasticity Research Group, 149 13th Street, Room 4309, Charlestown, Massachusetts 02129, USA

Nicholas G. Shenker, MRCP, Department of Rheumatology, Addenbrooke's Hospital, Cambridge University NHS Foundation Trust, Cambridge CB2 2QQ, United Kingdom

Peter A. Simkin, MD, Division of Rheumatology, University of Washington, Box 356428, Seattle, Washington 98195, USA

Aliaa Rehan Youssef, Faculty of Kinesiology, University of Calgary, 2500 University Drive NW, Calgary AB T2N 1N4, Canada

PART I

THE NEUROSCIENCE OF ARTICULAR PAIN

1

SPINAL MECHANISMS CONTRIBUTING TO JOINT PAIN

Hans-Georg Schaible

Department of Physiology, Friedrich-Schiller University of Jena, Teichgraben 8, D-07740 Jena, Germany

INTRODUCTION

Nociceptive input from the joint is processed in different types of spinal cord neurons. A proportion of these neurons are only activated by mechanical stimulation of the joint and other deep tissue (e.g., adjacent muscles). Other neurons are activated by mechanical stimulation of the joint, muscles, and skin. The majority of the neurons are wide dynamic range neurons (small responses to innocuous pressure to deep tissue and stronger and graded responses to noxious mechanical stimulation). Importantly, neurons with joint input show pronounced hyperexcitability during development of joint inflammation (enhanced responses to mechanical stimulation of the inflamed joint as well as to healthy adjacent deep structures, reduction of mechanical threshold in high threshold neurons, and expansion of the receptive field). Thus inflammation induces neuroplastic changes in the spinal cord, which alter nociceptive processing. This state of hyperexcitability is maintained during persistent

Pain in Osteoarthritis, Edited by David T. Felson and Hans-Georg Schaible

3

inflammation. The neurons are under strong control of descending inhibition, which increases during the acute phase of inflammation. Several transmitters and mediators contribute to the generation and maintenance of inflammation-induced spinal hyperexcitability including glutamate, substance P, neurokinin A, CGRP, and prostaglandins. The latter compounds show enhanced release and an altered release pattern during inflammation in the joint.

PAIN SENSATION IN THE JOINT

Sensory information from muscle and joint influences the motoric system and is involved in the sense of movement and position but usually this does not reach consciousness. The major conscious sensation in deep tissue such as joint and muscle is pain. In a normal joint, pain is most commonly elicited by twisting or hitting the joint. In awake humans, direct stimulation of fibrous structures with innocuous mechanical stimuli evoked pressure sensations. Pain was elicited when noxious mechanical, thermal, and chemical stimuli were applied to the fibrous structures such as ligaments and fibrous cartilage.[1,2] No pain was elicited by stimulation of cartilage, and stimulation of normal synovial tissue rarely evoked pain.[1]

Joint inflammation is characterized by hyperalgesia and persistent pain at rest that is usually dull and badly localized.[1,3,4] Hyperalgesia means that the application of noxious stimuli causes stronger pain than normal, and that pain is even evoked by mechanical stimuli whose intensity is normally not sufficient to elicit pain (i.e., movements in the working range and gentle pressure, e.g., during palpation). This heightened pain sensitivity results from peripheral sensitization (increase of sensitivity of nociceptive primary afferent neurons[5]) and central sensitization (hyperexcitability of nociceptive neurons in the central nervous system).

Pain resulting from degenerative osteoarthritis (OA) shows similarities and differences to inflammatory arthritic pain. Osteoarthritic pain is usually localized to the joint with OA but it can be referred (e.g., hip OA may cause knee pain). It varies in intensity and is usually worsened by exercise (weight-bearing, movement) and relieved at rest. It is usually episodic but may be constantly present in advanced OA. A particular quality of OA pain is pain at night.[6] The *site* of OA pain and the *nature* of OA pain are under discussion because the cartilage is not innervated[7] and because there is a poor correlation between radiological signs (narrow joint space and osteophytes) and the occurrence of joint pain.[6] Some recent studies used magnetic resonance imaging (MRI) and found that painful OA knee joints exhibit more MRI abnormalities than nonpainful OA joints. Pathological findings in MRI studies are synovial hypertrophy and synovial effusions as well as subchondral bone marrow edema lesions (which may increase intraosseal pressure).[8] These data and the observation of inflammatory cells in the sublining tissue[6] evoked a discussion to which extent OA pain is evoked by inflammatory mechanisms that appear from time to time (possibly corresponding to painful episodes in chronic OA). At later stages, capsular fibrosis and muscle contracture around the joint may contribute to OA pain. Quite clearly, however, factors such as obesity, perceived helplessness, and other psychological factors influence OA pain as well.[6]

SPINAL CORD NEURONS THAT RESPOND TO MECHANICAL STIMULATION OF THE JOINT

The articular nerves supplying the knee or elbow joint of rat, cat, and monkey enter the spinal cord via several dorsal roots, thus projecting to several spinal segments. Due to the widely distributed projection area, joint afferents influence sensory neurons and reflex pathways in several spinal segments. Within the gray matter, knee joint afferents project to the superficial lamina I and to the deep laminae V–VII.[7] Figure 1.1A shows the spinal termination fields of horseradish peroxidase-labeled knee joint afferents in the segment L7 in the cat spinal cord. Correspondingly, spinal cord neurons that are synaptically activated by joint afferents can be identified in the superficial and deep dorsal horn and also in the ventral horn.[9,10]

Receptive Fields and Activation Thresholds of Neurons with Joint Input

In both cat and rat, mechanonociceptive inputs from the joint are processed in dorsal horn neurons that respond solely to mechanical stimulation of deep tissue, or in neurons that respond to mechanical stimulation of both deep tissue and the skin. Receptive fields of single sensory neurons (regions from which neurons can be activated) are usually not restricted to the joint but more extended. Figure 1.1C shows the receptive field of a spinal cord neuron with convergent inputs from skin, deep tissue, and the knee joint. The neuron was activated by pressure applied to the knee joint (capsule, ligaments) and also by compression of the quadriceps muscle in the thigh and the gastrocnemius–soleus muscle in the lower leg, and in addition it had a cutaneous receptive field at the paw. However, many neurons have receptive fields that are restricted to the deep tissue. Figure 1.1D shows the receptive field of a spinal cord neuron with a receptive field in the deep tissue of the leg and in the knee joint. Some neurons have bilateral receptive fields.[7]

Concerning mechanical thresholds, neurons are either nociceptive-specific (NS) or wide-dynamic-range (WDR) neurons. Nociceptive-specific neurons respond only to intense pressure and/or to painful movements such as forceful supination and pronation. These stimuli elicit pain. WDR neurons respond to both innocuous pressure and noxious pressure, encoding stimulus intensity by

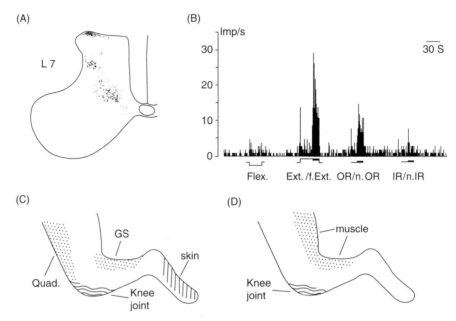

Figure 1.1. Spinal projection of primary afferent fibers of the knee joint and response properties of spinal cord neurons with input from the knee joint. (A) Spinal termination field of horseradish peroxidase-labeled primary afferent fibers of the posterior articular nerve of the knee joint in the gray matter of the segment L7 in the cat. (B) Responses of a wide dynamic range neuron with input from the knee joint to innocuous and noxious movements of the knee joint. The histograms show the number of action potentials per second that were elicited by the movements (bin width 1 s). Flex, flexion of the knee joint; Ext., extension of the knee joint; f.Ext, forced extension of the knee joint; OR, outward rotation of the knee joint (supination); n.OR, noxious outward rotation of the knee joint; IR, inward rotation of the knee joint (pronation); n.IR, noxious inward rotation of the knee joint. (C) Receptive field of a spinal cord neuron with input from the knee joint. This neuron was excited by pressure applied to the skin of the paw, the deep tissue of thigh (quadriceps muscle), and lower leg (gastrocnemius–soleus muscle) and the structures of the knee joint. (D) Receptive field of a spinal cord neuron that was only excited by pressure applied to deep tissue (muscles) and the knee joint. (Part A from Ref. 77; B–D from Ref. 10).

the frequency of action potentials. They may also be weakly activated by movements in the working range, but they show much stronger responses to painful movements. Figure 1.1B displays the response pattern of a WDR neuron with joint input. The neuron exhibited small responses to flexion, extension, and outward rotation (OR) of the knee in its physiological range, but pronounced responses were elicited by forced extension (f.Ext.) and by noxious outward rotation (n.OR) exceeding the working range of the joint. By and large, NS neurons have smaller receptive fields restricted to deep tissue in joint and muscle, and they do not have a receptive field in the skin.[5,7]

Supraspinal and Spinal Projections of Spinal Neurons with Joint Input

Neurons with joint input project to different supraspinal sites (cerebellum, spinocervical nucleus, thalamus, reticular formation) or to intraspinal (segmental) interneurons and motoneurons.[7] Ascending projections to the thalamus (in the spinothalamic tract) are important to activate the thalamocortical systems that generate the conscious pain sensation. In the cat, neurons were identified that have cell bodies in the ventral horn, belong to the spinoreticular tract, and are predominantly or exclusively excited by noxious stimulation of deep tissue.[11,12] Segmental projections are important for the generation of motor and sympathetic reflexes. Spinal and supraspinal motor reflexes regulate movements and exert protective functions including flexor reflexes upon nociceptive stimulation.[4] Noxious stimulation of joint afferents can evoke nociceptive withdrawal reflexes.[7,13] During acute chemical stimulation of the knee and during inflammation in the joint, spinal motor reflexes are enhanced.[13–15] Articular dysfunction and ligamentous strain may cause muscle spasms.[16] However, there is some evidence that the reflex pattern of γ-motoneurons changes in the course of inflammation such that inhibitory reflexes are generated.[15] The latter may create a new motoric balance and allow the leg with an inflamed knee to be kept in midposition. In midposition, the nociceptive outflow from the inflamed joint is at a minimum.

Inhibition by Heterotopic and Descending Inhibitory Systems

Neurons with joint input are inhibited by heterotopic noxious stimuli, in line with the concept of diffuse noxious inhibitory controls (DNICs). The latter means that painful stimulation at one site of the body may reduce the pain at another site of the body.[17] In addition, most spinal cord neurons with joint input are tonically inhibited by descending inhibitory systems that keep the spinal cord under continuous control.[18,19] The interruption of descending inhibition can lower the excitation threshold of spinal cord neurons for mechanical input from the knee, substantially increase the receptive fields of neurons, and cause (increased) ongoing discharges. Thus the response properties of neurons with joint input are controlled by the primary afferent input, by intrinsic properties of the spinal cord neurons, by local circuits, and by descending pathways.

HYPEREXCITABILITY OF SPINAL CORD NEURONS DURING INFLAMMATION IN THE JOINT

Experimental Models of Joint Inflammation

As described in the Introduction, pain and hyperalgesia are usually elicited during inflammation of the joint. Hence experimental models have been used to study neuronal mechanisms underlying these pain symptoms. Acute inflammation in the joint can be induced by the intra-articular injections of crystals such as urate and kaolin or by carrageenan. The injection of kaolin and carrageenan (K/C) into the joint produces an edema and granulocytic infiltration within 1–3 hours with a plateau after 4–6 hours. Awake animals show limping of the injected leg and enhanced sensitivity to pressure onto the joint. By contrast, the injection of Freund's complete adjuvant (FCA) into a single joint produces a monoarthritis that is present for 2–4 weeks. Usually the lesion is restricted to the injected joint, although bilateral effects are observed sometimes. Hyperalgesia (limping or guarding of the leg, enhanced sensitivity to pressure onto the joint) develops within a day, reaches a peak within 3 days, and is maintained to some degree up to several weeks. When FCA is injected at a high dose into the tail base or lymph node, a polyarthritis develops.[7] More recently, other models such as collagen-induced polyarthritis[20] and antigen-induced monoarthritis[21,22] are also being used in order to investigate inflammatory pain.

Generation of Spinal Hyperexcitability (Central Sensitization)

During the development of a K/C-induced inflammation in the joint, both NS and WDR neurons with joint input show within 1–3 hours enhanced responses to noxious stimuli applied to the inflamed joint. NS neurons exhibit a reduction in their mechanical threshold such that the application of innocuous stimuli to the inflamed joint is sufficient to excite the neurons. Figure 1.2A shows the generation of hyperexcitability in a spinal cord neuron with joint input. Initially, while the joint was normal, the neuron responded only to noxious pressure applied to the knee (and adjacent muscles in thigh and lower leg, Fig. 1.2B, left side). No responses were elicited by pressure onto the ankle and the paw. After injection of kaolin and carrageenan (K/C) into the knee joint, the responses to noxious compression of the knee increased markedly, and at a latency of about half an hour the neuron started also to respond to pressure applied to the ankle and the paw. Thus the receptive field expanded from the knee toward the paw (Fig. 1.2B, right side), and the previously high threshold neuron was then even activated by gentle innocuous pressure. The increased responses to stimuli applied to the inflamed joint result most likely from the enhanced synaptic input from afferent units that are sensitized during stimulation. However, the appearance of responses to stimulation of ankle and paw must result from a mechanism in the spinal cord because these regions were not inflamed. Thus nociceptive spinal cord neurons obviously develop a state of hyperexcitability in which the responsiveness to both inputs from inflamed and noninflamed areas is increased.[23–26] The increased responses to stimulation of the inflamed area are thought to be the neuronal mechanism of primary hyperalgesia (hyperalgesia at the site of inflammation), whereas the increased responses to stimuli applied to healthy tissue are thought to be the neuronal

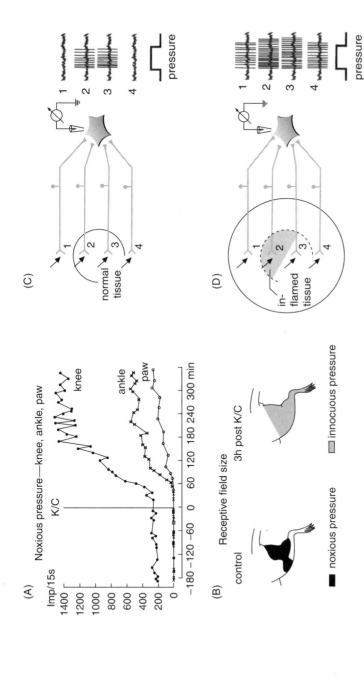

Figure 1.2. Development of inflammation-evoked hyperexcitability in a spinal cord neuron with input from the knee joint. (A) Histogram showing the responses (action potentials/response) of the neuron to noxious pressure applied to the knee joint, the ankle, and the paw before and after injection of kaolin and carrageenan (K/C) into the ipsilateral knee joint. (B) Receptive field (shaded area) of the neuron before (control) and during knee joint inflammation (3 h post K/C). (C,D) Model showing the responses and the receptive field of a spinal cord neuron before inflammation (C) and after development of hyperexcitability (D). Before inflammation the neuron was only excited by pressure to the initial receptive field (stimulation sites 2 and 3). After inflammation the neuron was activated from a larger area (stimulation sites 1–4). (Parts A and B from Ref. 25.)

mechanism underlying secondary hyperalgesia (hyperalgesia in healthy tissue adjacent to and remote from inflamed tissue).

Figure 1.2C,D shows the working hypothesis of how these changes are produced. When the tissue is normal, the neuron is only excited by stimuli applied to the restricted receptive field (circle in Fig. 1.2C) but not by stimuli applied to adjacent areas. When an inflammation develops in the receptive field (shaded area, Fig. 1.2D), primary afferents in this region are sensitized and they induce a process of spinal sensitization. When the spinal neuron is hyperexcitable, it shows stronger responses to stimuli applied to the original receptive field (stimulation sites 2 and 3), and in addition the neuron responds to inputs that are normally too weak to excite the neuron above threshold (stimulation sites 1 and 4). Hence the receptive field expands (Fig. 1.2D). The spinal "functional connection" between knee and paw and the change of synaptic effectiveness during inflammation was also shown in a recent study in which field potentials in the spinal cord were recorded. Electrical stimulation of the posterior articular nerve (PAN) of the knee joint evoked typical field potentials in lumbar spinal segments. The elicited N2 and N3 waves (generated by synaptic activation of dorsal horn neurons by thin myelinated PAN afferents) became gradually increased after induction of a local inflammation in the paw by capsaicin.[27] These data show that a disease process in an area may change synaptic processing from adjacent and even remote areas.

Central sensitization can persist during chronic inflammation. In rats with unilateral arthritis[28] as well as in rats suffering from chronic polyarthritis,[29] spinal cord neurons with joint input appear on average more sensitive and have expanded receptive fields. During chronic FCA-induced inflammation in the knee joint, secondary hyperalgesia at the ankle can also last several weeks, and for a long time this hypersensitivity is associated with enhanced responses of spinal cord neurons to A and C fiber inputs.[30]

Interestingly, the stimulation of primary afferents from deep tissue (muscle and joint) evokes more prolonged facilitation of a nociceptive flexor reflex than stimulation of cutaneous afferents,[13] and capsaicin injection into deep tissue elicits more prolonged hyperalgesia than injection of capsaicin into the skin,[31] suggesting that deep input is particularly able to induce long-term changes in the nociceptive system. However, spinal sensitization is counteracted to some extent by inhibitory influences. Descending inhibition[19] as well as heterotopic inhibitory influences (see above) are increased during inflammation,[32] at least in early stages.

While spinal cord recordings can only be done in experimental studies, human studies lend support to the concept of central sensitization. In humans it is possible to map areas of referred pain upon noxious stimulation at a restricted site. When a noxious stimulus, (e.g., intramuscular injection of 6% NaCl) is applied to a muscle, the area in which pain is felt extends far beyond the stimulation site. Interestingly, such areas were found to be significantly larger during pathological conditions such as osteoarthritis.[33] The enlargement of painful areas may correspond to the expansion of receptive fields of spinal cord neurons. By and large, the described neuronal changes in the spinal cord are likely to account for deep referred pain and secondary hyperalgesia that are induced in humans by noxious stimulation of deep tissue.[34] Based on this paradigm, numerous pathological conditions in humans such as inflammation and osteoarthritis seem to be associated with central sensitization, suggesting that the spinal cord is indeed in a state of hyperexcitability.

MOLECULAR MECHANISMS OF SPINAL SENSITIZATION

In general, the process of spinal sensitization depends on several preconditions. First, nociceptive spinal cord neurons have the potential for activity-dependent neuroplastic changes. For example, repetitive electrical stimulation of C fibers at the same current can induce wind-up of the synaptic responses to electrical nerve stimulation (a short-lived increase of responsiveness, however, not outlasting the stimulation protocol)[35] or a long-term potentiation (a persistent increase of synaptic responses to electrical stimulation outlasting the conditioning stimulus).[36] Second, both an increase of excitatory mechanism as well as a reduction of inhibition (e.g., by apoptosis of inhibitory interneurons under neuropathic conditions) may contribute to central sensitization.[37] Third, both neurons and glial cells may be involved in enhanced neuronal excitability.[20,38,39]

In the case of inflammation, peripheral nociceptive fibers play a key role in triggering the process of spinal sensitization. During developing inflammation, numerous nociceptive mechanosensitive joint afferents are sensitized to mechanical stimulation such that innocuous stimuli (palpation of the joint and movements in the working range) become sufficient to evoke action potentials. In addition, initially mechanoinsensitive nociceptive afferents are rendered mechanosensitive and contribute to the input into the spinal cord upon stimulation of the inflamed joint.[5,37] Numerous inflammatory mediators including classical inflammatory mediators such as bradykinin and prostaglandins,[5] as well as the cytokines interleukin-6[40] and TNF-α[21], have the potential to sensitize joint afferents for mechanical stimuli. As a consequence of peripheral sensitization, the intraspinal release of glutamate (the main transmitter of nociceptive afferents),[41] the neuropeptides substance P, neurokinin A, and CGRP (cotransmitters in primary afferents and interneurons), and spinal prostaglandins is enhanced, and these mediators are involved in the generation (and maintenance) of spinal hyperexcitability.

Excitatory Amino Acids (Glutamate)

As mentioned, glutamate is the major transmitter in the synaptic activation of spinal cord neurons with joint input. On the postsynaptic site, glutamate activates N-methyl-D-aspartate (NMDA) receptors and non-NMDA receptors.

The activation of non-NMDA receptors leads to basic excitation of neurons. By contrast, the activation of NMDA receptors leads to a calcium influx into neurons and causes processes of neuronal plasticity such as long-term changes of responses in many neuronal circuits. The ionophoretic application of antagonists at AMPA/kainate (non-NMDA) receptors close to neurons with joint input reduced the responses to innocuous and noxious pressure, whereas the application of NMDA receptor antagonists reduced only the responses to noxious mechanical stimulation. Thus, in our hands, NMDA receptors are only activated by noxious stimulation.[25]

The ionophoretic application of NMDA antagonists at AMPA/kainate and NMDA receptors to spinal cord neurons as well as systemic application of NMDA antagonists prevents the development of inflammation-evoked spinal hyperexcitability.[25] Figure 1.3 shows the effect of ketamine, an antagonist at NMDA receptors. In six control neurons without ketamine, the induction of inflammation in the knee joint by injection of kaolin/carrageenan (K/C) caused increases of the responses to noxious pressure applied to the injected knee and the noninjected ankle. When ketamine was administered before and during induction of inflammation, the development of inflammation in the knee joint did not cause changes of responses as long as the antagonist was applied (Fig. 1.3C,D). Importantly, antagonists at both receptor types can reduce responses of the neurons to mechanical stimulation of the joint also after inflammation is established, and this is even seen in a chronic model of inflammation.[25,42] Thus glutamate receptors play a key role in the generation and maintenance of inflammation-evoked spinal hyperexcitability even in the long-term range. In addition, NMDA receptors are involved in the regulation of spinal NOS isoforms during monoarthritis. During monoarthritis, the expression of nNOS, iNOS, and eNOS in the dorsal horn was increased, and ketamine reduced nNOS expression and increased iNOS and eNOS expression.[43] However, the functional consequences of these changes are to be determined.

Neuropeptides

Numerous joint afferents contain the neuropeptides substance P, neurokinin A, and CGRP that are coexpressed with glutamate. Noxious compression, but not innocuous compression, of the normal joint enhances the intraspinal release of these peptides above baseline.[44] This pattern of release changes when the joint is inflamed. During acute inflammation, release of neuropeptides occurs when the joint is stimulated at innocuous intensity. Thus under inflammatory conditions, a "cocktail" of transmitters and/or modulators is released in the spinal cord, which changes synaptic processing.[45–47] As a further indicator of spinal release of substance P during arthritis, movements of an arthritic joint was found to induce internalization of the neurokinin 1 receptor.[48] The

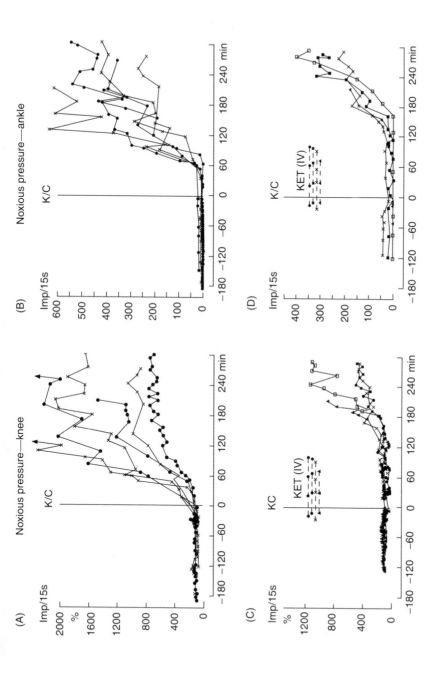

Figure 1.3. Blockade of the development of hyperexcitability in spinal cord neurons by intravenous (IV) administration of the NMDA receptor antagonist ketamine. (A,B) Changes of the responses of spinal cord neurons to noxious pressure applied to the knee joint and the ankle during development of inflammation in the knee joint after the injection of K/C into the ipsilateral knee joint. (C,D) Same experimental approach as in (A) and (B), but in these experiments ketamine was given IV during induction and in the initial period of inflammation in the knee joint. (From Ref. 25).

expression of substance P and of its (neurokinin 1) receptor was increased in the superficial dorsal horn during monoarthritis.[48]

Excitatory neuropeptides facilitate the responses of spinal cord neurons. The effect of substance P is shown in Figure 1.4A,B. The WDR neuron in Figure 1.4 showed graded responses to innocuous and noxious pressure applied to the knee joint. A short ionophoretic application of substance P to the spinal cord neuron caused reversible increases of ongoing discharges and responses to mechanical stimulation. In the NS neuron in Figure 1.4B, substance P caused an increase of responses to noxious pressure and a small response to innocuous pressure and to ankle stimulation.

Ionophoretic application of antagonists at neurokinin 1, neurokinin 2, and CGRP receptors attenuates the development of inflammation-evoked hyperexcitability. Figure 1.4C shows the effect of CP96,345, an antagonist at the neurokinin 1 receptor, on the development of inflammation-evoked hyperexcitability. Compared to control neurons (top graph, induction of inflammation in the absence of the antagonist), the neurons treated with spinal administration of the neurokinin 1 receptor antagonist showed a smaller increase of their responses after induction of inflammation (middle graph). The inactive enantiomer, CP96,344, did not attenuate the magnitude of inflammation-evoked hyperexcitability (bottom graph). The antagonists also reduce hyperexcitability when it is established.[49–51] Probably, the activation of these peptide receptors enhances the sensitivity of glutamatergic synaptic transmission.[52] However, it is important to point out that the antagonists at neuropeptide receptors are less antinociceptive than antagonists at glutamate receptors.

Prostaglandins

Spinal prostaglandins (PGs) are synthetized in dorsal root ganglion (DRG) neurons and in the spinal cord by both cyclooxygenases (COX) 1 and 2. PGE_2 receptors are located on primary afferent neurons and on spinal cord neurons, indicating that PGs can act presynaptically (influencing the release of synaptic mediators) and postsynaptically (influencing excitability).[53] During inflammation in the joint, there is a tonic release of PGE_2 within the dorsal and ventral horn.[54] This is likely to result from an upregulation of spinal COX-2 that is already increased at 3 hours after induction of knee joint inflammation (Fig. 1.5A,B). The application of PGE_2 to the spinal cord surface facilitates the responses of spinal cord neurons to mechanical stimulation of the joint, and the pattern of effects is similar to that observed during peripheral inflammation. When the COX inhibitor indomethacin was applied to the spinal cord before inflammation, the development of hyperexcitability was significantly attenuated compared to control rats in which only vehicle was applied to the spinal cord (Fig. 1.5C), indicating that spinal PGs are involved in the generation of inflammation-evoked spinal hyperexcitability.[55] Interestingly, however, the application of indomethacin to the spinal cord, after knee inflammation and

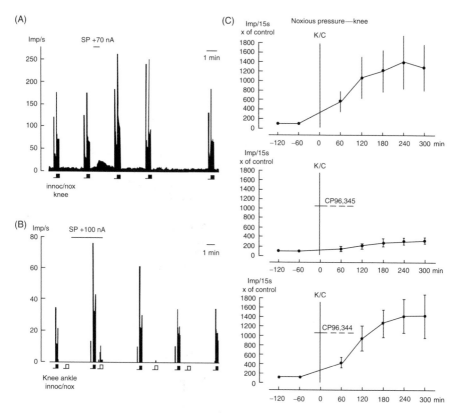

Figure 1.4. Effect of substance P on the responses of spinal cord neurons to mechanical stimulation of the knee joint and effect of a neurokinin 1 receptor antagonist on the development of inflammation-evoked hyperexcitability of spinal cord neurons. (A, B). The histograms (action potentials/second) show that ionophoretic application of substance P at 70 nA or 100 nA enhances responses to mechanical stimulation. In the neuron in (A), substance P also caused enhanced ongoing discharges. (C) Development of inflammation-evoked hyperexcitability in spinal cord neurons (responses to noxious pressure) in the absence of the antagonist (top), in the presence of the neurokinin 1 receptor antagonist CP96,345 at the spinal cord neurons (middle), and in the presence of the inactive enantiomer CP96,344 of the neurokinin 1 receptor antagonist (bottom). Parts A and B from Ref. 44; C from part Ref. 49.

spinal hyperexcitability are established, did not reduce enhanced responses of spinal cord neurons to mechanical stimulation of the inflamed knee joint,[55] thus raising the question of whether the continuous presence of PGE_2 is required for the maintenance of inflammation-evoked spinal hyperexcitability. By contrast, after systemic application, indomethacin reduced the responses of spinal cord neurons, showing that indomethacin still acted outside the spinal cord.[55]

Further support for a differential role of PGE_2 in the generation and maintenance of spinal hyperexcitability came from studies on the spinal effect

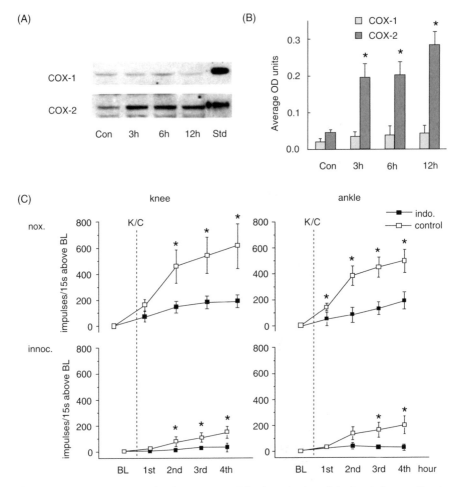

Figure 1.5. Upregulation of cyclooxygenase 2 in the spinal cord during inflammation in the knee joint and effect of spinal administration of indomethacin on the development of inflammation-evoked hyperexcitability of spinal cord neurones. (A,B). During inflammation in the joint, mainly spinal cyclooxygenase 2 (COX-2) shows an increase. (C) The spinal application of indomethacin, a blocker of COX-1 and COX-2, attenuates spinal hyperexcitability. Open squares show the inflammation-evoked changes of responses after kaolin/carrageenan injection in control neurons; filled squares show the changes of the responses during development of inflammation after topical administration of indomethacin to the spinal cord. Top graphs show responses to noxious pressure, bottom graphs responses to innocuous pressure. (Parts A and B from Ref. 54; Part C from Ref. 55).

of EP receptor agonists[56] and on the inhibition of the transcription factor NFκB in the spinal cord.[57] The enhancement of responses of spinal cord neurons to mechanical stimulation of the normal knee joint by spinal PGE_2 was mimicked by the spinal application of agonists at the EP1 receptor (which enhances calcium influx in neurons), and by agonists at the EP2 and EP4 receptors (which activate G_s proteins and adenylylcyclases). However, after inflammation and spinal hyperexcitability were established, only the EP1 receptor agonist further increased responses to mechanical stimulation of the inflamed knee, whereas the EP2 and EP4 agonists did not influence neuronal responses. On the other hand, spinal application of an agonist at the EP3 receptor (most isoforms are coupled to G_i proteins and reduce cAMP levels) had no influence on neuronal responses when the joint was normal but reduced the responses to mechanical stimulation of the knee when it was spinally applied during established inflammation.[56] Thus the status of the spinal cord may determine which EP receptor agonist causes an effect upon spinal application, and the level of cAMP could be an important molecular factor.

The activation of COX-2 depends on the activation of the transcription factor nuclear factor-κB (NFκB). In unstimulated tissue, NFκB is bound in the cytoplasma to IκBα and IκBβ, which prevent it from entering the nucleus. After stimulation, IκB kinase (IKK) phosphorylates IκB and causes its degradation, thus allowing the unbound NFκB to enter the nucleus. Hence IKK inhibitors reduce NFκB-mediated effects.[58,59] Recent reports indicate a role of spinal NFκB activation in spinal mechanisms of nociception.[60,61] A study on spinal mechanisms of joint nociception showed that spinal application of a specific IKK inhibitor before and early during development of inflammation totally prevented spinal hyperexcitability during developing joint inflammation, suggesting an important role of spinal NFκB in this process. However, during established inflammation, the IKK inhibitor did not reduce the responses of neurons to mechanical stimulation of the inflamed knee within 2.5 hours after spinal administration, thus suggesting that spinal hyperexcitability is not maintained by continuous NFκB activation.[57] The pattern of effect of the IKK inhibitor is similar to that of indomethacin (see above), and because NFκB inhibitors prevent the upregulation of spinal cyclooxygenases,[60,61] these data collectively suggest spinal PGE_2 is mainly important for the generation of inflammation-evoked spinal hyperexcitability but not for its maintenance.

It should be noted, however, that other prostaglandins are also synthesized in the spinal cord. The other major prostaglandin in the central nervous system including the spinal cord is PGD_2.[62] Electrophysiological recordings from spinal cord neurons with knee input showed that topical application of PGD_2 to the spinal cord at a high dose may cause a sensitization of spinal cord neurons for mechanical stimulation of the normal joint similar to PGE_2. This effect may result from synaptic facilitation due to an increase of the spinal release of substance P and CGRP from primary afferent neurons.[63–65] However, under conditions of joint inflammation, PGD_2 dose-dependently reduced responses of spinal cord neurons to stimulation of the inflamed knee joint, and

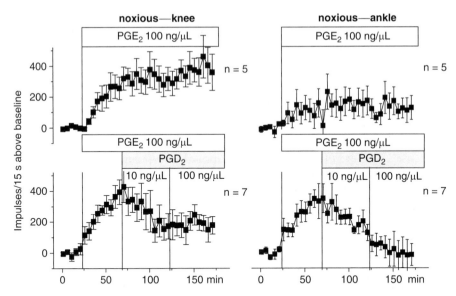

Figure 1.6. Effects of the coadministration of PGE_2 and PGD_2 on responses to mechanical stimulation of the normal knee and ankle joint. Increase of responses to noxious stimulation of the knee and ankle over predrug baseline (set to 0) by PGE_2 alone (top) and reduction of increased responses by coapplication of PGD_2 at two doses (bottom). Each symbol shows the average response of neurons at the time points indicated. (From Ref. 66).

spinal application of an antagonist at the DP1 receptor increased responses to stimulation of the inflamed knee.[66] Indeed, PGD_2 can reduce the enhanced discharges evoked by PGE_2.[66] This is shown in Figure 1.6. The spinal application of PGE_2 alone caused a pronounced and persistent facilitation of responses to noxious pressure onto the normal knee and ankle (Fig. 1.6, top). When instead PGD_2 and PGE_2 were coadministered starting 50 min after previous application of PGE_2 alone, responses to noxious stimulation were significantly reduced (Fig. 1.6, bottom). Thus PGD_2 seems to have potentially two opposite actions in the spinal cord depending on the state of the spinal cord. The reduction of enhanced responses by PGD_2 is in line with data showing that PGD_2 may have neuroprotective effects in the brain,[67] via DP1 receptors.[68] Possibly this inhibitory action is caused by activation of DP1 receptors on inhibitory spinal interneurons.[69]

CONCLUSION

The investigation of the spinal mechanisms of pain including joint pain is an active area of research, and it is very likely that further important spinal mechanisms of joint pain will be elucidated in the next few years. Of potential interest could be the role of glia cells, which produce a number of mediators including cytokines.[39,70]

While the spinal cord is an important site where neuronal plasticity such as central sensitization occurs, the conscious pain response is produced in the thalamocortical system. The thalamus and cortex contain nociceptive neurons that are activated by nociceptive deep input from muscle and joint. Most of these neurons have convergent inputs from skin and deep tissue, but small proportions of neurons respond only to noxious stimulation of muscle and tendon.[71–73] There is evidence that during arthritis neuroplastic changes are also induced at the thalamocortical level.[74–76] It is unknown whether these alterations mirror the altered spinal processing or whether additional elements of neuroplasticity are generated in the thalamus and cortex. In any case, the working of the nociceptive system is substantially modified under clinical pain conditions, and it is a continuous challenge to identify suitable target sites for pain therapy.

REFERENCES

1. Kellgren JH, Samuel EP. (1950). The sensitivity and innervation of the articular capsule. J Bone Joint Surg 32-B:84–91.
2. Lewis T. (1942). *Pain*. London: MacMillan.
3. Kellgren JH. (1939). Some painful joint condition and their relation to osteoarthritis. Clin Sci 4:193–205.
4. Lewis T. (1938). Suggestions relating to the study of somatic pain. Br Med J 1:321–325.
5. Schaible H-G. (2006). Basic mechanisms of deep somatic pain. In McMahon SB and Koltzenburg M (eds.), *Wall and Melzack's Textbook of Pain*, 5th ed. Amsterdam: Elsevier, Churchill Livingston, pp. 621–633.
6. Scott DL. (2006). Osteoarthritis and rheumatoid arthritis. In McMahon SB and Koltzenburg M (eds.) *Wall and Melzack's Textbook of Pain*, 5th ed. Amsterdam: Elsevier, pp. 653–667.
7. Schaible H-G, Grubb BD. (1993). Afferent and spinal mechanisms of joint pain. Pain 55:5–54.
8. Felson DT. (2005). The sources of pain in knee osteoarthritis. Curr Opin Rheumatol 17:624–628.
9. Schaible H-G, Schmidt RF, Willis WD. (1986). Responses of spinal cord neurones to stimulation of articular afferent fibres in the cat. J Physiol 372:575–593.
10. Schaible H-G, Schmidt RF, Willis WD. (1987). Convergent inputs from articular, cutaneous and muscle receptors onto ascending tract cells in the cat spinal cord. Exp Brain Res 66:479–488.
11. Fields HL, Clanton CH, Anderson SD. (1977). Somatosensory properties of spinoreticular neurons in the cat. Brain Res 120:49–66.

12. Meyers DER, Snow PJ. (1982). The responses to somatic stimuli of deep spinotha-lamic tract cells in the lumbar spinal cord of the cat. J Physiol 329:355–371.

13. Woolf CJ, Wall PD. (1986). Relative effectiveness of C primary afferent fibres of different origins in evoking a prolonged facilitation of the flexor reflex in the rat. J Neurosci 6:1433–1442.

14. Ferrell WR, Wood L, Baxendale RH. (1998). The effect of acute joint inflammation on flexion reflex excitability in the decerebrate, low spinal cat. Q J Exp Physiol 373:353–365.

15. He X, Proske U, Schaible H-G, Schmidt RF. (1988). Acute inflammation of the knee joint in the cat alters responses of flexor motoneurones to leg movements. J Neurophysiol 59:326–340.

16. Mense S. (1997). Pathophysiologic basis of muscle pain syndromes. Myofasc Pain Update in Diagnosis and Treatment 8:23–53.

17. LeBars D, Villanueva L. (1988). Electrophysiological evidence for the activation of descending inhibitory controls by nociceptive pathways. In Fields HL and Besson J-M (eds.) *Progress in Brain Research*, vol. 77, Amsterdam: Elsevier, pp. 275–299.

18. Cervero F, Schaible H-G, Schmidt RF. (1991). Tonic descending inhibition of spinal cord neurones driven by joint afferents in normal cats and in cats with an inflamed knee joint. Exp Brain Res 83:675–678.

19. Schaible H-G, Neugebauer V, Cervero F, Schmidt RF. (1991). Changes in tonic descending inhibition of spinal neurons with articular input during the development of acute arthritis in the cat. J Neurophysiol 66:1021–1032.

20. Inglis JJ, Notley CA, Essex D, Wilson AW, Feldmann M, Anand P, Williams R. (2007). Collagen-induced arthritis as a model of hyperalgesia. Functional and cellular analysis of the analgesic actions of tumor necrosis factor blockade. Arthritis Rheum 56:4015–4023.

21. Boettger MK, Hensellek S, Richter F, Gajda M, Stöckigt R, Segond von Banchet G, Bräuer R, Schaible H-G. (2008). Antinociceptive effects of TNF-α neutralization in a rat model of antigen-induced arthritis. Evidence for a neuronal target. Arthritis Rheum 58:2368–2378.

22. Segond von Banchet G, Petrow PK, Bräuer R, Schaible H-G. (2000). Monoarticular antigen-induced arthritis leads to pronounced bilateral upregulation of the expression of neurokinin 1 and bradykinin 2 receptors in dorsal root ganglion neurones of rats. Arthritis Res 2:424–427.

23. Dougherty PM, Sluka KA, Sorkin LS, Westlund KN, Willis WD. (1992). Neural changes in the acute arthritis in monkeys. I. Parallel enhancement of responses of spinothalamic tract neurons to mechanical stimulation and excitatory amino acids. Brain Res Rev 17:1–13.

24. Neugebauer V, Schaible H-G. (1990). Evidence for a central component in the sensitization of spinal neurons with joint input during development of acute arthritis in cat's knee. J Neurophysiol 64:299–311.

25. Neugebauer V, Lücke T, Schaible H-G. (1993). *N*-methyl-D-aspartate (NMDA) and non-NMDA receptor antagonists block the hyperexcitability of dorsal horn neurones during development of acute arthritis in rat's knee joint. J Neurophysiol 70:1365–1377.

26. Schaible H-G, Schmidt RF, Willis WD. (1987). Enhancement of the responses of ascending tract cells in the cat spinal cord by acute inflammation of the knee joint. Exp Brain Res 66:489–499.

27. Rudomin P, Hernández E. (2008). Changes in synaptic effectiveness of myelinated joint afferents during capsaicin-induced inflammation of the footpad in the anaesthetized cat. Exp Brain Res 187:71–84.

28. Grubb BD, Stiller RU, Schaible H-G. (1993). Dynamic changes in the receptive field properties of spinal cord neurons with ankle input in rats with unilateral adjuvant-induced inflammation in the ankle region. Exp Brain Res 92:441–452.

29. Menetrey D, Besson J-M. (1982). Electrophysiological characteristics of dorsal horn cells in rats with cutaneous inflammation resulting from chronic arthritis. Pain 13:343–364.

30. Martindale JC, Wilson AW, Reeve AJ, Chessell IP, Headley PM. (2007). Chronic secondary hypersensitivity of dorsal horn neurones following inflammation of the knee joint. Pain 133:79–86.

31. Sluka KA. (2002). Stimulation of deep somatic tissue with capsaicin produces long-lasting mechanical allodynia and heat hypoalgesia that depends on early activation of the cAMP pathway. J Neurosci 22:5687–5693.

32. Calvino B, Villanueva L, LeBars D. (1987). Dorsal horn (convergent) neurones in the intact anaesthetized arthritic rat. II. Heterotopic inhibitory influences. Pain 31:359–379.

33. Bajaj P, Bajaj P, Graven-Nielsen T, Arendt-Nielsen L. (2001). Osteoarthritis and its association with muscle hyperalgesia: an experimental controlled study. Pain 93:107–114.

34. Arendt-Nielsen L, Laursen RJ, Drewes AM. (2000). Referred pain as an indicator for neural plasticity. In Sandkühler J, Bromm B and Gebhart GF (eds.) *Progress in Brain Research*, Amsterdam: Elsevier, Vol. 129, pp. 343–356.

35. Mendell LM, Wall PD. (1965). Responses of single dorsal cord cells to peripheral cutaneous unmyelinated fibers. Nature 206:97–99.

36. Sandkühler J. (2000). Learning and memory in pain pathways. Pain 88:113–118.

37. Schaible H-G. (2006). Peripheral and central mechanisms of pain generation. In Stein C (ed.) *Handbook of Experimental Pharmacalogy*, Berlin: Springer-Verlag, Vol. 177, pp. 4–28.

38. Sun S, Cao H, Han M, Li TT, Pan HL, Zhao ZQ, Zhang YQ. (2007). New evidence for the involvement of spinal fraktalkine receptor in pain facilitation and spinal glial activation in rat model of monoarthritis. Pain 129:64–75.

39. Watkins LR, Maier SF. (2005). Glia and pain: past, present, and future. In Merskey H, Loeser JD, and Dubner R (eds.), *The Paths of Pain 1975–2005*. Seattle: IASP Press, pp. 165–175.

40. Brenn D, Richter F, Schaible H-G. (2007). Sensitization of unmyelinated sensory fibers of the joint nerve for mechanical stimuli by interleukin-6 in the rat. An inflammatory mechanism of joint pain. Arthritis Rheum 56:351–359.

41. Sorkin LS, Westlund KN, Sluka KA, Dougherty PM, Willis WD. (1992). Neural changes in acute arthritis in monkeys. IV. Time course of amino acid release into the lumbar dorsal horn. Brain Res Rev 17:39–50.

42. Neugebauer V, Lücke T, Grubb BD, Schaible H-G. (1994). The involvement of *N*-methyl-D-aspartate (NMDA) and non-NMDA receptors in the responsiveness of rat spinal neurons with input from the chronically inflamed ankle. Neurosci Lett 170:237–240.

43. Infante C, Diaz M, Hernandéz A, Constandil L, Pelissier T. (2007). Expression of nitric oxide synthase isoforms in the dorsal horn of monoarthritic rats: effects of competitive and uncompetitive *N*-methyl-D-aspartate antagonists. Arthritis Res Ther 9:R53.

44. Neugebauer V, Schaible H-G, Weiretter F, Freudenberger U. (1994). The involvement of substance P and neurokinin-1 receptors in the responses of rat dorsal horn neurons to noxious but not to innocuous mechanical stimuli applied to the knee joint. Brain Res 666:207–215.

45. Hope PJ, Jarrott B, Schaible H-G, Clarke RW, Duggan AW. (1990). Release and spread of immunoreactive neurokinin A in the cat spinal cord in a model of acute arthritis. Brain Res 533:292–299.

46. Schaible H-G, Jarrott B, Hope PJ, Duggan AW. (1990). Release of immunoreactive substance P in the cat spinal cord during development of acute arthritis in cat's knee: a study with antibody bearing microprobes. Brain Res 529:214–223.

47. Schaible H-G, Freudenberger U, Neugebauer V, Stiller U. (1994). Intraspinal release of immunoreactive calcitonin gene-related peptide during development of inflammation in the joint in vivo—a study with antibody microprobes in cat and rat. Neuroscience 62:1293–1305.

48. Sharif Naeini R, Cahill CM, Ribeiro-da-Silva A, Ménard HA, Henry JL. (2005). Remodelling of spinal nociceptive mechanisms in an animal model of monoarthritis. Eur J Neurosci 22:2005–2015.

49. Neugebauer V, Weiretter F, Schaible H-G. (1995). The involvement of substance P and neurokinin-1 receptors in the hyperexcitability of dorsal horn neurons during development of acute arthritis in rat's knee joint. J Neurophysiol 73:1574–1583.

50. Neugebauer V, Rümenapp P, Schaible H-G. (1996). The role of spinal neurokinin-2 receptors in the processing of nociceptive information from the joint and in the generation and maintenance of inflammation-evoked hyperexcitability of dorsal horn neurons in the rat. Eur J Neurosci 8:249–260.

51. Neugebauer V, Rümenapp P, Schaible H-G. (1996). Calcitonin gene-related peptide is involved in the generation and maintenance of hyperexcitability of dorsal horn neurons observed during development of acute inflammation in rat's knee joint. Neuroscience 71:1095–1109.

52. Ebersberger A, Charbel Issa P, Vanegas H, Schaible H-G. (2000). Differential effects of CGRP and CGRP 8-37 upon responses to NMDA and AMPA in spinal nociceptive neurons with knee input in the rat. Neuroscience 99:171–178.

53. Vanegas H, Schaible H-G. (2001). Prostaglandins and cyclooxygenases in the spinal cord. Prog Neurobiol 64:327–363.

54. Ebersberger A, Grubb BD, Willingale HL, Gardiner NJ, Nebe J, Schaible H-G. (1999). The intraspinal release of prostaglandin E_2 in a model of acute arthritis is accompanied by an upregulation of cyclooxygenase-2 in the rat spinal cord. Neuroscience 93:775–781.

55. Vasquez E, Bär K-J, Ebersberger A, Klein B, Vanegas H, Schaible H-G. (2001). Spinal prostaglandins are involved in the development but not the maintenance of inflammation-induced spinal hyperexcitability. J Neurosci 21:9001–9008.

56. Bär K-J, Natura G, Telleria-Diaz A, Teschner P, Vogel R, Vasquez E, Schaible H-G, Ebersberger A. (2004). Changes in the effect of spinal prostaglandin E_2 during inflammation—prostaglandin E (EP1-EP4) receptors in spinal nociceptive processing of input from the normal or inflamed knee joint. J Neurosci 24:642–651.

57. Ebersberger A, Buchmann M, Ritzeler O, Michaelis M, Schaible H-G. (2006). The role of spinal nuclear factor-κB in spinal hyperexcitability. NeuroReport 17:1615–1618.

58. Barnes PJ, Karin M. (1997). Nuclear factor-κB—a pivotal transcription factor in chronic inflammatory diseases. N Engl J Med 336:1066–1071.

59. Chen L-W, Egan L, Li Z-W, Greten FR, Kagnoff MF, Karin M. (2003). The two faces of IKK and NF-κB inhibition: prevention of systemic inflammation but increased local injury following intestinal ischemia-reperfusion. Nature Med 9:575–581.

60. Lee KM, Kang BS, Lee HL, Son SJ, Hwang SH, Kim DS, Park J-S, Cho H-J. (2004). Spinal NF-κB activation induces COX-2 upregulation and contributes to inflammatory pain hypersensitivity. Eur J Neurosci 19:3375–3381.

61. Tegeder I, Niederberger E, Schmidt R, Kunz S, Gühring H, Ritzeler O, Michaelis M, Geisslinger G. (2004). Specific inhibition of IκB kinase reduces hyperalgesia in inflammatory and neuropathic pain models in rats. J Neurosci 24:1637–1645.

62. Willingale HL, Gardiner NJ, McLymont N, Giblett S, Grubb BD. (1997). Prostanoids synthesized by cyclo-oxygenase isoforms in rat spinal cord and their contribution to the development of neuronal hyperexcitability. Br J Pharmacol 122:1593–1604.

63. Andreeva L, Rang HP. (1993). Effect of bradykinin and prostaglandins on the release of calcitonin gene-related peptide-like immunoreactivity from the rat spinal cord in vitro. Br J Pharmacol 108:185–190.

64. Jenkins DW, Feniuk W, Humphrey PP. (2001). Characterization of the prostanoid receptor types involved in mediating calcitonin gene-related peptide release from cultured rat trigeminal neurones. Br J Pharmacol 134:1296–1302.

65. Nakae K, Hayashi F, Hayashi M, Yamamoto N, Iino T, Yoshikawa S, Gupta J. (2005). Functional role of prostacyclin receptor in rat dorsal root ganglion neurons. Neurosci Lett 388:132–137.

66. Telleria-Diaz A, Ebersberger A, Vasquez E, Schache F, Kahlenbach J, Schaible H-G. (2008). Different effects of spinally applied prostaglandin D_2 (PGD_2) on responses of dorsal horn neurons with knee input in normal rats and in rats with acute knee inflammation. Neuroscience 156:184–192.

67. Grill M, Heinemann A, Hoefler G, Peskar BA, Schuligoi R. (2008). Effect of endotoxin treatment on the expression and localization of spinal cyclooxygenase, prostaglandin synthases, and PGD_2 receptors. J Neurochem 104:1345–1357.

68. Liang X, Wu L, Hand T, Andreasson K. (2005). Prostaglandin D_2 mediates neuronal protection via the DP1 receptor. J Neurochem 92:477–486.

69. Minami T, Okuda-Ashitaka E, Nishizawa M, Mori H, Ito S. (1997). Inhibition of nociceptin-induced allodynia in conscious mice by prostaglandin D_2. Br J Pharmacol 122:605–610.

70. Marchand F, Perretti M, McMahon SB. (2005). Role of the immune system in chronic pain. Nat Rev Neurosci 6:521–532.

71. Guilbaud G, Peschanski M, Gautron M, Binder D. (1980). Neurones responding to noxious stimulation in VB complex and caudal adjacent regions in the thalamus of the rat. Pain 8:303–318.

72. Hutchison WD, Lühn MA, Schmidt RF. (1992). Knee joint input into the peripheral region of the ventral posterior lateral nucleus of cat thalamus. J Neurophysiol 67:1092–1104.

73. Kniffki K-D, Mizumura K. (1983). Responses of neurons in VPL and VPL-VL region of the cat to algesic stimulation of muscle and tendon. J Neurophysiol 49:649–661.

74. Gautron M, Guilbaud G. (1982). Somatic responses of ventrobasal thalamic neurones in polyarthritic rats. Brain Res 237:459–471.

75. Lamour Y, Willer JC, Guilbaud G. (1983). Rat somatosensory (Sm I) cortex. II. Laminar and columnar organization of noxious and non-noxious inputs. Exp Brain Res 49:46–54.

76. Lamour Y, Willer JC, Guilbaud G. (1983). Altered properties and laminar distribution of neuronal responses to peripheral stimulation in the Sm I cortex of the arthritic rat. Brain Res 273:183–187.

77. Craig AD, Heppelmann B, Schaible H-G. (1988). The projection of the medial and posterior articular nerves of the cat's knee to the spinal cord. J Comp Neurol 276:279–288.

2

ACTIVATION OF SENSORY NEURONS IN THE ARTHRITIC JOINT

Blair D. Grubb

Department of Cell Physiology and Pharmacology,
University of Leicester, Leicester LE1 9HN, United Kingdom

INTRODUCTION

Joints are richly innervated with a range of sensory nerve fibers that convey information to the central nervous system about forces exerted on articular tissues by both low and high threshold mechanical stimuli. High threshold nociceptive afferents terminate primarily in the synovium and periosteum, and normally respond only to movement of the joint beyond the working limits. Following joint damage, two factors combine to alter the mechanical sensitivity of articular nociceptors. First, physical changes (joint effusion and tissue edema) alter the resting and movement-induced forces exerted on the joint tissues, and second, inflammatory mediators released within the damaged tissue sensitize articular nociceptive afferents by binding to receptors on the nerve endings. These factors result in a reduction of the mechanical threshold for activation of articular nociceptors such that manipulation of the joint within the normal range is easily sufficient to activate them. Acute and chronic animal

Pain in Osteoarthritis, Edited by David T. Felson and Hans-Georg Schaible
Copyright © 2009 Wiley-Blackwell.

models of joint inflammation have been used to study the mechanisms of articular nociceptor sensitization and a number of inflammatory mediators and their receptors have been implicated. The focus of this chapter is to introduce some of the important issues involved in the sensitization of nociceptive articular afferents.

JOINT INNERVATION

Joints are innervated by distinct articular nerves although additional innervation through accessory nerve is also known to be important. The network of primary afferent nerve fibers can detect both nonnoxious and noxious mechanical stimuli applied to the joint. In animal studies, most recordings from primary afferent articular nociceptors have been made in either rat or cat, where the anatomy of the articular nerves is well understood and the physiological characteristics of the primary afferent nerve fibers have been investigated. The precise location of articular nociceptors is an area of considerable interest and several studies have identified afferent nerve fibers in joint capsule, synovium, periosteum, proximal ligament, and tendon, suggesting that damage to any part of the joint structure can excite nociceptive afferents and thus elicit pain.[1]

The two main systems of classification for primary afferent fibers based on conduction velocity or fibers diameter, combined with the physiological properties, have long been established. Articular afferents can easily be classified using the same methods and data from several studies have established the range of afferent nerve fibers innervating joint structures. Detailed morphological analysis of articular nerves has shown that approximately 20% of articular afferent fibers are myelinated with the majority of this group falling into the group III (Aδ conduction velocity $= 2.5$–$20\,\mathrm{m \cdot s^{-1}}$.) category of finely myelinated nociceptors. In addition, a relatively small number of large diameter myelinated low threshold group II (Aβ conduction velocity $= 20$–$65\,\mathrm{m \cdot s^{-1}}$) fibers also innervate each joint. The remaining 80% of articular fibers are unmyelinated and studies suggest that approximately half of these are sensory group IV (C-fibers, conduction velocity $\leqslant 2.5\,\mathrm{m \cdot s^{-1}}$) while the remainder are efferent sympathetic neurons innervating the joint. Low threshold afferents typically have largely corpuscular endings with Ruffini, Golgi, and Paccinian endings all found in joint tissues.[2] The high threshold mechanonociceptive articular afferents show very little terminal specialization and can only be identified on the basis of beaded varicosities containing accumulations of mitochondria. These nerve fibers are often found in association with blood or lymphatic vessels, where they often form a dense network of axons running for considerable distances along each vessel.[3]

MECHANICAL RESPONSES OF ARTICULAR AFFERENTS

Articular afferents have also been characterized according to their response properties with a range of mechanical sensitivities, from those activated by innocuous manipulation or rotation of the joint, to those only activated by noxious manipulation of the joint or rotation/flexion of the joint beyond the normal working range. More precisely, the majority of articular afferents characterized as belonging to group II are low threshold mechanoreceptor and can be either slowly or rapidly adapting.[4] Interestingly, a few of these fibers are only activated by noxious stimuli applied to the joint, indicating that they may have a role in nociception. Articular afferents belonging to groups III and IV typically have much higher threshold than group II fibers and are most often activated by noxious movements or manipulations of the joint.[1] In addition, a further class of group III and IV nociceptors has been reported, the "silent nociceptors," which are mechanoinsensitive in the normal animal but which develop mechanical sensitivity following the development of joint inflammation.[5,6]

PHENOTYPE CLASSIFICATION OF PRIMARY AFFERENT NERVE FIBERS

Primary afferent nerve fibers have also been classified according to their neuropeptide phenotype, which provides a guide to the subclasses of nociceptors that exist. In very general terms, primary afferent neurons have been classified into three main groups: (1) large diameter nonnociceptive neurons and nerve fibers that bind the RT97 + ve antibody,[7] which recognizes phosphorylated epitopes on identified neurofilament proteins;[8] (2) isolectin B4 (IB4) positive neurons, which are nonpeptidergic nociceptive neurons;[9] and (3) calcitonin gene-related peptide expressing neurons,[10] classed as peptidergic nociceptive neurons that can be recognized using the selective CGRP antibodies. It should be noted that while CGRP is used to identify a distinct subpopulation of primary afferent nociceptors, many other neuropeptides are also expressed in primary afferent neurons innervating joint structures. These include substance P, which is present in about half of the CGRP-positive neurons, and many others including neurokinin A, galanin, opioid peptides, and neuropeptide Y. The proportions of peptidergic and nonpeptidergic nociceptors vary between different tissues. In joints, peptidergic nociceptors have been found to predominate with relatively few nonpeptidergic, IB4-positive nerve fibers present.[11-14] It has been suggested that this has relevance to the role of peptidergic nociceptors in inflammation.

Approximately 25% of all dorsal root ganglion neurons contain CGRP in the normal animal and neuroanatomical studies have clearly demonstrated CGRP-positive nerve terminals in a number of joint structures including synovium, intervertebral disks, ligaments, joint capsule, and soft tissues. When Freund's adjuvant monoarthritis is induced in the rat ankle joint, the proportion of CGRP-positive cell bodies in lumbar dorsal root ganglion (DRG) neurons increases markedly, presumably as a consequence of the increase in neuronal activation.[15] The precise functional consequence of this upregulation of CGRP expression in sensory nerves innervating the joint is unclear. It is known, however, that these neuropeptides are released from both the central and peripheral terminals of nociceptors, where they are involved in central transmission and peripheral neurogenic inflammation, respectively.

MODELS OF INFLAMMATION USED TO STUDY THE PROPERTIES OF ARTICULAR NOCICEPTORS

Osteoarthritis (OA) is a significant clinical problem for which suitable analgesic therapies are required. In recent years a number of animal models have been developed which share similarities with the human disease process. These include naturally occurring OA models in guinea pig and instability-induced OA in mice with a natural predisposition to spontaneous OA. In addition, there are also a number of surgically induced models of OA in dog, rat, and guinea pig.[16] Unfortunately, these models have been little used to study the effects of inflammation on the properties of articular afferents. The original studies, which were performed in the 1980s and early 1990s, were designed to look at the process of afferent sensitization without any specific disease model in mind. Most studies have used either (1) the carrageenan/kaolin model of acute arthritis, which produces noticeable changes in afferent activity in 1–2 hours and which is normally continued for up to 24 hours, and (2) the Freund's complete adjuvant-induced mono- or polyarthritis, where injections of heat-killed *Mycobacterium tuberculosis* or *Mycobacterium butyricum* induce an arthritic process lasting several days to months. The joint inflammation normally peaks early at 2–5 days and then declines and either resolves (monoarthritic model) or enters a second phase that can last several weeks (polyarthritic model).

More recently, however, the sodium monoiodoacetate (MIA) model of osteoarthritis has been used to study the effect of a number of inflammatory mediators on nociceptor sensitization. In this model, MIA is injected into the joint space and marked joint swelling is observed after around 14 days alongside a joint pathology that has similarities to human OA.[17,18]

ARTICULAR AFFERENTS AND INFLAMMATION

Following trauma to the joint, we experience an increased sensitivity to load bearing and to movement of the joint within the normal range (allodynia). In addition, there is also a markedly increased sensitivity to any further noxious mechanical stimulation (hyperalgesia). These conscious manifestations of the joint damage are brought about by changes in the sensitivity of primary afferent nerve fibers, by spinal processing of joint input, and by processing within higher centers.

Following the development of joint inflammation, low threshold group II articular afferents only show acute and relatively transient changes in their responses to joint manipulation, which resolve within a few hours. By contrast, articular afferents belonging to groups III and IV often start to show ongoing spontaneous activity in the absence of joint movement, and show enhanced responses to manipulation of the joint (rotation/extension/flexion of the joint) or capsular indentation using a blunt probe.[6,19,20] Furthermore, many units that were previously mechanoinsensitive develop receptive fields and may also show ongoing spontaneous activity. These alterations in the firing characteristics of group III and IV afferents are the result of a marked reduction in the mechanical threshold for activation of articular mechanoreceptors and this contributes, in part, to the psychophysical measures of allodynia and hyperalgesia experienced in humans.

MECHANISMS UNDERLYING ARTICULAR MECHANONOCICEPTOR SENSITIZATION

Inflammation is a complex process in which a number of inflammatory mediators are released in response to tissue damage. In acute inflammation, these inflammatory mediators are part of the normal process that is required for tissue repair and regeneration. A number of these inflammatory mediators are responsible for the sensitization of primary afferent articular mechanonociceptors and this serves to limit mobility and thus protect the joint so that it is not damaged further during the repair process.

In chronic disease, the inflammatory response may be protracted due to abnormal pathology in the joint tissues. In the case of OA, this is largely due to the destruction of cartilage and bone remodeling (osteophytes or bony spurs) that is a response of bone to local damage. The loss of the normal articulating surfaces and the abnormal bone pathology result in chronic inflammation that can last years. To understand the mechanisms underlying the sensitization of articular mechanonociceptors in chronic inflammation, it is vital to understand the inflammatory mediators that are present during each stage of the disease process. One problem is that the inflammation is not constant, but rather episodic and dependent on a number of factors including activity. This can mean that the inflammatory mediators present in the joint will vary, thus making the targeting of treatment potentially difficult. Since specific animal models of OA have seldom been used to study mechanisms of sensitization of articular mechanonociceptors, the information available regarding their sensitization has largely been generated using the animal models of joint inflammation mentioned previously.

Prostaglandins

An important group of inflammatory mediators that regulate the mechanical sensitivity of articular mechanonociceptors are the prostaglandins. Prostaglandins are formed when membrane phospholipids are broken down by the enzyme PLA_2 to form arachidonic acid. This is then converted by the enzyme cyclooxygenase (COX) to the biologically active prostaglandins, PGE_2, PGI_2, PGD_2, and $PGF_{2\alpha}$. There is good evidence from the literature that nonselective COX inhibitors (nonsteroidal anti-inflammatory drugs), such as indomethacin and the salicylic acid derivatives, reverse the sensitization of articular mechanonociceptors seen in animal models of arthritis.[21,22] This evidence, combined with ample evidence that COX inhibitors are clinically useful treatments for arthritis in humans, shows that the joint tissues are a major target for this class of drugs. Further studies have shown that PGE_2 (and the related PGE_1) and PGI_2 seem to be particularly important for the sensitization of nerve fibers since these compounds are able to either directly excite articular mechanonociceptors or sensitize them to mechanical stimuli.[23-27]

The COX enzyme exists in at least two forms in humans (possibly three in dog).[28] COX–1[29] is a constitutive enzyme that is present in a large number of cell types and is seen as the housekeeping isoform. COX-2[30] is only constitutively expressed in a small number of tissues (e.g., brain and spinal cord) but is readily upregulated in many tissues in response to damage.[31] In the periphery, an inflammatory insult will readily upregulate COX-2 expression, resulting in an increase in prostaglandin synthesis. While no afferent fiber studies have been published showing the roles of COX-1 and COX-2 in producing articular mechanonociceptor sensitization, the undeniable analgesic benefits of coxibs, the selective COX-2 inhibitors, suggests that prostaglandins synthesized through this pathway are responsible in large part for nociceptor sensitization in chronic joint inflammation in humans.

However, the use coxibs to treat chronic inflammatory disease, including OA and RA, has run into problems in recent years due to marked side effects. These drugs were developed as anti-inflammatory drugs that had a low gastric side-effect profile. However, in longitudinal studies a number of different side effects have been observed for different coxibs, which include cardiovascular effects, skin rashes, and hepatotoxicity. In the United Kingdom, this has resulted in the Medicines and Healthcare products Regulatory Agency (MHRA) issuing advice against the use of coxibs for the treatment of different forms of arthritis at present. This has been a major setback in the treatment of arthritic joint pain and it remains to be seen whether other approaches that inhibit the activity of prostaglandins can be identified (e.g., selective prostaglandin receptor inhibition). Much work has been done in recent years to determine which of the prostaglandin receptors might be the most suitable target for drug development, with the EP_4 receptor for prostaglandin E_2 being one of the more likely.[32,33]

Another approach is to broaden the action of NSAIDs to target other molecules in the inflammatory pathway. NSAID with nitric oxide releasing properties (NO-NSAIDs) and combined cyclooxygenase and lipoxygenase (COX-LOX) inhibitors are all under investigation for their ability to reduce inflammation and to limit the development of joint damage in animal models of arthritis. However, no studies to date have examined their ability to prevent peripheral nociceptor sensitization directly.[34]

Bradykinin and Serotonin

In addition to the prostaglandins, a number of other inflammatory mediators have been shown to excite and or sensitize articular mechanonociceptors. Bradykinin, for example, has been shown to directly excite the majority of group III and IV articular afferents in cat knee and rat ankle joint[35,36] and to sensitize them to movements.[37] In addition, it is well established that prostaglandins (PGE_2/PGI_2) may augment the excitatory or sensitizing actions of bradykinin.[26,27,35] Likewise, another important inflammatory mediator, serotonin, has been shown to excite approximately two-thirds of articular mechanonociceptors in the rat ankle and cat knee joint. This list is by no means extensive and there exists a large literature on the effects of leukotrienes, histamine, neuropeptides, and other inflammatory mediators on the sensitization of articular mechanonociceptors.[1]

TRPV1 Channel

An interesting paradox is that many joint, skin, and muscle afferents express the heat sensitive TRP channel (VR1) since they can respond to capsaicin. This means that joint afferents have the capacity to respond to damaging or potentially damaging heat stimuli, which they are unlikely to experience. One hypothesis[38] suggests that the sensitization of skin afferents by bradykinin produces a reduction in the thermal threshold for opening of the vanilloid receptor/channel complex that normally opens only in response to noxious heat. The threshold is reduced so far, indeed, that normal body temperature is sufficient to open these channels and excite the nociceptor. Such mechanisms could also be an explanation for the presence of these heat-responsive channels in deep tissues and could indicate that there is homogeneity in the mechanisms by which noxious stimuli are detected in different tissues.

In more recent studies, TRPV1 channels have been found in articular afferents[11,12] and there is now strong evidence that these channels contribute to the development of joint inflammation. This comes from studies using

TRPV1$^{-/-}$ animals, where the development of joint pathology, mechanical hyperalgesia, and joint swelling are all markedly attenuated in a model of FCA-induced arthritis in the mouse knee joint.[39–41] These data strongly suggest that the TRPV1 channel is activated, possibly through the above mechanism, during the development of joint inflammation. It has been suggested that this activation of TRPV1 contributes to the development of joint inflammation through the release of neuropeptides from TRPV1 expressing peptidergic afferents in joint tissues as part of a local neurogenic inflammatory response. In addition, TRPV1 expression has been reported to increase in a surgically induced model of OA[11] but not in an antigen-induced model of arthritis,[42] providing some further evidence for a role of TRPV1 in the development of arthritis.

Cannabinoid Receptors

The two cannabinoid receptors are expressed in mammals, one on sensory nerves (CB$_1$) and the other on immune cells (CB$_2$). Cannabinoid receptor agonists elicit analgesia in a number of experimental paradigms and there is good evidence from electrophysiological recordings from articular afferents[43] and from behavioral experiments[44] that this is mediated by CB$_1$ receptors in joints. Paradoxically, higher doses of the endocannabinoid, anandamide, have been shown to activate articular nociceptors,[45] possibly through activation of multiple receptors.

Cannabinoid receptor expression alters under certain circumstances with CB$_2$ receptor expression increasing following peripheral nerve damage, for example,[46] suggesting that the analgesic actions of cannabinoid receptor agonists may be different in diseased and normal tissues.[43] In humans, anandamide and other endocannabinoids have been found in synovial fluid aspirated from the knee joint of OA and RA patients undergoing knee arthroplasty but not in volunteers with normal knee joints. Furthermore, both CB$_1$ and CB$_2$ receptor mRNA are present in the synovium, suggesting that the cannabinoid system may play a role in endogenous pain regulation in arthritis.[47] Collectively, these data suggest that the endogenous cannabinoid system may serve to reverse the sensitization of articular nociceptors under certain circumstances, thus producing endogenous analgesia.

Interestingly, the actions of anandamide are not simply restricted to regulation of cannabinoid receptors but also include a direct action on TRPV1 ion channels. In osteoarthritic rat knee joints, both a CB$_1$ receptor antagonist, and a TRPV1 channel antagonist, block the desensitizing effect of the selective CB$_1$ agonist, ACEA (arachidonyl-2-chloroethylamide), on re-sponses of joint afferents to movements.[43] These data strongly suggest that there are interactions between the two proteins and that at least a component of the analgesic actions of endocannabinoids is mediated through direct or indirect regulation of TRPV1 channel activity.

Purinoceptors

P2X receptors are ligand-gated ion channels that are activated by ATP, an important inflammatory mediator released following tissue injury. Purinoceptors are present in sensory neurons[48] and their activation by ATP results in a rapidly desensitizing depolarization of the cell. The main P2X receptor subtype present in nociceptive fibers appears to be P2X3, although there is some evidence for the P2X2 subtype, or even P2X2/3 heteromultimers.[48] This has been confirmed in joints where P2X3 is the main subtype identified in immunocytochemical studies.[49,50] When ATP or α,β-methylene ATP is applied to the region of the joint, it elicits a short-lasting excitation of C and A-δ nerve fibers in the joint[51] and behavioral hyperalgesia.[52] indicating that P2X receptors, possibly the P2X3 receptor subtype, are responsible. P2X receptors may therefore contribute to the development of nociceptor sensitization and are a valid target for the treatment of arthritic pain.

Cytokines

Cytokines are important inflammatory mediators, produced by a range of cell type following tissue damage, that orchestrate the inflammatory response. In chronic joint disease, these regulate the release of a number of inflammatory mediators including prostaglandins and bradykinin. Two cytokines, IL1 and TNF-α, are targets for the treatment of inflammatory joint disease and drugs such as Anakinra, an IL1 receptor antagonist, and Enteracept, a soluble TNF-α receptor fusion protein, inhibit the actions of these molecules, reduce pain, and limit disease progression. No basic studies of their effect on nerve activity have been performed but they act high up in the inflammatory cascade and inhibiting their action prevents the release of a number of inflammatory mediators that sensitize joint nociceptors.

INFLUENCE OF JOINT MECHANICS

An important aspect of joint damage is the effusion that accumulates in the joint space. This is particularly important when considering the responses of joint mechanonociceptors to joint flexion or extension. Joint pressure is normally subatmospheric and lowest when the joint is in the resting or in the mid range position. However, up to 70 mL of effusate can be removed from an arthritic human knee joint,[53] which markedly increases the baseline pressure within the joint. More importantly, however, upon flexion or extension, joint pressure can increase dramatically, thus increasing stretching of the capsule and surrounding tissues. Since these are densely innervated by articular mechanonociceptors, there can be little doubt that these physical changes in the condition of the joint will also contribute to the enhanced firing of these articular afferents.

CONCLUSION

Considerable work has been undertaken in recent years to understand the inflammatory mediators that are responsible for the sensitization of articular nociceptors using a range of animal models. In order to progress this field in the future, it is important that "disease-relevant" models of OA are used where possible. One problem is that there is a poor relationship between radiological scores in OA and the pain scores reported by patients, and work is needed to understand why this is the case.

One area that has not been covered in this chapter in detail is the ion channel and receptor phenotype of articular afferents. An important question is whether articular afferents really are unique in terms of the basic mechanisms by which they detect and respond to mechanical stimuli and to inflammatory mediators. As neurons, it is clear that there are relatively few data that would allow one to distinguish a joint afferent from a skin or muscle afferent in terms of phenotype. By better understanding how joint nociceptors phenotypically differ from other peripheral nociceptors, we can understand and exploit any differences for the development of analgesic drugs.

In order to progress, we need to establish whether basic common principles apply to all nociceptors irrespective of the tissue that they innervate. We need a better understanding of the basic transduction mechanisms for thermal and mechanical stimuli, the mechanisms of sensitization including an appreciation of the G-protein coupled receptors, signaling pathways, and the ion channels that regulate nerve terminal excitability and firing. Only by combining electrophysiological measurements from single cells, molecular biology, protein biochemistry, and modern neuroanatomical and imaging techniques can we hope to start to understand the molecular mechanisms of articular mechanonociception in OA.

REFERENCES

1. Schaible H-G, Grubb BD. (1993). Spinal and afferent mechanisms of joint pain. Pain 55:5–54.
2. Johansson H, Sjolander P, Sojka P. (1991). Receptors in the knee joint ligaments and their role in the biomechanics of the joint. Crit Rev Biomed Eng 18:341–368.
3. Heppelmann B, Messlinger K, Neiss WF, Schmidt RF. (1990). Ultrastructural three-dimensional reconstruction of group III and group IV sensory nerve endings ("free nerve endings") in the knee joint capsule of the cat: evidence for multiple receptive sites. J Comp Neurol 292:103–116.

4. Dorn T, Schaible H-G, Schmidt RF. (1991). Response properties of thick myelinated group II afferents in the medial articular nerve of normal and inflamed knee joints of the cat. Somatosens Motor Res 8:127–136.

5. Grigg P, Schaible H-G, Schmidt RF. (1986). Mechanical sensitivity of group III and IV afferents from posterior articular nerve in normal and inflamed cat knee. J Neurophysiol 55:635–643.

6. Schaible H-G, Schmidt RF. (1988). Time course of mechanosensitivity changes in articular afferents during a developing experimental arthritis. J Neurophysiol 60:2180–2195.

7. Bergman E, Carlsson K, Liljeborg A, Manders E, Hokfelt T, Ulfhake B. (1999). Neuropeptides, nitric oxide synthase and GAP-43 in B4-binding and RT97 immunoreactive primary sensory neurons: normal distribution pattern and changes after peripheral nerve transection and aging. Brain Res 832:63–83.

8. Johnstone M, Goold RG, Fischer I, Gordon-Weeks PR. (1997). The neurofilament antibody RT97 recognises a developmentally regulated phosphorylation epitope on microtubule-associated protein 1B. J Anat 191:229–244.

9. Silverman JD, Kruger L. (1990). Selective neuronal glycoconjugate expression in sensory and autonomic ganglia: relation of lectin reactivity to peptide and enzyme markers. J Neurocytol 19:789–801.

10. McCarthy PW, Lawson SN. (1990). Cell type and conduction velocity of rat primary sensory neurons with calcitonin gene-related peptide-like immunoreactivity. Neuroscience 34:623–632.

11. Fernihough J, Gentry C, Bevan S, Winter J. (2005). Regulation of calcitonin gene-related peptide and TRPV1 in a rat model of osteoarthritis. Neurosci Lett 388:75–80.

12. Ioi H, Kido MA, Zhang J-Q, Yamaza T, Nakata S, Nakashima A, Tanaka T. (2006). Capsaicin receptor expression in the rat temporomandibular joint. Cell Tissue Res 325:47–54.

13. Ivanivicius SP, Blake DR, Chessell IP, Mapp PI. (2004). Isolectin B4 binding neurones are not present in the rat knee joint. Neuroscience 128:555–560.

14. Kuniyoshi K, Ohitori S, Ochiai N, Murata R, Matsudo T, Yamada T, Ochiai SS, Moriya H, Takahashi K. (2007). Characteristics of sensory DRG neurons innervating the wrist joints in rats. Eur J Pain 11:323–328.

15. Hanesch U, Pfrommer U, Grubb BD, Schaible H-G. (1993). Acute and chronic phases of unilateral inflammation in rat's ankle are associated with an increase in the proportion of calcitonin gene-related peptide-immunoreactive dorsal root ganglion cells. Eur J Neurosci 5:154–161.

16. Bendele AM. (2002). Animal models of osteoarthritis in an era of molecular biology. J Musculoskel Neur Interact 2:501–503.

17. Guingamp C, Gegout-Pottie P, Phillippe L, Terlain B, Nettler P, Gillet P. (1997). Mono-iodoacetate-induced experimental osteoarthritis: a dose-response study of the loss of mobility, morphology and biochemistry. Arthritis Rheum 40:1670–1679.

18. Scheulert N, McDougall JJ. (2006). Electrophysiological evidence that the vasoactive intestinal peptide receptor antagonist VIP_{6-28} reduces nociception in an animal model of osteoarthritis. Osteoarthritis Cartilage 14:1155–1162.

19. Coggeshall RE, Hong KAP, Langford LA, Schaible H-G. (1983). Discharge characteristics of fine medial articular afferents at rest and during passive movements of inflamed knee joints. Brain Res 272:185–188.

20. Guilbaud G, Iggo A, Tegner R. (1985). Sensory receptors in ankle joint capsules of normal and arthritic rats. Exp Brain Res 58:29–40.

21. Guilbaud G, Iggo A. (1985). The effect of acetylsalicylate on joint mechanoreceptors in rats with polyarthritis. Exp Brain Res 61:164–168.

22. Heppelmann B, Pfeffer A, Schaible H-G, Schmidt RF. (1986). Effects of acetylsalicylic acid and indomethacin on single groups III and IV sensory units from acutely inflamed joints. Pain 26:337–351.

23. Birrell GJ, McQueen DS, Iggo A, Coleman RA, Grubb BD. (1991). PGI_2-induced activation and sensitization of articular mechanoreceptors. Neuroscience Lett 124:5–8.

24. Grubb BD, Birrell GJ, McQueen DS, Iggo A. (1991). The role of PGE_2 in the sensitization of joint mechanoreceptors in normal and inflamed ankle joints of the rat. Exp Brain Res 84:383–392.

25. Heppelmann B, Schaible H-G, Schmidt RF. (1985). Effects of prostaglandins E1 and E2 on the mechanosensitivity of group III afferents from normal and inflamed cat knee joints. Adv Pain Res Ther 9:91–101.

26. Schaible H-G, Schmidt RF. (1988). Excitation and sensitization of fine articular afferents from cat's knee joint by prostaglandin E2. J Physiol 403:91–104.

27. Schepelmann K, Messlinger K, Schaible H-G, Schmidt RF. (1992). Inflammatory mediators and nociception in the joint: excitation and sensitization of slowly conducting afferent fibers of cat's knee by prostaglandin I2. Neuroscience 50:237–247.

28. Chandrasekharan NV, Dai H, Roos KLT, Evanson NK, Tomsik J, Elton TS, Simmons DL. (2002). COX-3, a cyclooxygenase-1 variant inhibited by acetaminophen and other analgesic/antipyretic drugs: cloning, structure, and expression. Proc Nat Acad Sci USA 99:13926–13931.

29. Funk CD, Funk LB, Kennedy ME, Pong AS, Fitzgerald GA. (1991). Human platelet/erythroleukemia cell prostaglandin G/H synthase: cDNA cloning, expression, and gene chromosomal assignment. FASEB J 5:2304–2312.

30. Hla T, Neilson K. (1992). Human cyclooxygenase-2 cDNA. Proc Natl Acad Sci USA 89:7384–7388.

31. Seibert K, Zhang Y, Leahy K, Hauser S, Masferrer J, Perkins W, Lee L, Isakson P. (1994). Pharmacological and biochemical demonstration of the role of cyclooxygenase 2 in inflammation and pain. Proc Natl Acad Sci USA 91: 12013–12017.

32. Lin C-R, Amaya F, Barrett L, Wang H, Takada J, Samad TA, Woolf CJ. (2006). Prostaglandin E2 receptor EP4 contributes to inflammatory pain hypersensitivity. J Pharmacol Exp Ther 319:1096–1103.

33. Southall MD, Vasko MR. (2001). Prostaglandin receptor subtypes, EP3C and EP4, mediate the prostaglandin E_2-induced cAMP production and sensitisation of sensory neurones. J Biol Chem 276:16083–16091.

34. Schaible H-G, Scmelz M, Tegeder I. (2006). Pathophysiology and treatment of pain in joint disease. Adv Drug Delivery Rev 58:323–342.

35. Birrell GJ, McQueen DS, Iggo A, Grubb BD. (1993). Prostanoid-induced potentiation of the excitatory and sensitising effects of bradykinin on articular mechanonociceptors in the rat ankle joint. Neuroscience 54:537–544.

36. Kanaka R, Schaible H-G, Schmidt RF. (1985). Activation of fine articular afferent units by bradykinin. Brain Res 327:81–90.

37. Neugebauer V, Schaible H-G, Schmidt RF. (1989). Sensitization of articular afferents to mechanical stimuli by bradykinin. Pflugers Arch 415:330–335.

38. Liang Y-F, Haake B, Reeh PW. (2001). Sustained sensitization and recruitment of rat cutaneous nociceptors by bradykinin and a novel theory of its excitatory action. J Physiol 532:229–239.

39. Barton NJ, McQueen DS, Thompson D, Gauldie SD, Wilson AW, Salter DM, Chessell IP. (2006). Attenuation of experimental arthritis in TRPV1R knockout mice. Exp Mol Pathol 81:166–170.

40. Keeble J, Russell F, Curtis B, Starr A, Pinter E, Brain SD. (2005). Involvement of transient receptor potential vanilloid 1 in the vascular and hyperalgesic components of joint inflammation. Arthritis Rheum 52:3248–3256.

41. Szabó A, Helyes Z, Sándor K, Bite A, Pintér E, Németh J, Bánvölgyi A, Bölcskei K, Elekes K, Szolcsányi J. (2005). Role of transient receptor potential vanilloid 1 receptors in adjuvant-induced chronic arthritis: in vivo study using gene-deficient mice. J Exp Pharmacol Ther 314:111–119.

42. Bär K-J, Schaible H-G, Bräuer R, Halbhuber K-J, Segond von Banchet G. (2004). The proportion of TRPV1 protein positive lumbar DRG neurones does not increase in the course of acute and chronic antigen-induced arthritis in the knee joint of the rat. Neurosci Lett 361:172–175.

43. Scheulert N, McDougall JJ. (2008). Cannabinoid-mediated antinociception is enhanced in rat osteoarthritic knees. Arthritis Rheum 58:145–153.

44. Croci T, Zarini E. (2007). Effect of cannabinoid CB_1 receptor antagonist rimonabant on nociceptive responses and adjuvant-induced arthritis in obese and lean rats. Br J Pharmacol 150:558–566.

45. Gauldie SD, McQueen DS, Pertwee R, Chessell IP. (2001). Anandamide activates peripheral nociceptors in normal and arthritic knee joints. Br J Pharmacol 132:617–621.

46. Wotherspoon G, Fox A, McIntyre P, Colley S, Bevan S, Winter J. (2005). Peripheral nerve injury induces cannabinoid receptor 2 protein in rat sensory neurones. Neuroscience 135:235–245.

47. Richardson D, Pearson RG, Kurian N, Latif ML, Garle MJ, Barrett DA, Kendall DA, Scammell BE, Reeve AJ, Chapman V. (2008). Characterisation of the cannabinoid receptor system in synovial tissue and fluid in patients with osteoarthritis and rheumatoid arthritis. Arthritis Res Ther 10:R43.

48. Grubb BD, Evans RJ. (1999). Characterization of cultured dorsal root ganglion neuron P2X receptors. Eur J Neurosci 11:149–154.

49. Ichikawa H, Fukanaga T, Jin HW, Fujita M, Takano-Yamamoto T, Sugimoto X. (2004). VR1-, VRL-1- and P2X3 receptor-immunoreactive innervation of the rat tempormandibular joint. Brain Res 1008:131–136.

50. Shinoda M, Ozaki N, Asai H, Nagmine K, Sugiura Y. (2005). Changes in P2X3 receptor expression in the trigeminal ganglion following monoarthritis of the temporomandibular joint in rats. Pain 116:42–51.

51. Dowd E, McQueen DS, Chessell IP, Humphrey PPA. (1998). P2X receptor-mediated excitation of nociceptive afferent in the normal and arthritic rat knee joint. Br J Pharmacol 125:341–346.

52. Oliveira MCG, Parada CA, Ferraz MC, Veiga A, Rodrigues LR, Barros SP, Tambeli H. (2005). Evidence for the involvement of endogenous ATP and P2X receptors in TMJ pain. Eur J Pain 9:87–93.

53. Jayson MIV, Dixon ASJ. (1970). Intraarticular pressure in rheumatoid arthritis of the knee. I. Pressure changes during passive joint distension. Ann Rheum Dis 261–265.

CHANGES IN THE NEURAL SUBSTRATE OF NOCICEPTION IN A RAT DERANGEMENT MODEL OF OSTEOARTHRITIS

James L. Henry

Michael G. DeGroote Institute for Pain Research and Care,
McMaster University, 1200 Main Street West HSC 1J11,
Hamilton, Ontario L8N 3Z5, Canada

INTRODUCTION

Statistics on joint pain may be surprising. An estimated one-quarter of all patients seen by primary care physicians present with musculoskeletal conditions,[1,2] and osteoarthritis (OA) is the most common presentation,[3] affecting approximately 12% of adults. An estimated 25% of persons over 55 years of age report having had knee pain on most days in a one month period during the previous year.[4] Approximately half of these have radiographic signs of OA in the knee.[5] It is estimated that by age 65 over 80% of adults will develop radiographic evidence of OA.[6] Pain is the primary symptom of OA,[7] pain is the major factor that leads OA patients to use health care facilities,[8] and pain is the leading cause of disability.[9–11] In contrast to other forms of arthritis, disability from pain rather than joint pathology is more pronounced in OA.[12] Despite a focus of research on physical signs of OA,[13,14] epidemiological studies have shown that baseline pain is a predictor of subsequent radiographic OA.[15,16]

Pain in Osteoarthritis, Edited by David T. Felson and Hans-Georg Schaible
Copyright © 2009 Wiley-Blackwell.

Given the prevalence and impact of the pain of OA, it is surprising that there is a lack of effective pain therapies that have a known mechanistic basis of action. Existing drug therapies are poor, with only moderate effectiveness.[14,17] Treatment of OA pain has largely been through NSAIDs and COX-2 inhibitors, but these are associated with a number of issues, including adverse side effects and variable efficacy, precluding their long-term use. Furthermore, anti-inflammatory drugs provide only partial relief of the pain, possibly because the pain is a mixture of nociceptive, inflammatory, and neuropathic origins.[18] Significant research resources are being applied to limiting cartilage loss and alterations in bone structure,[19,20] but until recently, there has been little scientific investigation focused on understanding the mechanisms underlying the initiation and the maintenance of the pain of OA. We still know little of what generates the pain of OA.

NEURAL BASIS OF PAIN

Pain is a product of the nervous system and may be divided into two general categories. One is transient and serves the physiologically important function of preventing or limiting tissue injury. It is brought about by direct activation of nociceptive sensory neurons and is generally considered acute nociceptive pain. The second category is associated with inflammation or damage to neurons and tends to be persistent or chronic. This latter pain is composed of multiple subtypes and is often characterized by nervous system plasticity. Such plasticity may be induced by one or more transient changes that can occur in the extracellular milieu, as neuronal function, protein expression, and trafficking can be regulated by factors taken up from this extracellular milieu.[21] These factors can generate signaling complexes that regulate the genetic material of the neurons[22,23] and, in particular, changes in the immune system, either in the central nervous system or in the peripheral nervous system, may play important roles in altering neuronal phenotype.[24]

Thus, as persistent pain may be due to long-term or permanent changes in neuronal phenotype, treating only the pathology after it has developed into a clinically significant condition may fail to treat the underlying pain. Phantom limb pain is a prime example of nervous system plasticity that persists even after treating the peripheral pathology.[25] It is not surprising then that studies on "joint-oriented" therapies have highlighted the transience of pain relief when only treating the physical joint in cases of chronic OA.[26] It can be argued that an approach aimed more at OA pain as a neurological disorder may lead to more effective treatment.

ORIGINS OF JOINT PAIN

Damage to the joint induces immediate changes in the nerve bundles innervating the joint.[27] Damage to sensory neurons results in changes in excitability as well as in action potential configuration recorded from the dorsal root gang-lia.[28–30] This can lead to abnormal sensory or painful input that is thought to be generated by a number of components of joint pathology including aberrant activation of nerve endings in the joint, synovial inflammation, ligament stretch, and bone remodeling. These form the basis for theories on the mechanisms of OA pain.[31–34] However, as we shall see later, current hypotheses on mechanisms of OA pain cannot account for the discordance of pathology and pain, or for the referred pain and the decrease in motor coordination that are experienced by people who suffer OA.

It is commonly thought that synovial products in the OA joint activate or sensitize peripheral terminals of small diameter sensory neurons that normally transmit the pain signal[35] (for reviews see Refs. 32, 36 and 37). Inflammation of the synovial membrane is a hallmark of OA and is also a predictive factor of pain in patients.[38] In normal joint tissue the cartilage synovial interface, the joint capsule, ligaments, periosteum, and subchondral bone are highly inner-vated by both myelinated and unmyelinated fibers.[39,40] A number of observa-tions implicate small diameter fiber growth into these areas, including the presence of hypertrophic chondrocytes, which produce growth factors,[41] the growth of blood vessels into the tide mark along with innervation of this new vasculature,[42] and the presence of these fibers within the cartilage in other painful pathological conditions.[43] Thus sprouting of new sensory nerve terminations has been suggested to give rise to the pain of OA.[44,45]

A torn anterior cruciate ligament (ACL) and the subsequent rips that develop in the menisci and the surrounding joint capsule not only mechanically destabilize the joint but also result in damage to the nerve fibers innervating these structures. This damage has been proposed to lead to pain through either Wallerian degeneration or neuroma formation. Schwann cells of an injured fiber recruit and activate inflammatory cells to clear away the cellular debris in the region of the injured fiber. This inflammatory response may generate ectopic activity in these fibers. However, the Schwann cell autocrine response is not limited to immune activation alone. Autocrine signaling also induces regrowth of injured fibers, and this signaling affects uninjured fibers traveling within the same nerve bundles to an equal extent. Neuroactive growth and trophic factors released by Schwann cells in response to the injury will therefore generate ectopic activity and growth in both injured and uninjured fibers. However, as the joint space now separates the torn ACL and as the rips in the menisci and joint capsule require extensive periods to heal (because of repetitive shear forces during use), there are no neural tubes for fiber regrowth.[46] The lack of these tubes contributes to neuroma formation, which is likely underway as nerve growth has been reported to accompany tissue repair.[47] In addition, production of autocrine angiogenic molecules within these structures and their presence within the synovial fluid[48] and cartilage matrix[49] extends the effects of de novo growth or neuroma formation to uninjured joint areas due to nonspecific signaling.

Both Wallerian degeneration and neuroma formation are to a large extent due to nonspecific autocrine signaling. The ACL is involved in motor loops; it contains efferent and afferent nerve fibers.[50] When lesions occur to these muscle fibers, the effects of nonspecific autocrine signaling are exacerbated as muscle fibers require higher tonic levels of growth factors for normal functioning.[51,52] In addition, unmyelinated fibers or fibers considered to be pain specific have higher susceptibilities to the neuroactive substances due to their lack of myelin, which are inhibitory to many autocrine signaling cascades in the developed peripheral nervous system.[53] Thus demyelination and/or secretion of autocrine products and also the formation of neuromas by regenerating sensory fibers may be a cause of OA pain.

These suggested origins of OA pain provide a reasonable view of possible mechanisms generating this type of pain. However, as we shall see later, none of the leading hypotheses can account for three important features of OA pain, and a result of this lack of full understanding of the genesis of OA pain is the lack of effective therapeutic approaches to manage this type of pain.[17] Thus an alternate view is proposed here: that OA pain is generated by changes in primary sensory neurons resulting from injury as well as secondary degeneration of neighboring fibers.

One of the important features of OA pain that is not addressed in current hypotheses is the discordance between radiographic signs and the degree of the pain—some patients with advanced OA in radiograms experience little or no pain, while others with severe joint pain exhibit mild or no structural evidence of OA.[54,55] In fact, rather than arising from nociceptors in the joint, others have suggested that the pain originates in bony osteophytes outside the joint capsule[56] or even in bone marrow near the joint.[57] We are also left with the fact that some patients continue to experience pain after total joint replacement.[58,59] If factors in the synovial fluid activate nociceptors, or if pain originates in ligaments, meniscus, or bone, then it should be expected that the more severe the pathology the more severe the pain, and this is often *not* the case. Therefore the alternate view is that the discordance may be because the pain is directly linked to damage to primary afferent neurons, resulting in a disorder (pain) that does not necessarily vary directly with joint pathology. The present project investigates whether primary sensory neurons undergo changes in an animal model of OA that match changes that have been reported to occur in injured primary afferent neurons.

A second issue that tends to be overlooked in hypotheses on OA pain is the referred pain that essentially all people with OA suffer. This can radiate from knee to hip, from hip to back, and even to the contralateral side.[60–63] Generation of pain from localized synovium, ligament, meniscus, or bone cannot account for such extensive referral of pain. It is suggested that referred pain is due to branching of peripheral or central terminal arborizations resulting from injury. Referred pain may also be due to changes in neighboring sensory neurons traveling in nerve bundles close to those directly innervating the joint; the process of cross-talk between axons would be through Wallerian degeneration. A similar concept is emerging to account for referred sensitivity in the viscera.[64]

A cascade of events may underlie the third issue, which is the motor instability that accompanies OA.[9,65,66] Motor instability may come through changes in mechanisms of proprioception. Disease progression results in a modification of both frequency and pattern of mechanoreceptor activation within the knee, due either to a change in the pattern of load distribution as a result of bone or ligament remodeling or to a voluntary change in the manner in which the knee is used due to pain.[67] Myelinated afferent fibers are particularly susceptible to nonspecific antigen recognition because of the high lipid to protein ratio of the myelin sheaths.[68] Thus activated immune cells in the synovial membrane attack the myelin sheath, inducing an autoimmune response. This autoimmune response is self-propagating as it leads to the exposure of the normally protected Po and P2 epitopes within the sheaths. The exposure of these epitopes leads to a secondary autoimmune response, which increases the number of immune cells present and by extension the levels of neuroactive substances that are released by these cells.[69] Damage to the myelin sheath leads to abnormal activity in afferent fibers and activation of the supporting glial cells.[70] This may also spread to the myelin sheath surrounding motoneurons, which may also result from secondary degenerative changes that occur in damaged neurons.[71] Thus changes in proprioceptive input as well as motor output may share a common etiology with the mechanisms giving rise to the pain of OA—due to compromised myelination of axons in mixed nerves.

MECHANISMS OF SENSORY FUNCTION

To understand the persistent pain of OA, it is important to focus on changes in the neural substrate of sensory function in order to formulate ways of accounting for the three clinical correlates of OA stated previously. Current hypotheses do not account for several of the observations associated with the pain of OA, and an alternate model is proposed that will be directly investigated in the present proposal. Our novel approach has focused on changes in the physiological properties of primary sensory neurons that innervate the joint and widely surrounding tissues, identified by recording intracellularly from the cell bodies of these neurons in the dorsal root ganglia (DRG). The common approaches are generally to investigate changes in sensitivity or activation thresholds of the peripheral terminals of neurons innervating the joint, or development of central sensitization of nociceptive or pain mechanisms at the spinal level.[72] The present chapter focuses uniquely on changes in the physiological properties of the primary sensory neuron itself.

STRUCTURE OF THE JOINT

The intra-articular joint includes several structures, including ligaments, that are highly innervated and vascularized especially the anterior cruciate ligament

(ACL). This prevents anterior displacement of the tibia in relation to the femur and menisci, structures that are also highly innervated and serve to distribute force evenly onto the articulating surfaces[73] and cartilage, which forms a cap over the articulating surfaces of the tibia and femur. There are two menisci: the medial meniscus, which is attached to the tibia, and the lateral meniscus, which is attached to the lateral collateral ligament. Following injury to the ACL, the menisci are often ripped, injuring nerve fibers, and once this occurs there is an approximate 70% chance of development of knee joint pain.[74,75]

SELECTION OF THE ANIMAL MODEL

There are several different types of animal model of OA. Studies on animal models of OA can be broken down into two groups. One group is designed to elucidate the mechanisms underlying different components of the joint pathology. These models are induced by modulation of gene[76] or protein expression,[77] injection of inflammatory cytokines,[78] or injection of photolytic enzymes.[79] The second type of study is designed to model OA for preclinical testing and is generally based on surgical induction[80] or excessive use of the joint.[81] These divergent groups are well suited to addressing the individual questions for which they were designed. However, translation of findings from the first group by the second into clinically relevant data is impaired by the lack of standardization within these preclinical models. In addition, the clinically established role of the nervous system in the development of OA cannot be effectively addressed by current preclinical models, as there is no existing body of research regarding long-term changes in nervous system function in these animals.

Thus the model selected for our studies is based on mechanical derangement of the knee joint. It was selected because this is the most prevalent etiology[82] and knee malalignment is the most potent risk factor for structural deterioration of the joint. The procedure involves transection of the ACL. This ligament is highly innervated,[83,84] is often ripped in sports injuries,[85] connects the tibia to the femur thus stabilizing the joint by preventing anterior displacement of the tibia, and may or may not[86,87] be involved in motor loops that protect the joint from overextension. The procedure also involves removal of the medial meniscus, another highly innervated structure,[88] which distributes load evenly onto the articulating surfaces[89] and which is often damaged during the development of OA.[74] Removal of this structure therefore results in an approximate 65% increase in the load on the articulating surfaces and thus increases the severity of the derangement.[73] As both structures are innervated, following surgery mechanical derangement of the joint is accompanied by nerve trauma and this may represent the mechanisms triggering changes in the physiology and structure of primary sensory neurons.[90]

CHANGES IN SPINAL NOCICEPTIVE MECHANISMS IN THE OA MODEL

We have found that in the Mosconi–Kruger[91] model of neuropathic pain, dorsal horn neurons exhibit expanded peripheral receptive fields[92,93] and we have found the same in our model of OA. These changes can be due to a number of factors, including changes in central sprouting, engagement of silent synapses in the spinal cord, sensitization of dorsal horn neurons, recruitment of additional primary afferent neurons, and a number of additional mechanisms. Therefore a series of experiments was done to identify changes in spinal nociceptive mechanisms in the rat derangement model of OA.

In initial studies, we confirmed that the model displays histological and imaging profiles resembling those in human knee OA and instituted forced mobilization on a slowly rotating treadmill to regulate the severity of the model.[94,95] In addition, it was important to determine whether the model exhibits any signs of pain associated with the arthritic joint. Articulation of the deranged knee induced a brief heterosegmental pronociceptive effect in the tail flick test. In a modified open field test, this pronociceptive effect led to a decrease in voluntary use of the joint. Tests on the treadmill confirmed that this decrease was not due to a reduction in the mechanical viability of the joint.[95]

CHANGES IN PRIMARY AFFERENT MECHANISMS IN THE OA MODEL

Damage to sensory nerve fibers can cause changes in myelination and in expression of sodium channels.[30,96,97] These changes can be detected through intracellular recording from the cell bodies of sensory neurons. Changes in myelination can be detected through measuring conduction velocity, through responses to paired pulse stimulation of the axons, and through measuring the maximum stimulation frequency that the neuron follows. Changes in sodium channels can be determined through changes in the configuration of the evoked action potential as well as the response to direct injection of depolarizing currents into the cell. Similar approaches have been applied to understand mechanisms of inflammatory pain and neuropathic pain in animal models, but to our knowledge this is the first attempt to understand mechanisms of pain in an animal model of OA by recording intracellularly from DRG neurons.

Our own pilot studies on DRG neurons were thus carried out to gain insight into any differences between DRG neurons in OA model animals compared to naïve and sham-operated animals. Action potentials from different DRG neuron types are uniquely identifiable on the basis of the criteria and a standard classification scheme proposed by Lawson et al.[98] Each DRG neuron type has a characteristic configuration, and this is used along with the other parameters to classify each neuron recorded according to the types listed by Lawson and colleagues. The unique configuration of each type of action potential reflects the unique set of ion channels that are involved in conducting the signal, and any difference in the configuration of any specific neuron type, between OA and control animals, will indicate a functional change in the particular ion channel. Initially, we were concerned that we would be unable to record from a reasonable number of cells in the DRG that originate in the joint, largely due to their relative paucity compared to the large number of other neurons.[99] What was quite unexpected, then, was that when we started recording from DRG neurons in OA animals, we found that the most obvious changes were NOT in sensory neurons from the knee but in neurons innervating other sites around the knee. Furthermore, it was NOT the small or high threshold afferents where most of the changes were observed, but low threshold A fibers, including the largest, fastest conducting muscle spindle afferents.[100,101]

These results constitute an entirely novel discovery that may have important implications for future research on mechanisms of OA pain, on the pursuit of new avenues to explore for innovative approaches to treating the pain of OA, and ultimately the life habits and quality of life for those who suffer the burden of OA pain. Our pilot studies have thus provided unexpected results: that the greatest changes are in the large diameter afferents, quite different from most of the mechanisms being proposed in the literature today.[100,101] The changes seen in our pilot studies may have important functional significance and have not been reported previously.

GENERAL CONCLUSIONS

As we were gathering these data we began discussing these results with local rheumatologists and they were not the least surprised that we saw changes in neurons innervating sites outside the joint and particularly proprioceptive afferents. They indicated that our results were consistent with three observations made in the clinic: that in addition to their joint pain, OA patients also report referred pain at sites outside the joint, that patients with OA exhibit altered proprioception, and that sensory function changes with respect to mechanical and thermal sensitivity. A local study being initiated in the School of Rehabilitation Sciences at McMaster University indicates also a loss of organization of sensory mapping in the periphery of OA subjects (Drs. Galea and Wessel, McMaster University, personal communication). Our pilot data suggest that significant changes are occurring in selected types of DRG neuron and that these changes are not consistent with expectation.

FUTURE DIRECTIONS

Our studies aim to explore new avenues to pursue in the search for effective treatment for the pain of OA by exploring fundamental mechanisms that generate changes in the neural substrate of nociception in the surgically induced derangement model of knee OA. Given the controversy about the type of primary afferent mediating different types of nociceptive signal,[102–104] data from these experiments will provide important information on the specific neuron types undergoing change and will provide an indication of mediators of change, whether these will be changes in Na^+, K^+, or other channels.[30,96]

Referred pain may arise from increased terminal distribution in the spinal cord. Changes in the pattern of the central arborization of primary sensory neurons, particularly to areas of spinal cord involved in processing of nociceptive information, has been suggested to account for the shift in sensory processing whereby light tactile stimulation elicits pain.[102–104] This involves retraction of small diameter afferents and sprouting of larger diameter afferents into areas vacated by the small fiber neurons.[105] Yet there is no detailed mapping of spinal arborization patterns of functionally identified single afferents in an animal model of OA. Characteristic arborizations for primary afferent neuron types are currently well understood. Changes induced in these projection patterns will provide important information on neural connections of normally nonnociceptive neurons to nociceptive relay sites in the dorsal horn of the spinal cord, providing novel insights into movement-evoked breakthrough pain and also the referred pain that characterize OA pain.[106]

Nerve injury induces changes in the phenotype of primary sensory neurons[107,108] and one might expect that this will be accompanied by a change in expression of neurotransmitters. There is no expectation that substance P expression occurs in DRG neuron types that normally do not express substance P, but given its implication in nociceptive mechanisms it is important to establish whether there is such a change.

Rodent models of OA have been in use since the late 1970s (see Ref. 109 for review), yet since that time little is known about disease progression in these models, because studies tend to focus on early changes or establishing and characterizing different types of model. In addition to the need to understand the mechanisms engaged at different stages of OA, it is also important to characterize progression of our model of OA before it may be fully utilized in preclinical studies on emerging novel therapeutic approaches. We have recently published reports on evaluation of our model,[94,110] using parameters of early stage[111] and late stage[112] OA. We reported that forced mobilization exercise accelerates progression of OA, as indicated using OARSI histopathology scores, in vivo microcomputed tomography, biochemical analysis of type II collagen breakdown, and hypertrophic chondrocyte markers in articular cartilage.[95,113]. Given the disconnect between signs of OA and the pain of OA, it is important to determine the effects of forced mobilization on changes in properties of sensory neurons in this model.

ACKNOWLEDGMENTS

The information obtained from electrophysiological studies on this model has been obtained by Neil Schwartz and Qi Wu. Generous financial support is acknowledged from the Canadian Arthritis Network and the Canadian Institutes of Health Research.

REFERENCES

1. Mazzuca SA, Brandt KD, Katz BP, Li W, Stewart KD. (1993). Therapeutic strategies distinguish community based primary care physicians from rheumatologists in the management of osteoarthritis. J Rheumatol 20:80–86.

2. Lawrence RC, Helmick CG, Arnett FC, Deyo RA, Felson DT, Giannini EH, Heyse SP, Hirsch R, Hochberg MC, Hunder GG, Liang MH, Pillemer SR, Steen VD, Wolfe F. (1998). Estimates of the prevalence of arthritis and selected musculoskeletal disorders in the United States. Arthritis Rheum 41:778–799.

3. Felson DT, Lawrence RC, Dieppe PA, et al. (2000). Osteoarthritis: new insights. Ann Intern Med 33:635–646.

4. Peat G, McCarney R, Croft P. (2001). Knee pain and osteoarthritis in older adults: a review of community burden and current use of primary health care. Ann Rheum Dis 60:91–97.

5. Hinton R, Moody RL, Davis AW, Thomas SF. (2002). Osteoarthritis: diagnosis and therapeutic considerations. Am Fam Physician 65:841–848.

6. Oddis CV. (1996). New perspectives on osteoarthritis. Am J Med 100:10S–15S.

7. Schumacher HR, Klippel JH, Koopman WJ. (1993). *Primer on the Rheumatic Diseases*, 10th ed. Atlanta, GA: Arthritis Foundation.

8. Bedson J, Mottram S, Thomas E, Peat G. (2007). Knee pain and osteoarthritis in the general population: what influences patients to consult? Fam Pract 24:43–453.

9. Guccione AA, Felson DT, Anderson JJ, et al. (1994). The effects of specific medical conditions on the functional limitations of elders in the Framingham Study. Am J Public Health 84:351–358.

10. Hootman JM, Helmick CG. (2006). Projections of US prevalence of arthritis and associated activity limitations. Arthritis Rheum 54:226–229.

11. Axford J, Heron C, Ross F, Victor CR. (2008). Management of knee osteoarthritis in primary care: pain and depression are the major obstacles. J Psychosom Res 64:461–467.

12. Carr AJ. (1999). Beyond disability: measuring the social and personal consequences of osteoarthritis. Osteoarthritis Cartilage 7:230–238.

13. Aigner T, Kim HA. (2002). Apoptosis and cellular vitality: issues in osteoarthritic cartilage degeneration. Arthritis Rheum 46:1986–1996.

14. Wieland HA, Michaelis M, Kirschbaum BJ, Rudolphi KA. (2005). Osteoarthritis–an untreatable disease? Nature Rev Drug Discov 4:331–344.

15. Hart DJ, Doyle DV, Spector TD. (1999). Incidence and risk factors for radiographic knee osteoarthritis in middle-aged women: the Chingford Study. Arthritis Rheum 42:17–24.

16. Felson DT. (2003). Epidemiology of osteoarthritis. In: Brandt KD, Doherty M, and Lohmander LS (eds.). *Osteoarthritis*. Oxford, UK: Oxford University Press, pp. 9–16.

17. Goldring MB, Goldring SR. (2007). Osteoarthritis. J Cell Physiol 213:626–634.

18. Bove SE, Laemont KD, Brooker RM, et al. (2005). Surgically induced osteoarthritis in the rat results in the development of both osteoarthritis-like joint pain and secondary hyperalgesia. Osteoarthritis Cartilage 14:1041–1048.

19. Hogenmiller MS, Lozada CJ. (2006). An update on osteoarthritis therapeutics. Curr Opin Rheumatol 18:256–260.

20. Ameye LG, Young MR. (2006). Animal models of osteoarthritis: lessons learned while seeking the "Holy Grail." Curr Opin Rheumatol 18:537–547.

21. Willis DE, van Niekerk EA, Sadaki Y, Mesngon M, Merianda TT, Williams GG, Kendall M, Smith DS, Bassell GJ, Twiss JH. (2007). Extracellular stimuli specifically regulate localized levels of individual neuronal mRNAs. J Cell Biol 178:965–980.

22. Hanz SE, Perlson D, Willis JQ, et al. (2003). Axoplasmic importins enable retrograde injury signaling in lesioned nerve. Neuron 40:1095–1104.

23. Perlson E, Hanz S, Ben-Yaakov K, Segal-Ruder Y, Fainzilber M. (2005). Vimentin-dependent spatial translocation of an activated MAP kinase in injured nerve. Neuron 45:715–726.

24. Woolf CJ, Salter MW. (2000). Neuronal plasticity: increasing the gain in pain. Science 288:1765–1769.

25. Flor HR. (2003). Remapping somatosensory cortex after injury. Adv Neurol 93:195–204.

26. Hunziker EB. (2002). Articular cartilage repair: basic science and clinical progress. A review of the current status and prospects. Osteoarthritis Cartilage 10:432–463.

27. Gomez-Barrena E, Nunez A, Martinez-Moreno E, Valls J, Munuera L. (1997). Neural and muscular electric activity in the cat's knee. Changes when the anterior cruciate ligament is transected. Acta Orthop Scand 68:149–155.

28. Devor M, Wall PD. (1990). Cross-excitation in dorsal root ganglia of nerve-injured and intact rats. J Neurophysiol 64:1733–1746.

29. Gurtu S, Smith PA. (1988). Electrophysiological characteristics of hamster dorsal root ganglion cells and their response to axotomy. J. Neurophysiol 59:408–423.

30. Oyelese AA, Rizzo MA, Waxman SG, Kocsis JD. (1997). Differential effects of NGF and BDNF on axotomy-induced changes in GABA(A)-receptor-mediated conductance and sodium currents in cutaneous afferent neurons. J Neurophysiol 78:31–42.

31. Felson DT. (2005). The sources of pain in knee osteoarthritis. Curr Opin Rhuematol 17:624–628.

32. McDougall JJ. (2006). Arthritis and pain: neurogenic origin of joint pain. Arthrit Res Ther 8:220–231.

33. Gwilym SE, Pollard TC, Carr AJ. (2008). Understanding pain in osteoarthritis. J Bone Joint Surg Br 90:280–287.

34. Hunter DJ, McDougall JJ, Keefe FJ. (2008). The symptoms of osteoarthritis and the genesis of pain. Rheum Dis Clin North Am 34:623–643.

35. Scheuelert N, McDougall JJ. (2006). Electrophysiological evidence that the vasoactive intestinal peptide receptor antagonist VIP6-28 reduces nociception in an animal model of osteoarthritis. Osteoarthritis Cartilage 14:1155–1162.

36. Niisalo S, Hukkanen M, Imai S, Tomowall J, Konttinen YT. (2002). Neuropeptides in experimental and degenerative arthritis. Ann NY Acad Sci 966:384–399.

37. Schaible HG, Ebersberger A, Von Banchet GS. (2002). Mechanisms of pain in arthritis. Ann NY Acad Sci 966:343–354.

38. Myers SL, Brandt KD, Ehlich JW, Braunstein EM, Shelbourne KD, Heck DA, Kalasinki LA. (1990). Synovial inflammation in patients with early osteoarthritis of the knee. J Rheumatol 17:1662–1669.

39. Schwab W, Funk RH. (1998). Innervation pattern of different cartilaginous tissues in the rat. Acta Anat (Basel) 163:184–190.

40. Schwab W, Bilgicyildirim A, Funk RH. (1997). Microtopography of the autonomic nerves in the rat knee: a fluorescence microscopic study. Anat Rec 247:109–118.

41. Poole RA. (1998). Pathophysiology of osteoarthritis. Osteoarthritis Cartilage 6:374–376.

42. Moskowitz RW. (2001). *Osteoarthritis: Diagnosis and Medical/Surgical Management*, 3rd ed. Philadelphia: Saunders.

43. Coppes MH, Marani E, Thomeer RT, Groen GJ. (1997). Innervation of "painful" lumbar discs. Spine 22:2342–2349.

44. Mapp PI, Avery PS, Mcwilliams DF, Bowyer J, Day C, Moores S, Webster R, Walsh DA. (2007). Angiogenesis in two animal models of osteoarthritis. Osteoarthritis Cartilage 16:61–69.

45. Suri S, Gill SE, de Camin SM, et al. (2007). Neurovascular invasion of the osteochondral junction in osteophytes in osteoarthritis. Arthritis Res Dev. 10.113b/ard.2006.063354.

46. Stoll G, Muller HW. (1999). Nerve injury, axonal degeneration and neural regeneration: basic insights. Brain Pathol 9:313–325.

47. Ackermann PW, Ahmed M, Kreicbergs A. (2002). Early nerve regeneration after Achilles tendon rupture—a prerequisite for healing? A study in the rat. J Orthop Res 20:849–856.

48. Smith MD, Triantafillou S, Parker A, Youssef PP, Coleman M. (1997). Synovial membrane inflammation and cytokine production in patients with early osteoarthritis. J Rheumatol 24:365–371.

49. Wang J, Verdonk P, Elewaut D, Veys EM, Verbruggen G. (2003). Homeostasis of the extracellular matrix of normal and osteoarthritic human articular cartilage chondrocytes in vitro. Osteoarthritis Cartilage 11:801–809.

50. Madey SM, Cole KJ, Brand RA. (1997). Sensory innervation of the cat knee articular capsule and cruciate ligament visualised using anterogradely transported wheat germ agglutinin-horseradish peroxidase. J Anat 190:289–297.

51. Eriksson NP, Lindsay RM, Aldskogius H. (1994). BDNF and NT-3 rescue sensory but not motoneurones following axotomy in the neonate. Neuroreport 5:1445–1448.

52. Munson JB, Shelton DL, McMahon SB. (1997). Adult mammalian sensory and motor neurons: roles of endogenous neurotrophins and rescue by exogenous neurotrophins after axotomy. J Neurosci 17:470–476.

53. Woolf CJ, Bloechlinger S. (2002). It takes more than two to Nogo. Science 297:1132–1134.

54. Davis MA, Ettinger WH, Neuhaus JM, Barclay JD, Segal MR. (1992). Correlates of knee pain among US adults with and without radiographic knee osteoarthritis. J Rheumatol 19:1943–1949.

55. Sharma L, Felson DT. (1998). Studying how OA causes disability: nothing is simple. J Rheumatol 25:1–4.

56. Kijowski R, Blandenbaker DG, Stanton PT, Fine JP, De Smet AA. (2006). Radiographic findings of osteoarthritis versus arthroscopic findings of articular cartilage degeneration in the tibiofemoral joint. Radiology 239:818–824.

57. Torres L, Dunlop DD, Peterfy C, et al. (2006). The relationship between specific tissue lesions and pain severity in persons with knee osteoarthritis. Osteoarthritis Cartilage 14:1033–1040.

58. Lehner B, Koeck FX, Capellino S, Schubert TE, Hofbauer R, Straub RH. (2007). Preponderance of sensory versus sympathetic nerve fibers and increased cellularity in the infrapatellar fat pad in anterior knee pain patients after primary arthroplasty. J Orthop Res DOI 10.1002/jor.20498.

59. O'Sullivan M, Tai CC, Richards S, Skyme AD, Walter WL, Walter WK. (2007). Iliopsoas tendonitis a complication after total hip arthroplasty. J Arthr. plasty 22:166–170.

60. Kosek E, Ordeberg G. (2000). Lack of pressure pain modulation by heterotopic noxious conditioning stimulation in patients with painful osteoarthritis before, but not following surgical pain relief. Pain 88:69–78.

61. Bajaj P, Bajaj P, Graven-Nielson T, Arendt-Nielson L. (2001). Osteoarthritis and its association with muscle hyperalgesia: an experimental controlled study. Pain 93:107–114.

62. Bradley LA, Kersh BC, DeBerry JJ, Deutsch G, Alarcon GA, McLain DA. (2004). Lessons from fibromyalgia: abnormal pain sensitivity in knee osteoarthritis. Novartis Found Symp 260:258–270, discussion 270–279.

63. Ben-Galim P, Ben-Galim T, Rand N, et al. (2007). Hip–spine syndrome: the effect of total hip replacement surgery on low back pain in severe osteoarthritis of the hip. Spine 32:2099–2102.

64. Bielefeldt K, Lamb K, Gebhart GF. (2006). Convergence of sensory pathways in the development of somatic and visceral hypersensitivity. Am J Pysiol Gastrointest Liver Physiol 291:G658–G656.

65. Barrett DS, Cobb AG, Bentley G. (1991). Joint proprioception in normal, osteoarthritic and replaced knees. J Bone Joint Surg Br 73B:536–543.

66. Barrack RL, Skinner HB, Cook SD, Haddad RJ Jr. (1983). Effect of articular disease and total knee arthroplasty on knee joint-position sense. J Neurophys 50:6847–6854.

67. Hurley MV. (1999). The role of muscle weakness in the pathogenesis of osteoarthritis. Rheum Dis Clin North Am 25:283–298.

68. Bongarzone ER, Pasquini JM, Soto EF. (1995). Oxidative damage to proteins and lipids of CNS myelin produced by in vitro generated reactive oxygen species. J Neurosci Res 41:213–221.

69. Watkins LR, Maier S. (2002). Beyond neurons: evidence that immune and glial cells contribute to pathological pain states. Physiol Rev 82:981–1011.

70. Wu G, Ringkamp M, Murinson BB, Pogatzki EM, Hartke TV, Weerahandi HM, Campbell JN, Griffin JW, Meyer RA. (2002). Degeneration of myelinated efferent fibers induces spontaneous activity in uninjured C-fiber afferents. J Neurosci 22:7746–7753.

71. Ling SM, Conwit RA, Talbot L, et al. (2007). Electromyographic patterns suggest changes in motor unit physiology associated with early osteoarthritis of the knee. Osteoarthritis Cartilage 15:1134–1140.

72. Schaible HG, Grubb BD. (1993). Afferent and spinal mechanisms of joint pain. Pain 55:5–54.

73. Noyes FR, Bassett RW, Grood ES, Butler DL. (1980). Arthroscopy in acute traumatic hemarthrosis of the knee. Incidence of anterior cruciate tears and other injuries. J Bone Joint Surg Am 62:687–695,757.

74. Mitsou A, Vallianatos P. (1988). Meniscal injuries associated with rupture of the anterior cruciate ligament: a retrospective study. Injury 19:429–431.

75. Bhattacharyya T, Gale D, Dewire P, et al. (2003). The clinical importance of meniscal tears demonstrated by magnetic resonance imaging in osteoarthritis of the knee. J Bone Joint Surg Am 85:4–9.

76. Munoz-Guerra MF, Delgado-Baeza E, Sanchez-Hernandez JJ, Garcia-Ruiz JP. (2004). Chondrocyte cloning in aging and osteoarthritis of the hip cartilage: morphometric analysis in transgenic mice expressing bovine growth hormone. Acta Orthop Scand 75:210–216.

77. Johnson K, Terkeltaub R. (2004). Upregulated ank expression in osteoarthritis can promote both chondrocyte MMP-13 expression and calcification via chondrocyte extracellular PPi excess. Osteoarthritis Cartilage 12:321–335.

78. Hui W, Rowan AD, Richards CD, Cawston TE. (2003). Oncostatin M in combination with tumor necrosis factor alpha induces cartilage damage and matrix metalloproteinase expression in vitro and in vivo. Arthritis Rheum 48:3404–3418.

79. Kikuchi T, Sakuta T, Yamaguchi T. (1998). Intra-articular injection of collagenase induces experimental osteoarthritis in mature rabbits. Osteoarthritis Cartilage 6:177–186.

80. Liu W, Burton-Wurster N, Glant TT, Tashman S, Sumner DR, Kamath RV, Lust G, Kimura JH, Cs-Szabo G. (2003). Spontaneous and experimental osteoarthritis in dog: similarities and differences in proteoglycan levels. J Orthop Res 21:730–737.

81. Pap G, Eberhardt R, Sturmer I, Machner A, Schwarzberg H, Roessner A, Neumann W. (1998). Development of osteoarthritis in the knee joints of Wistar rats after strenuous running exercise in a running wheel by intracranial self-stimulation. Pathol Res Pract 194:41–47.

82. Creamer P, Lethbridge-Cejku M, Hochberg MC. (1998). Where does it hurt? Pain localization in osteoarthritis of the knee. Osteoarthritis Cartilage 6:318–323.

83. Haus J, Halata Z. (1990). Innervation of the anterior cruciate ligament. Int Orthop 14:293–296.

84. Krauspe R, Schmidt M, Schaible HG. (1992). Sensory innervation of the anterior cruciate ligament. An electrophysiological study of the response properties of single identified mechanoreceptors in the cat. J Bone Joint Surg Am 74:390–397.

85. Shirakura K, Terauchi M, Kizuki S, Moro S, Kimura M. (1995). The natural history of untreated anterior cruciate tears in recreational athletes. Clin Orthop 317:227–236.

86. Friden T, Roberts D, Ageberg E, Walden M, Zatterstorm R. (2001). Review of knee propioception and the relation to extremity function after anterior cruciate ligament rupture. J Orthop Sports Phys Ther 31:567–576.

87. Solomonow M, Krogsgaard M. (2001). Sensorimotor control of knee stability. A review. Scand J Med Sci Sports 11:64–80.

88. Mach DB, Rogers SD, Sabino MC, Luger NM, Schwei MJ, Pomonis JD, Keyser CP, Clohisy DR, Adams DJ, O'Leary P, Mantyh PW. (2002). Origins of skeletal pain: sensory and sympathetic innervation of the mouse femur. Neuroscience 113:155–166.

89. Iwasaki A, Inoue K, Hukuda S. (1995). Distribution of neuropeptide-containing nerve fibers in the synovium and adjacent bone of the rat knee joint. Clin Exp Rheumatol 13:173–178.

90. Michaelis M, Liu X, Janig W. (2000). Axotomized and intact muscle afferents but no skin afferents develop ongoing discharges. J Neurosci 20:2742–2748.

91. Mosconi T, Kruger L. (1996). Fixed-diameter polyethylene cuffs applied to the rat sciatic nerve induced a painful neuropathy: ultrastructural morphometric analysis of axonal alterations. Pain 64:37–57.

92. Pitcher GM, Henry JL. (2000). Cellular mechanisms of hyperalgesia and spontaneous pain in a spinalized rat model of peripheral neuropathy: changes in myelinated afferent inputs implicated. Eur J Neurosci 12:2006–2020.

93. Pitcher GM, Henry JL. (2004). Nociceptive response to innocuous mechanical stimulation in a spinalized rat model of peripheral neuropathy: NK-1 receptor activation and myelinated afferent inputs implicated. Exp Neurol 186:173–197.

94. Appleton CTG, Pitelka V, Henry JL, Beier F. (2007). Global analysis of gene expression in early experimental osteoarthritis. Arthritis Rheum 56:1854–1868.

95. Appleton CTG, McErlain DD, Pitelka V, Schwartz N, Bernier SM, Henry JL, Holdsworth DW, Beier F. (2007). Forced mobilization accelerates pathogenesis: characterization of a preclinical surgical model of osteoarthritis. Arthritis Res Ther 9:R13.

96. Fjell J, Cummins TR, Dib-Hajj SD, et al. (1999). Differential role of DGNF and NGF in the maintenance of two TTX-resistant sodium channels in adult DRG neurons. Mol Brain Res 67:267–282.

97. Abdulla FA, Smith PA. (2002). Changes in Na^+ channel currents of rat dorsal root ganglion neurons following axotomy and axotomy-induced autotomy. J Neurophysiol 88:2518–2529.

98. Lawson SN, Crepps BA, Perl ER. (1997). Relationship of substance P to afferent characteristics of dorsal root ganglion neurones in guinea-pig. J Physiol 505:177–191.

99. Prats-Galino A, Puigdellivol-Sanchez A, Ruano-Gil D, Molander C. (1999). Representations of hindlimb digits in rat dorsal root ganglia. J Comp Neurol 408:137–145.

100. Wu Q, Henry JL. (2006). Electrophysiological properties of dorsal root ganglion neurons in vivo in a derangement rat model of osteoarthritis. Soc Neurosci Abst 738:24.

101. Wu Q, Henry, JL. (2007). Increased kinetics of TTX-sensitive sodium channels in AƎ sensory neurones in a rat model of osteoarthritis: in vivo intracellular recording. Soc Neurosci Abst 820:7.

102. Koltzenburg M, Torebjork HE, Wahren LK. (1994). Nociceptor modulated central sensitization causes mechanical hyperalgesia in acute chemogenic and chronic neuropathic pain. Brain 117:579–591.

103. Hughes DI, Scott DT, Todd AJ, Riddell JS. (2003). Lack of evidence for sprouting of Abeta afferents into the superficial laminas of the spinal cord dorsal horn after nerve section. J Neurosci 23:9491–9499.

104. Yoshimura M, Furue H, Nakatsuka T, Matayoshi T, Katafuchi T. (2004). Functional reorganization of the spinal pain pathways in developmental and pathological conditions. Novartis Found Symp 261:116–124.

105. White FA, Kocsis JD. (2002). A-fiber sprouting in spinal cord dorsal horn is attenuated by proximal nerve stump encapsulation. Exp Neurol 177:385–395.

106. Ferreira-Gomes J, Adaes S, Castro-Lopes JM. (2008). Assessment of movement-evoked pain in osteoarthritis by the knee-bend and cat walk tests: a clinically relevant study. J Pain PMID: 18650131.

107. Peters CM, Ghilardi JR, Keyser CP, et al. (2005). Tumor-induced injury of primary afferent sensory nerve fibers in bone cancer pain. Exp Neurol 193:85–100.

108. Obata K, Yamanaka H, Fukuoka T, et al. (2003). Contribution of injured and uninjured dorsal rot ganglion neurons to pain behavior and the changes in gene expression following chronic constriction injury of the sciatic nerve in rats. Pain 101:65–77.

109. Schwartz ER. (1987). Animal models: a means to study the pathogenesis of osteoarthritis. J Rheum 14:101–103.

110. Appleton CTG, McErlain DD, Henry JL, Holdsworth DW, Beier F. (2007). Molecular and histological analysis of a new rat model of experimental knee osteoarthritis. Ann NY Acad Sci 1117:165–174.

111. Boyd SK, Muller R, Matayas JR, Wohl GR, Zernicke RF. (2000). Early morphometric and anisotropic change in periarticular cancellous bone in a model of experimental knee osteoarthritis quantified using microcomputed tomography. Clin Biomech 15:624–631.

112. Boyd SK, Muller R, Leonard T, Herzog W. (2005). Long-term periarticular bone adaptation in a feline knee injury model for post-traumatic experimental osteoarthritis. Osteoarthritis Cartilage 13:235–242.

113. McErlain DD, Appleton CTG, Litchfield RB, Pitelka V, Henry JL, Beier F, Holdsworth DW. (2008). Study of subchondral bone adaptations in a rodent surgical model of OA using in vivo micro-computed tomography. Osteoarthritis Cartilage 16:458–469.

4

INFLAMMATORY MEDIATORS AND NOCICEPTION IN OSTEOARTHRITIS

Bruce L. Kidd

*Barts & The London School of Medicine & Dentistry,
London E1 2AD, United Kingdom*

Jason J. McDougall

*Department of Physiology and Pharmacology, University of Calgary,
3330 Hospital Drive NW, Calgary, Alberta T2N 4N1, Canada*

Julia J. Inglis

*Kennedy Institute of Rheumatology, Imperial College
London, London W6 8LH, United Kingdom*

INTRODUCTION

Pain is not an aubiquitous feature of osteoarthritis (OA), but in symptomatic individuals a wide spectrum of both stimulus dependent and independent pain is apparent. It remains unclear whether such pain arises in consequence of a

Pain in Osteoarthritis, Edited by David T. Felson and Hans-Georg Schaible
Copyright © 2009 Wiley-Blackwell.

single mechanism or many, or whether different mechanisms play a role at different stages of the disease.

As with all chronic pain states, symptoms are strongly influenced by sensitization of pain (or nociceptive) pathways, although the relative influence of peripheral versus central mechanisms remains uncertain. It is clear, however, that over and above any direct mechanical effect, there is a critical mediator-driven interaction between the damaged joint and the nociceptive system that potentially leads both to direct excitation as well as to longer term sensitization.

This chapter focuses on the evidence for a causal role in OA pain for mediators that have been classically associated with inflammation including prostaglandins, cytokines, growth factors, and neurally derived peptides. All have been shown to be present at some stage in human OA.

MODELS OF OSTEOARTHRITIS

Human psychophysical studies provide objective evidence for the presence of nociceptive sensitization in symptomatic patients with OA and for the reversibility of such processes.[1,2] These studies have not investigated the role of specific mediators, although the analgesic efficacy of non steroidal anti-inflammatory agents (NSAIDs) points to an important role for prostaglandins in symptomatic disease. The analgesic efficacy of intra-articular steroids is also consistent with a role for inflammatory mediators in this disorder.

The paucity of data from human studies regarding OA pain mechanisms has led to a search for surrogate animal models. Classically, animal models of OA have focused primarily on cartilage/bone destruction and remodeling rather than pain.[3] This has changed more recently with an interest in developing models that show at least some overlap with clinical features observed in human disease. The goal of this work has been to produce models that are reproducible, predictive, and able to provide mechanistic insight into disease mechanisms. Broadly, the models developed to date fall into three categories, including chemical, mechanical, and degenerative.

Chemical Models

These models involve intra-articular injection of substances including mono-sodium iodoacetate (IOA), collagenase, or papain into a joint such as the knee.[4–7] They characteristically produce severe and rapidly progressive joint damage, with behavioral changes occurring within days of the procedure. One drawback of these chemically induced models is that they have a substantial early inflammatory component that is not necessarily always apparent in human OA.[8]

Sodium Monoiodoacetate Model

A common model used in OA pain research involves the intra-articular injection of the glycolysis inhibitor sodium monoiodoacetate.[9] Since articular cartilage derives its metabolism via a glycolytic pathway, sodium monoiodoacetate causes gradual but profound loss of articular chondrocytes. Although this model is not ideal for disease modification research, it has been used as a model of OA pain.[7] Following sodium monoiodoacetate injection, there is an initial inflammatory reaction in the joint which resolves into a more degenerative type lesion,[6] thereby providing an opportunity to study different phases of the evolving pathology. Standard analgesics, including NSAIDs, are effective in reducing pain-related behaviors in this model, suggesting an important contribution from prostaglandins in both early and late stages of disease. Furthermore, cannabinoids, vasointestinal peptide (VIP), and blocking various elements of the arachadonic acid pathway have all been shown to be analgesic in this model.[10–14] An increase in TRPV1 expression and CGRP expression has been found in the nerves innervating the diseased joint.[15] In addition, a substantial induction of ATF-3 expression in the dorsal root ganglion (DRG) occurs with this model, indicating a neuropathic component, although whether this is relevant to human disease is unclear.[8]

Mechanical Models

Since OA is known to develop post-trauma,[16] a number of surgically induced joint instability models have been developed (Fig. 4.1). Transection of articular ligaments and/or meniscal tears causes a gradual deterioration in articular cartilage, synovial hypertrophy, and subchondral bone loss.[17,18] Animal behavioral experiments have shown that joint pain and secondary allodynia are common sequelae of injury-induced OA, confirming their utility in OA pain assessment.[19] It should be noted, however, that functional gait analysis as a surrogate measure of pain may not be ideal for these surgical models since it is impossible to determine whether observed kinematic changes are due to pain perception or merely a consequence of joint instability.

Medial Meniscotibial Ligament Transection

A surgical technique that induces a slowly progressive course of joint degeneration in mice has recently been described which involves destabilization of the medial meniscus (DMM).[20] In this model, transection of the medial meniscotibial ligament results in instability of the medial meniscus leading to a slowly progressive degeneration of the articular cartilage with little or no synovitis. As is the case with symptomatic OA, both NSAIDs and opioids are analgesic in this model even with an apparent lack of inflammatory infiltrate. In contrast to

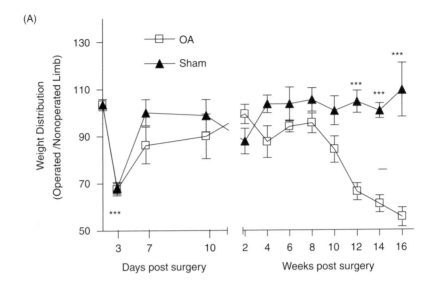

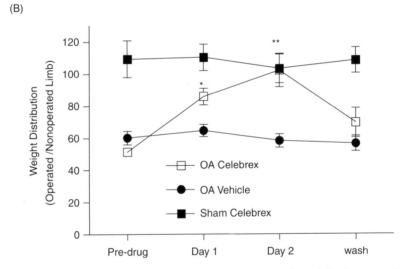

Figure 4.1. Pain-related behaviors in a surgically induced model of osteoarthritis. (A) Degeneration of the articular cartilage in mice was induced by transection of the medial meniscotibial ligament, producing instability of the medial meniscus. Changes in weight distribution were used as a surrogate measure of pain and were assessed in mice presurgically and postsurgically induced OA, or sham operated mice. (Data expressed as a percentage of operated limb compared to unoperated limb.) (B) Weight distribution assessed in mice displaying pain behaviors at 14 weeks post surgery, or sham controls, treated with celecoxib (30 mg/kg), or vehicle. Data presented as mean $\pm$ SEM. $*p < 0.05$, $**p < 0.01$, $***p < 0.001$.

many other OA models, behavioral pain scores only become abnormal late in disease. There are obviously parallels with human disease, where there is an overall increasing probability of pain reporting with time, albeit with relatively modest correlations between symptoms and radiographic damage.[21] Interestingly, increased mu-opioid receptor expression in the peripheral nerve has been reported in the DMM model, suggesting an important local effect of opioids in this model.

Naturally Occurring Models

Naturally occurring models potentially provide the most realistic method for the study of OA disease progression and pain. The Dunkin Hartley strain of guinea pig, for example, exhibits mild degenerative changes in the joint which become progressively worse as the animal ages.[22] Electrophysiological studies have revealed increased nociceptor activity in the Dunkin Hartley guinea pig, suggesting that this model may be ideally suited for OA pain assessment.[23] Similarly, the SRT/ort, C57bl/6, and BALB/c mouse strains all develop OA naturally, with overt histological changes being observed at about 1–2 years of age.[24–26] The plethora of available transgenic and knockout mice implies that these models may prove to be very important for investigating the genetic variability in pain sensitivity to OA.

PERIPHERAL SENSITIZATION

Far from being a hard-wired system, nociceptive pathways exhibit considerable plasticity such that they can respond in a variety of ways to a given stimulus. Whereas minor injuries produce short-lived excitation of specialized high threshold nociceptors with brief, spatially localized pain, more severe tissue injury or damage produces not only direct nociceptor excitation but also altered nociceptive responsiveness to subsequent stimuli (peripheral sensitization).[27] Under these circumstances, the response to a noxious stimulus becomes exaggerated and normally innocuous stimuli may produce pain.

The terminals of nociceptive fibers express multiple receptors that characteristically become active across relatively narrow ranges of stimulus intensity. The sensitivity of these receptors is governed by a critical interaction with the local microenvironment as well as by factors related to previous stimuli. The cellular mechanisms by which these changes occur involve early post-translational changes to receptors/ion channels and later, longer-lasting transcription-dependent mechanisms involving changes to the chemical phenotype of the cell.[28] (Fig. 4.2)

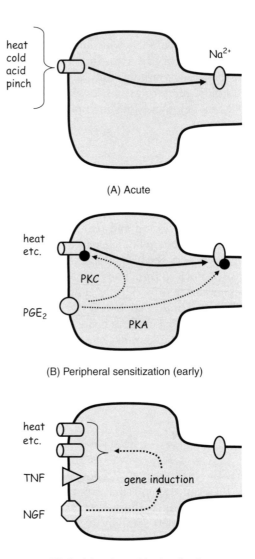

(A) Acute

(B) Peripheral sensitization (early)

(C) Peripheral sensitization (late)

Figure 4.2. Peripheral sensitization. Contribution of peripheral nociceptors to pain. (A) Acute pain: noxious stimuli activate a variety of high threshold receptors (represented by a single marker) with resultant propagation of axon potentials via sodium and other ion channels (solid arrow). (B) Early phase sensitization: mediators, including prostaglandin E_2, activate kinases to phosphorylate receptors/ion channels and lower threshold for activation (dotted arrow) (C) Late phase sensitization: gene induction in response to growth factors resulting in changes to cell phenotype. (Adapted from Ref. 10.)

Acute Inflammatory Mediators

While some mediators such as bradykinin contribute to pain by directly activating nociceptors, others are generally considered to be sensitizing agents. This may arise as a result of changes to the sensitivity of receptor molecules or via modulation of voltage-gated ion channels. Prostaglandins, for example, increase cellular cAMP levels and may enhance nociceptor sensitization by lowering the activation threshold for sodium channels via a protein kinase A pathway.[29] Within the joint, experimental application of prostaglandin E_2 has been shown to sensitize nociceptors to mechanical and chemical stimuli with a time course that matches the development of pain-related behavior in awake animals.[30] Consistent with human symptomatic disease, cyclooxygenase 2 (COX-2) inhibitors have been shown to be highly analgesic in experimental OA models.[15] Inhibition of prostaglandin synthesis (by blocking prostaglandin E synthase), or treatment with antagonists of the PGE_2 (EP4) receptor, reduces pain-related behaviors in the iodoactetate induced OA model.[10,11] Interestingly, inhibition of prostacyclin synthesis also reduces pain scores, indicating that other components of the arachadonic acid pathway play a role in the generation of pain in this model.[13]

Cytokines

Cytokines play an important role in the initiation and maintenance of many chronic diseases as mediators of cell-to-cell interactions. In addition to their enhancing and inhibitory effects on immune and inflammatory cells, cytokines exert considerable influence over sensory neurons. Similar to other mediators, cytokines may act directly on nociceptors or more commonly indirectly, stimulating the release of agents such as prostaglandins. During acute phases, cytokines appear to induce sensitization via receptor associated kinases and phosphorylation of ion channels, whereas in chronic inflammation, transcriptional upregulation of receptors and secondary signaling becomes more important.[31,32]

Most studies of the long-term role of cytokines have focused on the proinflammatory cytokines, including tumor necrosis factor alpha (TNF-α), interleukin-1 (IL-1), IL-6, and IL-8. Intradermal injections of these agents generally produce both mechanical and thermal hyperalgesia. TNF-α antiserum reduces hyperalgesia in inflammatory models[33] and the use of novel anti-TNF therapies in rheumatoid arthritis is accompanied by substantial reductions in pain scores. This is reflected in animal models in which anti-TNF is potently analgesic at time points prior to its anti-inflammatory actions.[32,34] Modest reductions in pain scores have also been observed following ant IL-1 therapy. Experimental studies using IL-6 knockout mice have shown reduced mechanical and thermal hyperalgesia in response to inflammatory stimuli[35] or following chronic nerve constriction.[36]

Nerve Growth Factors

Nerve growth factor (NGF) has been found in synovial fluid from patients with OA and RA and is produced by cultured synovial membranes when stimulated by cytokines including IL-1β.[37,38] NGF belongs to a family of neurotrophin growth factors that make significant and long-lasting contributions to the changes of neuron sensitivity. NGF mRNA and/or protein has been identified in various cell types including fibroblasts, keratinocytes, Schwann cells, and a range of immune cells. A large number of inflammatory mediators act to increase NGF production, particularly IL-1β and TNF-α[33]. During the acute stages of an inflammatory response, NGF, acting via neuronal trkA receptors, produces tyrosine phosphorylation of intracellular targets including ion channels. Over the longer term, NGF exerts a more global influence by regulating gene expression leading to long-lasting changes in neuron function.[39]

In studies using primary cultures of adult dorsal root ganglion neurons, treatment with NGF has been shown to increase both VR-1 mRNA expression and capsaicin-evoked release of CGRP in a dose-dependent fashion.[40] Other studies have shown NGF regulation of mRNA for the neuropeptides substance P and CGRP as well as the tetrodotoxin resistant sodium channel SNS/PN3. More recently, NGF has also been shown to exert longer term influences on nociceptor activity in a transcription-independent fashion via the p38 mitogen-activated protein kinase (MAPK).[41]

The importance of NGF in mediating inflammation-induced hyperalgesia has been highlighted by a number of studies showing very significant reductions of enhanced behavioral responses using a variety of anti-NGF strategies including the use of novel sequestration antibodies.[42] Consistent with this, increased levels of NGF have been reported in animal models of inflammation and in human disorders including arthritis, cystitis, and asthma.[42] In human subjects, NGF produces cutaneous hyperalgesia at the injection site and widespread deep pain that persists for several days. In animal models, anti-NGF therapy has been shown to be effective against hyperplasia, cachexia, and inflammation, indicating a key function of NGF in many aspects of arthritis.[33,43]

NEUROGENIC INFLAMMATION

The immune system acts in concert with the nervous and endocrine systems to constitute an interactive, communicative network. The central nervous system influences the immune responses systemically via humoral substances such as cortisol following activation of the hypothalamic–pituitary–adrenal (HPA) axis. A second and potentially more selective mechanism by which neuroimmune interactions may occur is via local sensory and autonomic nerves. Such interactions, which are well documented in disorders affecting the respiratory and gastrointestinal systems,[44–46] may also influence the clinical features of many rheumatic disorders. For example, a neurogenic role in the production of symmetrical joint disease has been suggested following the observation that inflammation in one joint can result in a neurogenically mediated response in the contralateral joint.[47]

Neuropeptides

Neuropeptides are a group of neurotransmitters that are contained within the terminals of small diameter sensory neurons and autonomic nerves. Depolarization of the nerve terminal via local axon reflexes causes the peripheral release of neuropeptides, which can then bind to the free nerve ending leading to an alteration in afferent sensitivity. Inflammatory neuropeptides such as substance P (SP), calcitonin gene related peptide (CGRP), and vasoactive intestinal peptide (VIP) are created in the dorsal root ganglia of primary afferent neurons and then transported peripherally in the axoplasmic flow, where they are stored in vesicles in the nerve terminal. During arthritis and joint injury, the neuronal levels of these neuropeptides increase dramatically, implying an involvement in joint inflammation and pain processing.[48–50]

The 28 amino acid neuropeptide VIP enhances joint nociceptor sensitivity to mechanical stimuli,[51] with pain behavioral studies showing that intra-articular VIP administration leads to reduced hind-paw pain thresholds.[52] Consistent with this, treatment of OA knee joints with the VIP receptor antagonist VIP_{6-28} reduces afferent firing rate and ameliorates pain sensitivity, implying a potential novel therapy for OA pain.[51,52] Similarly, local administration of SP to rat knees sensitizes articular receptors to joint movement although there is no direct effect on spontaneous nociceptor activity.[53]

Other neuropeptides have also been linked to joint pain modulation. Nociceptin/orphanin FQ (N/OFQ) is an opioid-like neuropeptide that has been immunolocalized in the peripheral and central nervous systems.[54–56] Intrathecal and intracerebroventricular injection of N/OFQ alters pain sensitivity in animal models,[57,58] indicating a central site of action, although peripheral effects have also been reported.[59,60] Low dose N/OFQ causes peripheral sensitization of knee joint afferents with concomitant hyperalgesia and allodynia.[59–61] This effect appears to be mediated by the secondary release of SP since it can be blocked by a selective neurokinin-1 antagonist.[60]

Cannabinoids

Cannabinoids are a family of lipid mediators derived from the hemp plant *Cannabis sativa*, which are known to have a multitude of physiological effects including pain control. Cannabinoids bind to two G protein-coupled receptors, namely, CB_1 and CB_2.[62,63] In addition to plant-derived phytocannabinoids,

cannabinoids can also be produced naturally in the body (endocannabinoids). The endocannabinoid anandamide acts on both CB_1 and CB_2 receptors to cause peripheral sensitization when administered in very high concentrations.[64] In contrast, activation of knee joint CB_1 receptors with a selective CB_1 agonist reduces nociceptor firing rate and this antinociceptive effect is enhanced in OA knees.[65] Interestingly, the pain relieving effect of cannabinoids in joints involves cross-talk with transient receptor potential vanilloid channel-1 (TRPV1) since joint afferent desensitization can be inhibited by treatment with a TRPV1 antagonist.[65]

CENTRAL SENSITIZATION

Sustained or repetitive activity within peripheral fibers leads to substantial changes to the function and activity of spinal and supraspinal nociceptive pathways (central sensitization). Although primarily mediated by neurotransmitters, activity within these more central pathways can be modified substantially by the same inflammatory mediators that play a role in peripheral sensitization. Under these circumstances the mediators are derived from nonneuronal cells including both astrocytes and microglia.[66]

Central sensitization involves exaggerated responses to normal stimuli together with expansion of receptive field size producing tenderness and referred pain in areas away from the site of injury.[67] Functional imaging studies of the brain following noxious stimuli using fMRI and PET show a complex pattern with discrete areas of activity throughout both cerebral hemispheres (cortical sensitization).[68] The consequences of cortical sensitization remain unclear but may produce the state of hypervigilance and other more general phenomena observed in patients with chronic pain (Fig. 4.3).

Both astrocytes and microglia have been shown to be activated in animal models of arthritis.[34,69] Activated microglia produce IL-1, IL-6, IL-10, TNF, and TGF and synthesize several complement components that have been implicated in the sensitization of sensory neurons.[70,71] Other pathways

Figure 4.3. Central sensitization. Contribution of spinal cord neurons to pain. (A) Acute pain: activation of AMPA receptors by glutamate (open oval). Note that the NMDA receptor is blocked by a magnesium ion (hatched oval). (B) Early phase sensitization: activation of NMDA receptor following expulsion of magnesium ion to extracellular space and mediated by substance P (SP) acting on NK1 receptors (black circles and triangle, respectively). (C) Late phase sensitization: gene induction with enhanced production of prostaglandins and other local mediators acting via relevant receptors (hatched and open circles, respectively). Modulation by descending facilitatory/inhibitory pathways (hatched and black squares, respectively)

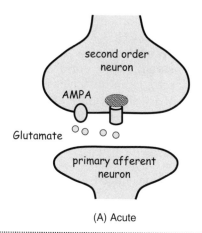

(A) Acute

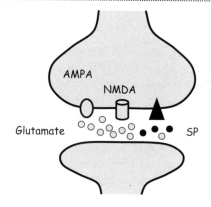

(B) Central sensitization (early)

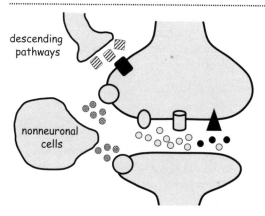

(C) Central sensitization (late)

mediating intercellular communication in the spinal cord include the chemokines fractalkine (CX3CL1) and CCL2, as well as Toll-like receptors. Fractalkine is a membrane-bound protein released from central nociceptive afferents and from transmission neurons in the dorsal horn in response to cytokine stimulation. Glial cells express receptors for both chemokines. Modulation of fractalkine and CCL2 activity significantly affects hyperalgesia, implicating these chemokines in central mechanisms of pain.[71]

A further mechanism of central nociceptive sensitization involves activation of purinergic receptors belonging to P2RX and P2Y types by ATP. These receptors are expressed on neural cells of different lineages as well as on microglia and immune cells, including T and B lymphocytes.[72]

CONCLUSION

Pain and disability arising from OA present major challenges to both the sufferer and to society. The enigma of why only some individuals with radiological disease experience symptoms can now at least partially be resolved by appreciating the pivotal role of the nervous system. Sensitization of nociceptive receptors and channels results in seemingly innocuous stimuli becoming painful and may cause ongoing symptoms under resting conditions. Many of those mediators that are classically associated with inflammation have profound and complex effects on these processes, both at the periphery and at more central levels. The potent analgesic actions of NSAIDs, and the more recent experiences with anti-TNF therapy, testify to the efficacy of inflammatory mediators in this regard.

Although many mediators have been described as being associated with OA, relatively little research has been undertaken to date to assess whether these same mediators interact with pain pathways. The emergence of relevant animal models and the increasing understanding of nociceptive mechanisms offer exciting challenges for the future.

REFERENCES

1. Bajaj P, Bajaj P, Graven-Nielsen T, Arendt-Nielsen L. (2001). Osteoarthritis and its association with muscle hyperalgesia: an experimental controlled study. Pain 93:107–114.

2. Kosek E, Ordeberg G. (2000). Lack of pressure pain modulation by heteotropic noxious conditioning stimulation in patients with painful osteoarthritis before, but not following, surgical pain relief. Pain 88:69–78.

3. Brandt KD. (2002). Animal models of osteoarthritis. Biorheology 39(1–2):221–235.

4. Pritzker KP. (1994). Animal models for osteoarthritis: processes, problems and prospects. Ann Rheum Dis 53:406–420.

5. Rudolphi K, Gerwin N, Verzijl N. (2003). Pralnacasan, an inhibitor of interleukin-1beta converting enzyme, reduces joint damage in two murine models of osteoarthritis. Osteoarthritis Cartilage 11:738–746.

6. Combe R, Bramwell S, Field MJ. (2004). The monosodium iodoacetate model of osteoarthritis: a model of chronic nociceptive pain in rats? Neurosci Lett 370:236–240.

7. Fernihough J, Gentry C, Malcangio M, et al. (2004). Pain related behaviour in two models of osteoarthritis in the rat knee. Pain 112:83–93.

8. Ivanavicius SP, Ball AD, Heapy CG, Westwood FR, Murray F, Read SJ. (2007). Structural pathology in a rodent model of osteoarthritis is associated with neuropathic pain: increased expression of ATF-3 and pharmacological characterisation. Pain 128:272–282.

9. Kalbhen DA. (1987). Chemical model of osteoarthritis—a pharmacological evaluation. J Rheumatol 14(Suppl 14):130–131.

10. Xu D, Rowland SE, Clark P, Giroux A, Cote B, Guiral S, Salem M, Ducharme Y, Friesen RW, Methot N, Mancini J, Audoly L, Riendeau D. (2008). MF63 {2-(6-chloro-1H-phenanthro[9,10-d]imidazol-2-yl)isophthalonitrile}, a selective microsomal prostaglandin E synthase 1 inhibitor, relieves pyresis and pain in preclinical models of inflammation. J Pharmacol Exp Ther 326(3):754–763.

11. Clark P, Rowland SE, Denis D, Mathieu MC, Stocco R, Poirier H, Burch J, Han Y, Audoly L, Therien AG, Xu D. (2008). MF498 [N-{[4-(5,9-diethoxy-6-oxo-6,8-dihydro-7H-pyrrolo[3,4-g]quinolin-7-yl)-3-methylbenzyl]sulfonyl}-2-(2-methoxyphenyl) acetamide], a selective E prostanoid receptor 4 antagonist, relieves joint inflammation and pain in rodent models of rheumatoid and osteoarthritis. J Pharmacol Exp Ther 325(2):425–434.

12. Schuelert N, McDougall JJ. (2008). Cannabinoid-mediated antinociception is enhanced in rat osteoarthritic knees. Arthritis Rheum Jan 58(1):145–153.

13. Pulichino AM, Rowland S, Wu T, Clark P, Xu D, Mathieu MC, Riendeau D, Audoly LP. (2006). Prostacyclin antagonism reduces pain and inflammation in rodent models of hyperalgesia and chronic arthritis. J Pharmacol Exp Ther 319(3):1043–1050.

14. McDougall JJ, Watkins L, Li Z. (2006). Vasoactive intestinal peptide (VIP) is a modulator of joint pain in a rat model of osteoarthritis. Pain 123(1–2):98–105.

15. Fernihough J, Gentry C, Bevan S, Winter J. (2005). Regulation of calcitonin gene-related peptide and TRPV1 in a rat model of osteoarthritis. Neurosci Lett 388(2):75–80.

16. McDaniel WJ, Dameron TB. (1980). Untreated ruptures of the anterior cruciate ligament. J Bone Joint Surg 62A:696–705.

17. Pond MJ, Nuki G. (1973). Experimentally-induced osteoarthritis in dog. Ann Rheum Dis 32:387–388.

18. Gilbertson EMM. (1975). Development of periarticular osteophytes in experimentally induced osteoarthritis in the dog. Ann Rheum Dis 34:12–25.

19. Bove SE, Laemont KD, Brooker RM, Osborn MN, Sanchez BM, Guzman RE, et al. (2006). Surgically induced osteoarthritis in the rat results in the development of

both osteoarthritis-like joint pain and secondary hyperalgesia. Osteoarthritis Cartilage 14(10):1041–1048.

20. Glasson SS, Askew R, Sheppard B, et al. (2004). Characterization of and osteoarthritis susceptibility in ADAMTS-4-knockout mice. Arthritis Rheum 50:2547–2558.

21. Kidd BL. (2006). Osteoarthritis and joint pain. Pain 123:6–9.

22. Bendele AM, Hulman JF. (1988). Spontaneous cartilage degeneration in guinea pigs. Arthritis Rheum 31(4):561–565.

23. McDougall JJ, Schuelert N. (2007). Age alters the ability of substance P to sensitize joint nociceptors in guinea pigs. J Mol Neurosci 31(3):289–296.

24. Mason RM, Chambers MG, Flannelly J, Gaffen JD, Dudhia J, Bayliss MT. (2001). The STR/ort mouse and its use as a model of osteoarthritis. Osteoarthritis Cartilage 9(2):85–91.

25. Wilhelmi G. (1977). [Preventive effect of tribenoside in spontaneous arthrosis of the mouse]. Z Rheumatol 36(3–4):112–119.

26. Stoop R, van der Kraan PM, Buma P, Hollander AP, Billinghurst RC, Poole AR et al. (1999). Type II collagen degradation in spontaneous osteoarthritis in C57Bl/6 and BALB/c mice. Arthritis Rheum 42(11):2381–2389.

27. Raja S, Meyer R, Kingkamp M. (1999). Peripheral neural mechanisms of nociception. In Wall P and Melzac R (eds.). *Textbook of Pain*. Edinburgh: Churchill Livingstone, pp. 11–58.

28. Woolf CJ, Costigan M. (1999). Transcriptional and posttranslational plasticity and the generation of inflammatory pain. Proc Natl Acad Sci 96:7723–7730.

29. England S, Bevan SJ, Docherty RJ. (1996). Prostaglandin E2 modulates the tetrodotoxin-resistant sodium current in neonatal rat dorsal root ganglion neurones via the cyclic AMP—protein kinase A cascade. J Physiol 495:429–440.

30. Schaible H-G, Grubb BD. (1993). Afferent and spinal mechanisms of joint pain. Pain 55:5–54.

31. Opree A, Kress M. (2000). Involvement of the proinflammatory cytokines tumor necrosis factor-α, IL-1β and IL-6 but not IL-8 in the development of heat hyperalgesia: effects on heat-evoked calcitonin gene-related peptide release from rat skin. J Neurosci 20:6289–6293.

32. Inglis JJ, Nissim A, Lees DM, Hunt SP, Chernajovsky Y, Kidd BL. (2005). The differential contribution of tumour necrosis factor to thermal and mechanical hyperalgesia during chronic inflammation. Arthritis Res Ther 7(4):R807–R816.

33. Woolf CJ, Allchorne A, Safieh-Garabedian B, Poole S. (1997). Cytokines, nerve growth factor and inflammatory hyperalgesia: the contribution of tumor necrosis factor α. Br J Pharmacol 121:417–424.

34. Inglis JJ, Notley CA, Essex D, Wilson AW, Feldmann M, Anand P, Williams R. (2007). Collagen-induced arthritis as a model of hyperalgesia: functional and cellular analysis of the analgesic actions of tumor necrosis factor blockade. Arthritis Rheum 56(12):4015–4023.

35. Xu X, Hao J, Andell-Jonsson S, Poli V, Bartfai T, Wiesenfeld-Hallin Z. (1997). Nociceptive responses in interleukin-6-deficient mice to peripheral inflammation and peripheral nerve section. Cytokine 9:1028–1033.

36. Murphy PG, Ramer MS, Borthwick L, Gauldie J, Richardson PM, Bisby MA. (1997). Endogenous interleukin-6 contributes to hypersensitivity to cutaneous stimuli and changes in neuropeptides associated with chronic contriction in mice. Eur J Neurosci 11:2243–2253.

37. Manni L, Lundeberg T, Fiorito S, Bonini S, Vigneti E, Aloe L. (2003). Nerve growth factor release by human synovial fibroblasts prior to and following exposure to tumor necrosis factor-alpha, interleukin-1 beta and cholecystokinin-8: the possible role of NGF in the inflammatory response. Clin Exp Rheumatol 21(5):617–624.

38. Iannone F. (2002). Increased expression of nerve growth factor (NGF) and high affinity NGF receptor (p140 TrkA) in human osteoarthritic chondrocytes. Rheumatology (Oxford) 41:1413–1418.

39. Levine JD, Reichling DB. (1999). Peripheral mechanisms of inflammatory pain. In Wall PD and Melzac R (eds.), *Textbook of Pain*. Edinburgh: Churchill Livingstone, pp. 59–84.

40. Winston J, Toma H, Shenoy M, Pasricha P. (2001). Nerve growth factor regulates VR-1 mRNA levels in cultures of adult dorsal root ganglia neurons. Pain 89:181–186.

41. Ji RR, Samad TA, Jin SX, Schmoll R, Woolf CJ. (2002). p38 MAPK activation by NGF in primary sensory neurons after inflammation increases TRPV1 levels and maintains heat hyperalgesia. Neuron 36(1):57–68.

42. McMahon SB, Bennett DL. (1999). Trophic factors and pain. In Wall PD and Melzac R (eds.). *Textbook of Pain*. Edinburgh: Churchill Livingstone, pp. 105–128.

43. Shelton DL, Zeller J, Ho WH, Pons J, Rosenthal A. (2005). Nerve growth factor mediates hyperalgesia and cachexia in auto-immune arthritis. Pain 116(1-2):8–16.

44. Maggi CA. (1997). The effects of tachykinins on inflammatory and immune cells. Regul Peptides 70:75–90.

45. Joos GF, Pauwels RA. (2000). Pro-inflammatory effects of substance P: new perspectives for the treatment of airways disease? TIPS 21:131–133.

46. Chavolla-Calderon M, Bayer MK, Fontan JJP. (2003). Bone marrow transplantation reveals an essential synergy between neuronal and hemopoietic neurokin production in pulmonary inflammation. J Clin Invest 111:973–980.

47. Kidd BL, Cruwys SC, Garrett NE, et al. (1995). Neurogenic influences on contralateral responses during rat monarthritis. Brain Res 688:72–76.

48. McDougall JJ, Bray RC, Sharkey KA. (1997). A morphological and immunohistochemical examination of nerves in normal and injured collateral ligaments of rat, rabbit and human knee joints. Anat Rec 248:29–39.

49. Ahmed M, Bjurholm A, Schultzberg M, Theodorsson E, Kreicbergs A. (1995). Increased levels of substance P and calcitonin gene-related peptide in rat adjuvant arthritis. A combined immunohistochemical and radioimmunoassay analysis. Arthritis Rheum 38(5):699–709.

50. Heppelmann B, Shahbazian Z, Hanesch U. (1997). Quantitative examination of calcitonin gene-related peptide immunoreactive nerve fibres in the cat knee joint. Anat Embryol 195:525–530.

51. Schuelert N, McDougall JJ. (2006). Electrophysiological evidence that the vasoactive intestinal peptide receptor antagonist VIP(6-28) reduces nociception in an animal model of osteoarthritis. Osteoarthritis Cartilage 14:1155–1162.

52. McDougall JJ, Watkins L, Li Z. (2006). Vasoactive intestinal peptide (VIP) is a modulator of joint pain in a rat model of osteoarthritis. Pain 123:98–105.

53. Heppelmann B, Pawlak M. (1997). Sensitisation of articular afferents in normal and inflamed knee joints by substance P in the rat. Neurosci Lett 223:97–100.

54. Neal CR, Mansour A, Reinscheid R, Nothacker HP, Civelli O, Watson SJ Jr. (1999). Localization of orphanin FQ (nociceptin) peptide and messenger RNA in the central nervous system of the rat. J Comp Neurol 406(4):503–547.

55. Riedl M, Shuster S, Vulchanova L, Wang J, Loh HH, Elde R. (1996). Orphanin FQ/nociceptin-immunoreactive nerve fibers parallel those containing endogenous opioids in rat spinal cord. Neuroreport 7(8):1369–1372.

56. Schuligoi R, Amann R, Angelberger P, Peskar BA. (1997). Determination of nociceptin-like immunoreactivity in the rat dorsal spinal cord. Neurosci Lett 224(2):136–138.

57. Darland T, Grandy DK. (1998). The orphanin FQ system: an emerging target for the management of pain? Br J Anaesth 81(1):29–37.

58. Darland T, Heinricher MM, Grandy DK. (1998). Orphanin FQ/nociceptin: a role in pain and analgesia, but so much more. Trends Neurosci 21(5):215–221.

59. McDougall JJ, Pawlak M, Hanesch U, Schmidt RF. (2001). Peripheral modulation of rat knee joint afferent mechanosensitivity by nociceptin/orphanin FQ. Neurosci Lett 288(2):123–126.

60. McDougall JJ, Hanesch U, Pawlak M, Schmidt RF. (2001). Participation of NK1 receptors in nociceptin-induced modulation of rat knee joint mechanosensitivity. Exp Brain Res 137:249–253.

61. McDougall JJ, Larson SEM. (2006). Nociceptin/orphanin FQ evokes knee joint pain in rats via a mast cell independent mechanism. Neurosci Lett 398:135–138.

62. Matsuda LA, Lolait SJ, Brownstein MJ, Young AC, Bonner TI. (1990). Structure of a cannabinoid receptor and functional expression of the cloned cDNA. Nature 346(6284):561–564.

63. Munro S, Thomas KL, Abu-Shaar M. (1993). Molecular characterization of a peripheral receptor for cannabinoids. Nature 365(6441):61–65.

64. Gauldie SD, McQueen DS, Pertwee R, Chessell IP. (2001). Anandamide activates peripheral nociceptors in normal and arthritic rat knee joints. Br J Pharmacol 132(3):617–621.

65. Schuelert N, McDougall JJ. (2008). Cannabinoid-mediated antinociception is enhanced in rat osteoarthritic knees. Arthritis Rheum 58(1):145–153.

66. Watkins LR, et al. (2005). Glia: novel counter-regulators of opioid analgesia. Trends Neurosci 28(12):661–669.

67. Coderre T, Katz J, Vaccarino A, Melzack R. (1993). Contribution of central neuroplasticity to pathological pain: review of clinical and experimental evidence. Pain 52:259–285.

68. Gracely RH, Petzke F, Wolf JM, Clauw DJ. (2002). Functional magnetic imaging evidence of augmented pain processing in fibromyalgia. Arthritis Rheum 46:1333–1343.

69. Sun S, Cao H, Han M, Li TT, Pan HL, Zhao ZQ, Zhang YQ. (2007). New evidence for the involvement of spinal fractalkine receptor in pain facilitation and spinal glial activation in rat model of monoarthritis. Pain 129(1–2):64–75.

70. Griffin RS. (2007). Complement induction in spinal cord microglia results in anaphylatoxin C5a-mediated pain hypersensitivity. J Neurosci 27(32):8699–8708.

71. Scholz J, Woolf CJ. (2007). The neuropathic pain triad: neurons, immune cells and glia. Nat Neurosci 10(11):1361–1368.

72. Trang T, Beggs S, Salter MW. (2006). Purinoceptors in microglia and neuropathic pain. Pflugers Arch 452(5):645–652.

5

PHANTOMS IN RHEUMATOLOGY

Candida S. McCabe

*The Royal National Hospital for Rheumatic Diseases, Bath BA1 1RL,
United Kingdom and School for Health, University of Bath,
Claverton Down BA2 7AY, United Kingdom*

Richard C. Haigh

*Department of Rheumatology, Royal Devon & Exeter Hospital
(Wonford), Exeter EX2 5DW, United Kingdom*

Nicholas G. Shenker

*Department of Rheumatology, Addenbrooke's Hospital, Cambridge
University NHS Foundation Trust, Cambridge CB2 2QQ, United Kingdom*

Jenny Lewis

*The Royal National Hospital for Rheumatic Diseases,
Bath BA1 1RL, United Kingdom*

David R. Blake

*The Royal National Hospital for Rheumatic Diseases, Bath BA1 1RL,
United Kingdom and School for Health, University of Bath,
Claverton Down BA2 7AY, United Kingdom*

INTRODUCTION

This chapter examines rheumatology pain and how it may relate to amputee phantom limb pain (PLP), specifically as experienced in rheumatoid arthritis, fibromyalgia, and complex regional pain syndrome (CRPS). Clinical findings, which suggest cortical sensory reorganization, are discussed and illustrated for each condition. It is proposed that this sensory reorganization generates pain and altered body image in rheumatology patients in the same manner as has previously been hypothesized for amputees with PLP, that is, via a motor/sensory conflict. The correction of this conflict through the provision of appropriate visual sensory input, using a mirror, is tested in a population of patients with CRPS. Its analgesic efficacy is assessed in those with acute, intermediate, and chronic disease. The hypothesis is then taken to its natural conclusion whereby motor/sensory conflict is artificially generated in healthy volunteers and chronic pain patients to establish whether sensory disturbances can be created where no pain symptomology exists and exacerbated when it is already present. The findings of our studies support the hypothesis that a mismatch between motor output and sensory input creates sensory disturbances, including pain, in rheumatology patients and healthy volunteers. We propose the term ominory to describe the central monitoring mechanism and the resultant sensory disturbances as a dissensory state. Finally, we discuss the implications for this cortical model of pain for the generation and perpetuation of pain in osteoarthritis and the therapeutic approaches that maybe trialed to relieve it.

PAIN

Increasing pain and stiffness of the joints is something that is widely regarded as a natural consequence of aging and many of these problems can be attributed to osteoarthritis (OA), which is the leading of cause of joint pain and disability in older adults.[1,2] OA may affect any synovial joint but commonly occurs in the knees, hips, hands, and spine with most people over the age of 70 years having some of their joints affected.[1,3] Pain in OA is typified by the sufferer describing stiffness on initial movement, increasing pain with prolonged movement, and disturbed sleep due to pain.[4] There is a reduction in the range of movement in the affected joint and associated muscle weakness. Research to date, on the generation and perpetuation of OA and pain, has focused on the individual structures of the synovial joint and the role these structures and the biochemical pathways that serve them may play (see Ref. 5 for overview). However, there is not a close correlation between the degree of structural damage and the level of reported pain,[6,7] which suggests other mechanisms may contribute to OA pain.

Pain is the predominant complaint of patients with a rheumatological condition. It may be intermittent or continuous and vary in nature depending on the cause and course of the disease. In the majority of cases, clinical findings provide supporting evidence for the source of this pain such as swollen joints in rheumatoid arthritis (RA) or bony overgrowth in osteoarthritis. However, there are some conditions in rheumatology where a patient's pain cannot be matched to physical findings or relieved by traditional therapeutic measures. It is pain of this nature that this chapter addresses, specifically the types of pain experienced in RA, fibromyalgia, and complex regional pain syndrome, and how these may relate to amputee phantom limb pain. Finally, we examine how this central mechanism model may relate to OA pain.

AMPUTEE PHANTOM LIMB PAIN

Phantom limb pain (PLP) is a phenomenon that occurs in approximately 70% of patients after amputation.[8] For the amputee, "these pain memories are vivid, perceptually integrated experiences which incorporate both emotional and sensory aspects of the preamputation pain."[9] Tingling is the most common complaint but pins and needles, shooting, burning, or crushing pain have all been reported.[10] Phantom sensations are also described by 90–100% of amputees.[11] Postoperatively, an amputee will perceive a phantom limb that has all the same sensations and mobility of the real limb prior to amputation and is so strikingly real to the individual that it feels an integral part of them. The phantom appears to "inhabit the body"[11] when the eyes are open and moves appropriately with other limbs. It initially feels perfectly normal in size and shape but may alter over time so that the phantom gradually becomes less apparent and may eventually fade away.[12] For those people who wear a prosthesis, the phantom limb can appear to fill it or telescope up into the remaining stump.[11]

It has been proposed that it is a combination of the duration and intensity of preoperative pain that determines whether long-term central nervous system processes are altered with resulting persistent phantom sensations.[12] A long-lasting mild sensation such as a watch on a wrist or a sock on a foot may be just as effective at developing somatosensory memories as the intense short-term pain of gangrene.

Referred sensations (RSs) have also been described in amputees. These are somatosensory feelings that are perceived to emanate from a body part other than but in association with the body part being stimulated. They have been reported not only following limb amputation[13] but also in somatosensory deafferentation,[14] local anesthesia,[15] stroke,[16] and spinal cord injury.[17] Collectively these studies have shown that the referred sites (the body part not physically touched) are nonrandom and often closely correspond to the cortical topographical map representing the body structure first described by Penfield and Rasmussen.[18] In the case of an amputated upper limb, patients report sensation in their phantom when parts of the face are lightly stroked.[13] This is thought to be because the hand is positioned adjacent to the face on Penfield's map. These aberrant somatosensory, but reliable sensations were interpreted as resulting from central sensory reorganization following disconnection or dysfunction of sensory pathways.

In conclusion, amputees report a variety of sensations that are not supported by conventional notions of clinical pathology. The nature of the sensations described provide the first link to the rheumatology patient with unexplained pain.

PAIN IN RHEUMATOLOGY

Rheumatoid Arthritis

Rheumatoid arthritis (RA) affects 1% of the population and is a chronic disabling disease that occurs two-thirds more frequently in women than men.[19] The peak age of onset is between 40 and 50 years, its etiology is uncertain, and there is as yet no cure. The main symptoms of this disease are pain, stiffness, fatigue, and joint swelling, but other organs in the body may also be involved.[20] The pain that these patients experience is "chronic, unpredictable and frequently severe,"[21] resulting in progressive disability over time.

A key feature of RA is a pattern of remissions and flares that are a result of the fluctuations in disease activity. During these flares the joints, particularly the small joints of the hands and feet, become swollen and tender. This swelling is due to increased activity in the joint caused by an inappropriate inflammatory response. As a result of prolonged or frequent episodes of this inflammation, the synovium lining the joint becomes permanently thickened and bony erosions may occur.[20]

Pain is synonymous with RA and the types of pain that sufferers of this disease experience are complex and varied. The descriptions that they use may alter depending on the time of day, the duration of their disease, the joints that are involved, and whether those joints are moving or at rest.[22]

A less well reported quality of pain that some RA patients describe is where they feel their joints to be excessively more swollen than they look. They describe all the sensations associated with swollen joints but they are clinically not swollen and indeed when the subjects look at the affected joints they too are aware that they are not swollen.[23] Interestingly, this perception of swelling is not isolated to the joints; the patient will report that he/she feels the whole digit to be affected (Fig. 5.1). These sensations are similar to the effects you may have after an injection in your mouth at the dentist. The anesthetic leaves you feeling that your lip is huge and yet you look in the mirror and find that it is actually its normal size.

The characteristics of this "phantom swelling" and how it differs from routine reports of RA joint swelling were identified in a cross-sectional study

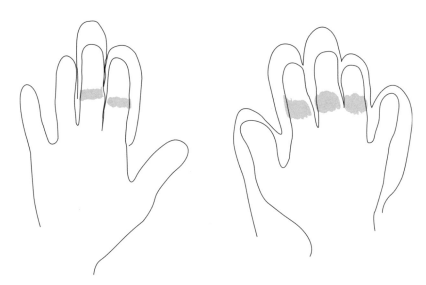

Figure 5.1. Rheumatoid arthritis patient's drawing of "phantom swelling" affecting the hands. The shaded areas depict perceived swelling over the joints, and the outer lines, perceived swelling of the digits.

involving ten patients with RA.[24] Five of the subjects reported phantom swelling and five did not. The two groups did not differ significantly in age, disease duration, or disease activity, as measured by inflammatory markers and joint activity. Using a modified McGill Pain Questionnaire (MPQ), each subject was asked to describe the sensations he/she currently experienced in all the joints at rest and on movement. A semistructured interview was used to collect additional information on duration and severity of disease in each joint and the impact of vision on the sensations that they reported.

Subjects with phantom swelling reported that their affected joints felt excessively hot ("burning," "scalding") and hugely swollen ("massive"). Their remaining RA affected joints were described in exactly the same manner as the control group described theirs—"warm" and "slightly puffy." When the phantom swollen joints were viewed by the subjects, the perception of swelling disappeared but the lesser sensation of "slight puffiness" in their other joints remained on visualization. Phantom swelling was only present in those joints that had been most severely affected by RA and for the longest duration, which is very reminiscent of Katz and Melzack's theory that it takes a certain duration and intensity of pain to alter central processing resulting in persistent sensations.

Interestingly, the nature and cause of stiffness in RA, another pain-related symptom, is not well explained, even though it is a well established and defining symptom of the disease.[25] Objective measures of stiffness do not relate to the subjective experience and, indeed, compared with non arthritic controls, objective stiffness can be reduced in RA joints.[26] We therefore hypothesized that the central nervous system is capable of generating a feedback-dependent state that can result in pathological sensations such as pain and stiffness in RA, which are to some extent independent of the initial peripheral pathology. We sought clinical evidence to support this proposal by investigating the clinical presentation of perceived stiffness in RA patients who had undergone limb amputation but nevertheless retained an experience of a phantom limb.[27]

Three patients with a current diagnosis of RA and lower limb amputation were identified from the local Artificial Limb Centre database and investigated to determine the nature and pattern of pain and stiffness in their phantom and intact limb. In addition to standard physical examination, pain and stiffness severity were measured using Visual Analogue Scales for both limbs. The duration and timing of stiffness was also recorded for each limb. In all three cases, the pattern of perceived RA stiffness was similar for the intact and phantom limb. All three patients described stiffness in their phantom limb (PL), which mirrored that of physical RA joint symptoms in terms of quality, frequency, diurnal variation, location, distribution, and response to medication (nonsteroidal anti-inflammatory drugs, corticosteroid, opiate, and disease modifying drugs). Unilateral exercise (or attempted exercise) relieved stiffness only in the limb being exercised. Thus the extent to which the subjective experience of perceived stiffness could be dissociated from the assumed original peripheral source was strikingly illustrated in RA patients with phantom limbs.

Accordingly, we proposed that the experience of peripherally located stiffness results from impairment to central brain processes. Conditions are present in RA to produce inaccurate sensory information, which may lead to conflict with planned output from motor systems. These include peripheral and central proprioceptive abnormality, cortical reorganization, neurogenic inflammation, and circulating cytokines with central effects. Such conflict of information is ultimately perceived as "stiffness" by the patient with RA.

RA is not the only rheumatological condition where phantom swelling and stiffness are described. Clinical experience has long shown that patients with fibromylagia also report stiffness and perceive body areas to be subjectively swollen when, objectively, they are not.

Fibromyalgia

Fibromyalgia (FMS) is a chronic pain condition where sufferers report widespread pain, fatigue, and psychological distress—all of which have a major impact on their daily lives.[28] Although hyperalgesia and allodynia are commonly reported at specific trigger points, these sensations often spread far beyond these areas with sufferers describing generalized sensitivity.[29] For the majority of patients, there is no known initiating event or observable physical pathology and symptoms are frequently resistant to therapeutic initiatives.

In addition to the symptoms just described, it has long been observed, but only recently systematically recorded, that these patients also experience phantom swelling sensations in the same manner as those with RA (C. McCabe and D. Blake, unpublished work 2001). The sensation most commonly affects the hands, bilaterally from the wrist to the ulna styloid, or the feet, bilaterally from the toes to the ankle joints. Subjects are most aware of the perceived swelling when they have their eyes closed and it decreases or disappears completely when they view the affected area. With regular viewing on a daily basis, the sensation can be diminished permanently. When phantom swelling is reported, it is commonly associated with patients feeling that they are clumsy or less aware of where their limbs are in space. This reduction in limb position sense will be discussed further toward the end of this chapter.

Phantom swelling in RA and FMS are clear examples of sensations being reported without supporting underlying clinical pathology, and complex regional pain syndrome is another such condition where the cause of the characteristic symptomology is ambiguous.

Complex Regional Pain Syndrome

Complex regional pain syndrome (CRPS) is a painful, debilitating condition. This diagnostic term embraces several syndromes including reflex sympathetic dystrophy, causalgia, and algodystrophy. The pain that a patient with CRPS will report shares many similar characteristics to amputee phantom limb pain—mislocalized, intense, and burning. Clinical features include sensory disturbances such as burning pain with allodynia and hyperalgesia, motor disturbances such as weakness, tremor, and muscle spasms, and changes in vascular tone, temperature, and edema.[30] Over time, functional loss and trophic changes may occur. The syndrome can occur spontaneously or following trauma (CRPS Type 1) or in association with peripheral nerve damage (CRPS Type 2).

A characteristic feature of CRPS is that signs and symptoms spread beyond the site of initial insult. Severe pain may occur seemingly out of proportion to the original pathology. It may persist over long periods and is frequently resistant to a wide range of treatments. Theories abound on the cause of this pain and its underlying pathology. Traditionally, interrupting the sympathetic supply to the painful area was thought to treat such pain. However, the effectiveness of this approach is not supported by randomized controlled trials.[31]

Neural plasticity occurs in a variety of pain syndromes.[32,33] We predicted that referred sensations would be present in patients with CRPS Type 1 as evidence of sensory cortical reorganization.[34] The resultant sensory mislocalizations could then provide the inappropriate sensory feedback required to create painful sensations. Furthermore, we hypothesized that these referred sensations would be perceived to emanate from the body structures immediately adjacent to the stimulated site and in keeping with their topographical location on the Penfield homunculus as in phantom and allied pain states. We specifically selected those patients with CRPS Type 1 as we wished to discover

TABLE 5.1. Location, Direction, and Type of Sensations[a] Referred in Subjects with a Diagnosis of CRPS Type 1 (Cases 1–5)

Patient	Pain Site	Disease Duration	Area Touched (1) Referral Site (2, 3)	Direction of Referral	Type of Sensation	Loss of Referred Sensation	Resolution of CRPS (weeks)
Case 1 28 yr F (Fig. 5.2a)	Left hand	3 wk	L 3rd fingertip (1) L lower jaw (2)	1–2	Light touch and pinprick	3 wk	6
Case 2 34 yr F (Fig. 5.2b)	Left ankle	8 wk	L forefoot (1) L patella (2)	1–2 and 2–1	Light touch and pinprick	3 wk	4
Case 3 24 yr M (Fig. 5.2c)	Left knee	3 yr	L patella (1) L forefoot (2)	1–2 and 2–1	Light touch	No change	Chronic
Case 4 41 yr F (Fig. 5.2d)	Right foot	6 yr	R forefoot (1) R patella (2)	2–1	Light touch	4 wk	Chronic
Case 5 57 yr F (Fig. 5.2e)	Left hand	4 yr	L shoulder (1)	1–2	Pulling, light touch, and hand movement	No change	Chronic
(Fig. 5.2f)			L ear (2) L hand (3) L cheek (1) L hand (2)	1–3 1–2	Light touch		

[a]Loss of detection of referred sensations is shown in relation to current disease duration and future status (resolved or chronic).

TABLE 5.2. Demographics of Total Study Population to Compare and Contrast Similarities and Differences in Age, Disease Duration, and Levels of Pain Between Subjects Who Experienced Referred Sensations and Those Who Did Not

Case	Age	Gender	Disease Duration	Affected Limb	Pain Level on Movement[a] at Presentation
1[b]	28 yr	F	3 wk	Left hand	8
2[b]	34 yr	F	8 wk	Left ankle	8
3[b]	24 yr	M	3 yr	Left knee	8
4[b]	41 yr	F	6 yr	Right foot	9
5[b]	57 yr	F	4 yr	Left hand	5
Mean[b]	*36.8 yr*	*4F:1M*	*2.6 yr*		*7.6*
6	38 yr	F	6 wk	Left ankle	9
7	35 yr	F	5 m	Right arm	5
8	40 yr	F	1 yr	Right arm	6
9	38 yr	F	3 yr	Left leg	5
10	27 yr	M	2 yr	Left leg	8
11	51 yr	F	2 yr	Right arm	7.5
12	68 yr	F	1 yr	Left arm	5
13	54 yr	M	4 yr	Left foot	9
14	38 yr	F	7 yr	Left foot	10
15	22 yr	F	4 yr	Left foot	9
16	59 yr	F	10 yr	Left foot	9.5
Mean	*42.7 yr*	*9F:2M*	*3.1 yr*		*8*

[a]Visual analogue 10 cm scale.

[b]Referred sensations reported.

whether central reorganization occurs even where there is no evidence of local peripheral nerve damage.

Over two years, 16 subjects (13 female, 3 male) who met the entry criteria were recruited. Only five showed evidence of referred sensations (Table 5.1). There was no difference in age, disease duration, levels of pain, or severity of disease (Table 5.2) between those who presented with CRPS and those who did not. All five patients reported referred sensations during examination with their eyes closed (Fig. 5.2). They were experienced in real time and disappeared when stimulation ceased or vision was permitted. When the subjects viewed the area being touched, the sensations were either diminished (Case 5) or not present and when the symptoms of CRPS resolved (Cases 1, 2, and 4), referred sensations were lost. Sensations were referred in a modality-specific manner with touch referred in all cases and pinprick also referred in two (Cases 1 and 2). Vibration was never referred. All referred sites were located on body parts immediately adjacent, on Penfield's homunculus, to the stimulated site.

The location of the referred sites, in our study population, was consistent with previous reports in other pain conditions[13,35] and fit particularly well with predicted cortical changes that have been shown to occur within the

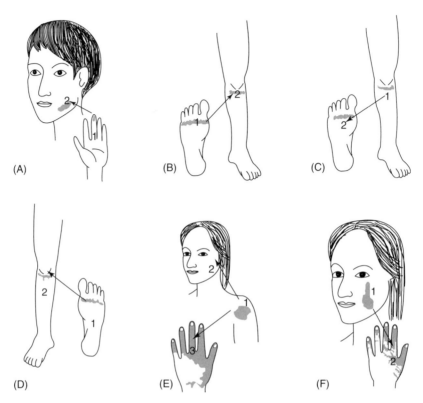

Figure 5.2. Artist's impression of Cases 1–5 illustrating location of stimulus and direction of referred sensations (area touched = 1, referred site(s) = 2,3 Parts (A)–(D)) correspond to Cases 1–4; (E) and (F) correspond to Case 5. Shaded area (1) depicts area stimulated by examiner; shaded areas 2 and 3 depict where referred sensation was felt. The arrows illustrate direction of referral.

somatosensory body map in amputees.[36] Ramachandran and Hirstein[37] proposed that due to the location and speed with which referred sensations occur in amputees, such "ectopic representations" following functional remapping were probably due to the unmasking of latent synapses within the cortex, as previously described in primates.[38,39] These synapses are suppressed when there is simultaneous input from two connected receptors but with reduced or impaired sensory activation in one area, the connection becomes disinhibited. Recent imaging studies, using magnetoencephalography, in six patients with upper limb CRPS Type 1 have also shown changes in the cortical somatosensory map, although it was not reported whether these were associated with referred sensations.[40] There was a significantly shorter distance between the areas representing the thumb and little finger on the somatosensory cortex contralateral to the affected limb than the ipsilateral side. Interestingly, there was no significant correlation between the distance of thumb and finger and the level or duration of pain. Hand dominance was also not an influencing factor.

Alternatively, referral of sensations may occur at the spinal level. A large body of evidence shows that sensitization of wide dynamic range neurons at level V of the dorsal horn results in ipsilateral and contralateral enlarged receptive fields that do not rely on a cortical homunculus.[41] In addition, experimental models of peripheral neuropathic pain all demonstrate bilateral spinal cord changes after unilateral nerve damage.[42] However, all of our patients had CRPS Type 1 and therefore had no precipitating neural trauma. Their sensations were not referred bilaterally, either from the stimulated site to its contralateral partner (i.e., left hand to right hand) or mirrored on the contralateral side (i.e., from stimulated site to referral site on the unaffected limb). In addition, the speed of referral in terms of disease duration, response time on stimulation, and resolution as the condition improved, combined with the magnitude of the sensations, all detract from a purely spinal route. Contemporary theories suggest that CRPS is a disorder involving both CNS and peripheral nervous system components.[43,44] This is based on the evidence that some patients respond positively to sympathetic blockade, thereby implicating involvement of the sympathetic nervous system; but conversely, sympathetically maintained pain involves the deep somatic tissue (as demonstrated by our patients' reports of increased pain on movement), which is the domain of the autonomic system. Therefore isolating one clear route for referred sensations is at present problematic.

THE POWER OF VISION AND MIRROR VISUAL FEEDBACK

Visual feedback strongly influences the experience of referred sensations in patients with CRPS. Recent studies have shown this also to be the case in amputees where stimulation of the intact limb evoked sensory changes in the phantom only when the subjects' eyes were closed.[45] Touch and vision are inextricably linked. Touch is known to influence vision such as dispelling the visual illusion of a three-dimensional object when it is drawn on a flat surface. Equally, in some clinical conditions such as somatosensory loss after stroke, visual feedback of the affected limb during testing can significantly improve reported perception.[46] In addition, recent findings by Taylor-Clark et al.[47] showed that the enhancing effect of vision modulated somatosensory cortical processing. Gregory[48] points out that vision evolved from the simpler processes for touch and that it is possible that the somatosensory map is inverted (the feet above the hand) in order to correspond with the inverted visual image on the retina. This ensures that the link between vision and touch is as short as possible. Consequently, when our subjects viewed their limbs being stimulated, it would appear that the more powerful sense of vision overruled the referred sensations.

It has already been stated that vision is able to dismiss the sensation of phantom swelling in RA and FMS, but in recent studies on PLP vision has been shown to also provide an analgesic benefit. Ramachandran and

Roger-Ramachandran[49] superimposed the image of amputees' normal limbs, by means of a mirror, on the space that their phantom limbs occupied. Viewing the mirror image of their residual limb, the amputees moved their normal limbs and attempted to move their abnormal side. Subjects reported that sensation in their abnormal limb returned toward normal during the exercises and their pain diminished. Harris[32] subsequently hypothesized that the reason for this analgesic effect was that PLP is generated by a discordance in motor intention and predicted proprioceptive feedback and that when this mismatch is corrected, through appropriate visual feedback via the mirror, pain is relieved.

Objective evidence of the cortical effects of this mismatch was provided by Fink and colleagues[50] using position emission tomography (PET) imaging and healthy volunteers. They demonstrated that when congruent and incongruent movements were performed, while viewing only one limb in a mirror, cortical activity varied depending on the movement. When the limbs moved incongruently and yet were seen, by means of mirror imaging, to move congruently, cortical activity was unilateral, unlike visually observed congruent and actual congruent movement, where bilateral cortical activity was produced. When unilateral cortical activity occurred, it was in the right dorsolateral prefrontal cortex and it was this area that Fink et al.[50] concluded was specifically involved in the monitoring of conflict between motor intention and its sensory/perceptual consequences.

The existence of referred sensations in CRPS and evidence of changes in cortical representation[40] suggest that pain in CRPS may also be driven by a mismatch between motor output and sensory input as Harris[32] proposed for PLP. We hypothesized that if this were the case then the provision of appropriate sensory input should correct the mismatch and reduce pain. Modifying Ramachandran's methodology[49] for the relief of PLP, we too used a mirror to provide congruent visual feedback, from the moving unaffected limb, to restore the integrity of cortical processing aiming to relieve pain and restore function in the affected limb.[50]

Eight subjects were recruited, aged 24–40 years (mean 33 years), with disease duration of 3 weeks to 3 years (three subjects with early disease of ≤8 weeks; two intermediate, 5 months and 1 year; and the remaining three longstanding disease of ≥2 years). All presented with a single limb affected by allodynia, hyperalgesia, reduced movement with related pain, and stiffness and vasomotor disturbances (Table 5.3).

All subjects reported no relief of pain on movement when both limbs were visualized without a device or when a nonreflective surface was viewed (Fig. 5.3). Indeed, movement exacerbated pain. All three subjects with early CRPS (≤8 weeks) reported a striking reduction in their visual analogue scale for pain, during and after visual feedback of their reflected moving, unaffected limb as provided by the mirror (Fig. 5.4). A marked analgesic effect was observed within a few minutes of mirror usage, followed by an abrupt return of pain when the mirror was removed initially. With repeated usage (4–9 × daily, week 1), the period of analgesia progressively extended from a few minutes to

TABLE 5.3. Patient Characteristics and the Effect of the Control and Intervention Phases on their Pain at Presentation

	At Presentation						Follow up[a]								
	Characteristics			Control Phase 1: Looking at Both Limbs (No Device)		Control Phase 2: Painful Limb Hidden	Intervention: Mirror Visual Feedback	Frequency of Mirror Usage × per Day (Duration of each treatment 10 min)							At 6 weeks	
Subject[b] (Painful Limb)	Symptom Duration	Mean Temperature Difference (°C) [Nonpainful–Painful Limb]		Pain VAS at Rest	Pain VAS on Movement	Pain VAS on Movement	Pain VAS on Movement				Week			Pain VAS	Mean Temperature Difference (°C)	Treatment Duration (weeks)
								1	2	3	4	5	6			
Case 1 (left leg) 38 yr F	6 weeks	1.1		9	9	9	2	8	3	3	3	2	0	0	0.2	6
Case 2 (left arm) 28 yr F	3 weeks	2.0		7	8	8	3	4	4	3	3	2	0	0	0.4	6
Case 3 (left leg) 34 yr F	8 weeks	2.7		6	8	8	2	9	4	3	0	0	0	0	0.8	4
Case 4 (right arm) 35 yr F	5 mths	1.9		0	5[d]	5[d]	3[d]	5	4	5	4	5	4	2[d]	0.3	6
Case 5 (right arm) 40 yr F	1 year	0.5		4	6	6	6	5	4	5	4	4	3	1	0.4	6
Case 6 (left leg) 24 yr M	2 years	1.4		7	8	8	8	5	5	5	0	0	0	8	1.3	Unresolved
Case 7[e] (left leg) 38 yr F	3 years	Not performed		4	5	5	5	4	4	0	0	0	0	5	Not performed	Unresolved
Case 8 (left leg) 27 yr M	2 years	2.1		7	8	8	8	4	4	0	0	0	0	8	2.6	Unresolved

[a]The frequency of mirror use on follow-up and final pain scores at 6 weeks with infrared thermal differences and unaffected limbs.

[b]M, male; F, female.

[c]Region of interest constant significant difference if >0.4 °C (Ref. 13).

[d]Stiffness.

[e]Case 7 had widespread ulceration on her left leg, which made thermal image interpretation impossible.

85

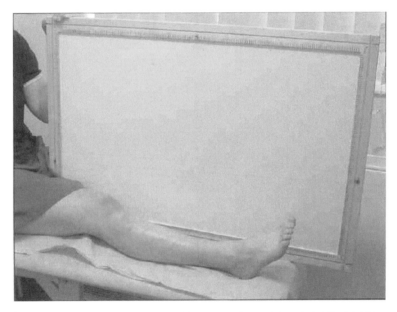

Figure 5.3. Subject viewing nonreflective surface with painful limb hidden.

hours, requiring less mirror use over the 6 week study period. At 6 weeks there was a reversal of vasomotor changes as measured by infrared thermal imaging, a return to normal function, and no pain at rest or on movement. All three subjects felt they no longer required analgesic relief from the mirror and had stopped prior to assessment at 6 weeks (Case 3, week 4; Cases 1 and 2, week 6).

The two subjects with intermediate disease duration, 5 months and 1 year (Cases 4 and 5), reported that the mirror immediately eased their movement-related stiffness but there was no analgesic effect in Case 5. They both reported that this reduction in stiffness facilitated movement and the effect lasted for increasing periods after mirror usage. Although no objective data was collected on function, both subjects felt that, by 6 weeks, function had improved to such an extent that they were able to return to their usual manual occupations. Interestingly, despite the lack of analgesic effect during the mirror visual feedback procedure, Case 5 reported reduced pain at the 6 week follow-up (VAS 6/10 at presentation to 1/10 at 6 weeks). Reversal of infrared thermal (IRT) imaging temperature differences were recorded in Case 4 at 6 weeks and Case 5 remained with no significant difference between the two affected limbs.

No subjective relief of pain and stiffness or reversal of IRT temperature differences were observed in the three subjects with chronic disease (≥ 2 years), and they had all discontinued mirror usage by the end of week 3 due to lack of analgesic effect.

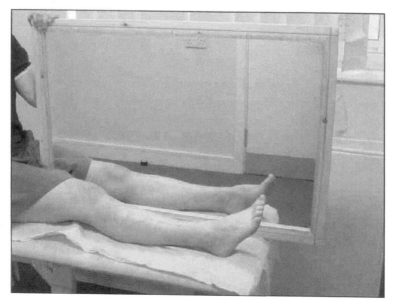

Figure 5.4. Subject viewing nonpainful limb in mirror with painful limb hidden.

These observations suggest that congruent visual feedback of the moving unaffected limb, via a mirror, significantly reduces the perception of pain in early CRPS and stiffness in the intermediate stages of the disease.[51] This supports the hypothesis that the CNS is capable of generating a feedback-dependent state that can produce pathological levels of pain. In CRPS, this might involve a mismatch between different interdependent modalities, such as a disruption of normal interaction between motor intention and sensory feedback. In those with an inherent vulnerability to this incongruence it can lead, in some, to referred, intractable pain following trauma or, in others, promote CRPS with a central nervous system origin. This might explain why some types of CRPS occur without discrete peripheral injury.

If the correction of a sensory/motor mismatch produces an analgesic response, then the reverse should also be true. That is, when expected sensory input is deliberately falsified, sensory abnormalities should be generated in healthy volunteers and exacerbated in patients with chronic pain of unknown etiology.

GENERATING PAIN

In two recent studies,[52,53] we invited healthy volunteers and patients with fibromyalgia (FMS) to move their upper and lower limbs while undergoing normal and altered visual sensory feedback as provided via a mirror. Motor/

sensory conflict was at its optimum when the subjects moved their limbs in opposing directions while viewing, via the mirror, their limbs apparently moving together. The primary aim of these studies was to comprehensively capture, using a qualitative methodology, the range of sensory experiences that subjects described as they underwent these maneuvers. Each assessment was conducted first with the subjects viewing the control side (a whiteboard) and moving their limbs congruently and incongruently and then repeating the movements while viewing the intervention side (a mirror).

In the first study,[52] 41 healthy volunteers (9 males, 32 females) were recruited, aged from 23 to 65 years (mean 40.4 years). They reported sensory changes at all stages of the protocol, control (congruent movement $n = 6$ (15%), incongruent movement $n = 4$ (10%)) and intervention. However, the maximum number of reports occurred when the subjects moved their limbs incongruently but perceived, via mirror imaging, that they were moving them congruently (congruent movement $n = 10$ (25%), incongruent movement $n = 23$ (56%)). The healthy volunteers reported discomfort ("pins and needles," "shooting pain"), changes in temperature and/or weight ("floaty sensation" or "my arm was so heavy I was unable to lift it"), perceived loss of or additional limbs, and disorientation ("dizzy," "strange") (Table 5.4). Altered

TABLE 5.4. Type and Incidence of Sensory Changes Reported by Healthy Volunteers[a] in Hidden Limb During Congruent and Incongruent Movement While Viewing a Whiteboard (Control) and Mirror (Intervention)

Type of Sensation	Whiteboard Congruent Movement	Whiteboard Incongruent Movement	Mirror Congruent Movement	Mirror Incongruent Movement
Discomfort/ pain	1 (2%)	1 (2%)	4 (10%)	7 (17%)
Temperature change	0	0	0	2 (5%)
Weight change	2 (5%)	0	3 (7%)	6 (15%)
Perceived "loss" of limb	4 (10%)	2 (4.9%)	8 (20%)	11 (27%)
Perceived "extra" limb	0	0	1 (2%)	9 (22%)
Disorientation	3 (7%)	4 (10%)	15 (37%)	13 (32%)
Total number of subjects experiencing any sensory disturbances	6 (15%)	4 (10%)	10 (24%)	23 (56%)

[a]$n = 41$ (male = 8, female = 33)

TABLE 5.5. Details of the Incidence of Symptoms Reported by Subjects with Fibromyalgia (FMS) and Healthy Volunteers (HVS) at Each Stage of the Protocol in Relation to the Total Study Populations

| | Whiteboard | | | | Mirror | | | | | |
| | Congruent Movement | | Incongruent Movement | | Congruent Movement | | Incongruent Movement | | At Any Stage in the Protocol | |
FMS n = 29 HVs n = 29	FMS	HV	FMS	HV	FMS	HV	FMS	HV	FMS	HV
Pain	8 (28%)	1 (3%)	9 (31%)	1 (3%)	7 (24%)	4 (14%)	9 (31%)	3 (10%)	18 (62%)	4 (14%)
Temperature	4 (14%)	0 (0%)	1 (3%)	0 (0%)	3 (10%)	0 (0%)	2 (7%)	1 (3%)	5 (17%)	1 (3%)
Weight change	8 (28%)	1 (3%)	6 (21%)	0 (0%)	7 (24%)	2 (7%)	10 (34%)	4 (14%)	15 (52%)	4 (14%)
Perceived loss of limb	7 (24%)	2 (7%)	8 (28%)	1 (3%)	17 (59%)	4 (14%)	15 (52%)	7 (24%)	19 (66%)	9 (31%)
Perceived extra limb	0 (0%)	0 (0%)	0 (0%)	0 (0%)	1 (3%)	0 (0%)	3 (10%)	5 (17%)	4 (14%)	5 (17%)
Peculiarity	5 (17%)	2 (7%)	13 (45%)	2 (7%)	12 (41%)	9 (31%)	14 (48%)	10 (34%)	18 (62%)	13 (45%)
Phantom stiffness	0 (0%)	0 (0%)	0 (0%)	0 (0%)	0 (0%)	0 (0%)	1 (3%)	0 (0%)	1 (3%)	0 (0%)
Total number of subjects experiencing any sensation	18 (62%)	4 (14%)	22 (76%)	2 (7%)	22 (76%)	10 (34%)	20 (69%)	13 (59%)	26 (90%)	14 (48%)

sensations were described predominantly in the hidden limb, although this sometimes automatically conferred sensations onto the visualized limb, such as a hidden limb felt heavier and therefore the visualized limb was perceived as lighter. All altered sensations faded rapidly after limb movement had ceased and the hidden limb was visualized by the subject.

In the second study,[53] 29 adult subjects diagnosed as suffering from FMS were recruited (one male) aged from 27 to 74 years (mean 47.9 years, SD 11.1). Twenty six (89.7%) subjects reported sensory changes at some stage in the protocol in addition to, or worse than, baseline; only three (10.3%) describing no effect. FMS subjects reported the same range of symptoms as those previously described by healthy volunteers and subjects related to these symptoms as being very similar to those they experience in a flare of their condition. However, when data were compared to an age matched cohort of healthy volunteers, the FMS population generated a higher frequency of report at all stages of the protocol than that of the maximum report in the healthy volunteer population (Table 5.5). In addition, the FMS population demonstrated a greater vulnerability to the generation of these symptoms than the healthy volunteers (HVs) (FMS 89.7% compared to HV 48%). Our findings suggest that visually mediated changes between motor output and predicted somatosensory feedback are sufficient to produce the additional somaesthetic disturbances, and exacerbation of preexisting symptoms, seen in the FMS population. This happens in a similar manner in healthy volunteers but importantly less frequently and to a lesser extent. This allows us to propose a preexisting motor/sensory conflict in the FMS population.

CONCLUSION

Our clinical observations and research studies support the conjecture put forward by Harris[32] that when motor intentions to move a limb or series of joints no longer matches the corresponding sensory feedback, then the subsequent "misrouting of information" activates a central monitoring mechanism that flags up such incongruity as pain. However, we would now like to extend Harris's[32] theory and propose that this monitoring mechanism is one of many monitoring mechanisms that act as alerts to warn the body that there is a problem with information processing and that pain may be only one of a broad range of sensory disturbances that subsequently occur. These central mechanisms we have termed ominory from the Latin word *ominor* meaning to prophesy, to predict, or foreboding. Our studies have focused on the mechanism that monitors motor/sensory conflict but a separate ominory mechanism could generate motion sickness when there is discordance between body position, balance, and equilibrium. These mechanisms may be triggered by externally induced conflict (e.g., incongruent movement while viewing the mirror) or internally (e.g., disease damage in RA leading to inaccurate execution of movement and/or altered proprioception). The key feature of these mechanisms is that when they are triggered they generate sensory disturbances such as nausea with motion sickness, pain in a phantom limb, and phantom swelling and stiffness in RA and FMS. These resultant states we have termed dissensory from the Latin word *dissensio* meaning conflict or disagreement. These are feedback-dependent states, which will continue to trigger the ominory mechanism, and ultimately either via duration or intensity of this state the subject will suffer pain. If, however, an intervention is targeted to correct the initial source of conflict, the ominory mechanism is suppressed and ideally pain is prevented or alleviated as with mirror visual feedback in early CRPS or the individual visualizing the phantom swollen joints in RA and FMS.

We propose that the threshold at which a person either triggers the ominory mechanism or becomes aware of the subsequent sensory disturbances is individually determined, but there will be some who are more sensitive than others. This we assume will relate to the standard variables of genetic factors, age, gender, and sex hormone state. This was demonstrated by our healthy volunteer study: not all subjects experienced sensory disturbances. In addition, our patient data shows that where sensory disturbances are already present, a far lower stimulus is required to intensify the problem. Simply hiding a limb from view was sufficient to exacerbate sensory disturbances in those with FMS.

So far we have only addressed three rheumatological conditions—RA, FMS, and CRPS—but the same ominory mechanism may apply to the pain of osteoarthritis (OA) and indeed the development of pathological changes in the joint.

It is known that proprioception reduces with age and with OA.[54] In the OA knee it has been demonstrated that this reduction in proprioception occurs in the affected and contralateral knee joint and that such a reduction may indeed predispose an individual to the onset of OA.[55] Furthermore, joints located at a distance from the knee also demonstrate a reduction in proprioception,[56] thereby suggesting that problems with the motor control system are not confined to the affected area alone but may be more widely present. Interestingly, the loss or reduction of one sense is known to have a negative effect on multisensory integration that is required for effective spatial integration,[57,58] and perhaps this makes the aging adult more vulnerable to the onset of changes in motor sensory integration and ultimately OA. The range in patient reported pain in OA may be more related to the individual vulnerability to cortically derived pain from changes in the motor control system than directly related to the structural changes within a joint. However, once these structural changes do occur, one could imagine this would maintain and perpetuate the problems with proprioception and so the cycle would continue.

Therapies as just discussed[49,51] and others[59-61] that have been devised to correct this sensorimotor incongruence in other chronic pain conditions have proved to give enhanced motor control and analgesic benefit. They have been designed to target all stages of motor planning progression from enhancement of premotor planning to the provision of corrective sensory feedback, but to date the studies have been small and there is little long-term follow-up data. In OA, increasing emphasis is being given to exercise-based therapies, which may be working through enhanced proprioception.[62,63]

It needs to be established what role this newly defined cortical model of pain has in the generation and/or the perpetuation of pain-related symptoms in OA. It may indeed also play a part in the pathogenesis and/or progression of the disease. Work to date in other chronic pain conditions has approached this from a number of different angles, and this may be a sensible model to follow in OA. Clinical studies have been designed to identify any preexisting motor sensory mismatch and to test the efficacy of novel therapies created to correct this discrepancy. Some of these studies have been supported by imaging techniques and others have relied on detailed histories and qualitative descriptors. Both designs appear to contribute equally valuable data. Highly sophisticated imaging studies have been used to look in detail at the movement trajectory of a single limb and identify at what point problems may arise, and others have focused on changes within the motor and sensory cortices. More laboratory based work has studied the impact of such a discrepancy on other key body systems such as the autonomic and immune systems. This may also be relevant in OA. Finally, once common characteristics are identified, it would be helpful to identify those individuals who are at greatest risk of developing a sensorimotor discrepancy so that interventions may be put in place early to reduce or prevent the disabling consequences of OA.

In conclusion, a mismatch between motor output and sensory input triggers a warning, ominory mechanism in rheumatology patients and healthy volunteers. This generates the dissensory state and the individual will experience sensory disturbances that may include pain.

ACKNOWLEDGMENTS

David R. Blake holds an endowed Chair—The Glaxo Wellcome Chair in Locomotor Sciences. An Arthritis Research Campaign ICAC award supports The Royal National Hospital for Rheumatic Diseases, Bath.

Copyright was granted by Oxford University Press for work previously published by Candida S. McCabe et al. in *Rheumatology*.

REFERENCES

1. Murray CJL, Lopez AD (eds.). (1996). *The Global Burden of Disease: A Comprehensive Assessment of Mortality and Disability from Diseases, Injuries, and Risk Factors in 1990 and Projected to 2002*. Geneva: World Health Organization.

2. Elders MJ. (2000). The increasing impact of arthritis on public health. J Rheumatol 60(S):6e8.

3. Petersson I. (1996). Occurrence of osteoarthritis of the peripheral joints in European populations. Ann Rheum Dis 55:659–661.

4. Dieppe PA, Lohmander LS. (2005). Pathogenesis and management of pain in osteoarthritis. Lancet 365:965–973.

5. Brandt KD, Rodin EL, Dieppe PA, van de Putte L. (2006). Yet more evidence that osteoarthritis is not a cartilage disease. Ann Rheum Dis 65:1261–1264.

6. Creamer P, Hochberg MC. (1997). Why does osteoarthritis of the knee hurt—sometimes? BJ Rheum 36:726–728.

7. Lawrence JS, Bremmer JM, Bier F. (1966). Osteo-arthrosis. Prevalence in the population and relationship between the symptoms and X-ray changes. Ann Rheum Dis 25:1–24.

8. Halbert J, Crotty M, Cameron ID. (2002). Evidence for the optimal management of acute and chronic phantom pain: a systematic review. Clin J Pain 18:84–92.

9. Hill A, Niven CA, Knussen C. (1995). Pain memories in phantom limbs: a case study. Pain 66:381–384.

10. Melzack R. (1971). Phantom limb pain: implications for treatment of pathologic pain. Anesthesiology 35:409–419.

11. Melzack R. (1990). Phantom limbs and the concept of a neuromatrix. Trends Neurosci 13(3):88–92.

12. Katz J, Melzack R. (1990). Pain memories in phantom limbs: review and clinical observations. Pain 43:319–336.

13. Ramachandran VS, Stewart M, Rogers-Ramachandran D. (1992). Perceptual correlates of massive cortical reorganisation. Neuroreport 3(7):583–586.

14. Clarke S, Regli L, Janzer RC, Assal G, de Tribolet N. (1996). Phantom face: conscious correlate of neural reorganization after removal of primary sensory neurones. Neuroreport 7(18):2853–2857.

15. Gandevia SC, Phegan CML. (1999). Perceptual distortions of the human body image produced by local anaesthesia, pain and cutaneous stimulation. J Physiol 514(2):609–616.

16. Turton AJ, Butler SR. (2001). Referred sensations following stroke. Neurocase 7:397–405.

17. Moore CL, Stern CE, Dunbar C, Kostyk SK, Gehi A, Corkin S. (2000). Referred phantom sensations and cortical reorganisation after spinal cord injury in humans. Proc Natl Acad Sci USA 97(26):14703–14708.

18. Penfield W, Rasmussen TL. (1950). *The Cerebral Cortex of Man: A Clinical Study of Localization of Function.* New York: MacMillan.

19. Walker DJ. (1995). Rheumatoid arthritis. In Butler RC and Jayson MIV (eds.). *Collected Reports on the Rheumatic Diseases.* Arthritis and Rheumatism Council, pp. 39–44.

20. Gordon DA, Hastings DE. (1995). Clinical features of rheumatoid arthritis: early, progressive and late disease. In Klippel JH and Dieppe PA (eds.). *Practical Rheumatology.* London: Times Mirror International Publishers, pp. 169–182.

21. Parker JC, Smarr KL, Buescher KL, Phillips LR, Frank RG, Beck NC, Anderson SK, Walker SE. (1989). Pain control and rational thinking. Implications for rheumatoid arthritis. Arthritis Rheum 32(8):984–990.

22. Papageorgiou AC, Badley EM. (1989). The quality of pain in arthritis: the words patients use to describe overall pain and pain in individual joints at rest and on movement. Rheumatology 16(1):106–112.

23. Blake DR, McCabe CS, Skevington SM, Haigh R. (2000). Cortical origins of pathological pain. Lancet 355:1365.

24. McCabe CS. (1999). An exploratory study into the experience of pain in rheumatoid arthritis. MSc thesis. University of Bath, Bath, UK.

25. Arnett FC, Edworthy SM, Bloch DA, McShane DJ, Fries JF, Cooper NS, et al. (1988). The American Rheumatism Association revised criteria for the classification of rheumatoid arthritis. Arthritis Rheum 31:315–324.

26. Helliwell PS, Howe A, Wright V. (1988). Lack of objective stiffness in rheumatoid arthritis. Ann Rheum Dis 47:754–758.

27. Haigh RC, McCabe CS, Halligan P, Blake DR. (2003). Joint stiffness in a phantom limb: evidence of central nervous system involvement in rheumatoid arthritis. Rheumatology 42:888–892.

28. Wolfe F, Smythe HA, Yunus MB, Bennett RM, Bombardier C, Golenberg DL, Tugwell P, Campbell SM, Abeles M, Clark P. (1990). The American College of Rheumatology 1990 criteria for the classification of fibromyalgia. Report of the multicenter Criteria Committee. Arthritis Rheum 33:160–172.

29. Staud R, Vierck CJ, Cannon RL, Mauderli AP, Price DD. (2001). Abnormal sensitisation and temporal summation of second pain (wind up) in patients with fibromyalgia syndrome. Pain 91:165–175.

30. Scadding JW. (1999). Complex regional pain syndrome. In Wall PD and Melzack R (eds.). *Textbook of Pain*, 4th ed. Edinburgh: Churchill Livingstone, pp. 835–850.

31. Jaded AR, Carroll D, Glynn CJ, McQuay H. (1995). Intravenous regional sympathetic blockade for pain relief in reflex sympathetic dystrophy: a systematic review and a randomised, double-blind crossover study. J Pain Symptom Manage 10(1):13–19.

32. Harris AJ. (1999). Cortical origins of pathological pain. Lancet 354:1464–1466.

33. Lenz F, Byl NN. (1999). Reorganisation in the cutaneous core of the human thalamic principal somatic sensory nucleus (ventral caudal) in patients with dystonia. J Neurophysiol 3204–3211.

34. McCabe CS, Haigh RC, Halligan PW, Blake DR. (2003). Referred sensations in complex regional pain syndrome type 1. Rheumatology 42:1067–1073.

35. Flor H, Braun C, Elbert T, Birbaumer N. (1997). Extensive reorganization of primary somatosensory cortex in chronic back pain patients. Neurosci Lett 224(1):5–8.

36. Halligan PW, Marshall JC, Wade DT, Davey J, Morrison D. (1993). Thumb in cheek? Sensory reorganisation and perceptual plasticity after limb amputation. Neuroreport 4:233–236.

37. Ramachandran VS, Hirstein W. (1998). The perception of phantom limbs. The D.O. Hebb lecture. Brain 121:1603–1630.

38. De Felipe J, Conley M, Jones EG. (1986). Long-range focal collateralisation of axons arising from corticocortical cells in monkey sensory-motor cortex. J Neurosci 6:3749–3766.

39. Jones EG. (1990). The role of afferent activity in the maintenance of primate neocortical function. J Exp Biol 153:155–156.

40. Juottonen K, Gockel M, Silen T, Hurrir H, Hari R, Forss N. (2002). Altered central sensorimotor processing in patients with complex regional pain syndrome. Pain 98:315–323.

41. Ji RR, Woolf CJ. (2001). Neuronal plasticity and signal transduction in nociceptive neurons: implications for the initiation and maintenance of pathological pain. Neurobiol Dis 8(1):1–10.

42. Koltzenberg M, Wall PD, McMahon SB. (1999). Does the right side know what the left is doing? TINS 24(3):122–127.

43. Baron R, Fields HL, Janig W, Kitt C, Levine JD. (2002). National Institutes of Health workshop: reflex sympathetic dystrophy/complex regional pain syndromes—state of the science. Anaesth Analg 95:1812–1816.

44. Janig W, Baron R. (2002). Complex regional pain syndrome is a disease of the central nervous system. Clin Auton Res 12:150–164.

45. Hunter JP, Katz J, Davis KD. (2003). The effect of tactile and visual sensory inputs on phantom limb awareness. Brain 126:579–589.

46. Halligan PW, Marshall JC, Hunt M, Wade DT. (1997). Somatosensory assessment: can seeing produce feeling? J Neurol 244(3):199–203.

47. Taylor-Clark M, Kennett S, Haggard P. (2002). Vision modulates somatosensory cortical processing. Curr Biol 12(3):233–236.

48. Gregory RL. (1998). *Eye and Brain. The Psychology of Seeing.* Oxford, UK: Oxford University Press, p. 53.

49. Ramachandran VS, Roger S, Ramachandran D. (1996). Synaesthesia in phantom limbs induced with mirrors. Proc R Soc Lond 263:377–386.

50. Fink GR, Marshall JC, Halligan PW, Frith CD, Driver J, Frackowiak RS, Dolan RJ. (1999). The neural consequences of conflict between intention and the senses. Brain 122(3):497–512.

51. McCabe CS, Haigh RC, Ring EFR, Halligan PW, Wall PD, Blake DR. (2003). A controlled pilot study of the utility of mirror visual feedback in the treatment of complex regional pain syndrome (type 1). Rheumatology 42:97–101.

52. McCabe CS, Haigh RC, Halligan PW, Blake DR. (2005). Simulating sensory–motor incongruence in healthy volunteers: implications for a cortical model of rheumatology pain. Rheumatology 44:509–516.

53. McCabe C, Bodamyali T, Cohen H, Blake DR. (2007). Somaesthetic disturbances in fibromyalgia are exaggerated by sensory–motor conflict: implications for chronicity of the disease? Rheumatology 46:1587–1592.

54. Sharma L, Pai YC, Holkamp K, Rymer WZ. (1997). Is knee joint proprioception worse in the arthritis knee versus the unaffected knee in unilateral knee osteoarthrits? Arthritis Rheum 40(8):1518–1525.

55. Lund H, Juul-Kristenses B, Christensesn H, Bliddal H, et al. (2004). Impaired proprioception of both knees and elbows in patients with knee osteoarthritis compared to healthy controls. Osteoarthritis Cartilage 12:S25.

56. Hurley MV. (1997). The effects of joint damage on muscle function, proprioception and rehabilitation. Man-Ther 2(1):11–17.

57. Calvert GA, Spence C, Stein BE. (2004). *The Handbook of Multisensory Processing.* Cambridge, MA: MIT Press.

58. Driver J, Grossenbacher PG. (1996). Mulitmodal constraints on tactile spatial attention. In Innui T and McClelland JL (eds.). *Attention and Performance XVI.* Cambridge, MA: MIT Press, pp. 209–236.

59. Moseley GL. (2004). Graded motor imagery is effective for long-standing complex regional pain syndrome: a randomised controlled trial. Pain 108:192–198.

60. Moseley GL. (2005). Is successful rehabilitation of complex regional pain syndrome simply sustained attention to the affected limb? A randomised clinical trial. Pain 114(1-2):54–61.

61. Flor H. (2002). The modification of cortical reorganisation and chronic pain by sensory feedback. Appl Psychophysiol Biofeedback 27(3):215–222.

62. Roddy E, Zhang W, Doherty M, Arden NK, Barlow J, et al. (2005). Evidence-based recommendations for the role of exercise in the management of osteoarthritis of the hip or knee—the MOVE concensus. Rheumatology 44(1):67–73.

63. Hurley MV, Scott DL. (1998). Improvements in quadriceps sensorimotor function and disability of patients with knee osteoarthritis following a clinically practicable exercise regime. Br J Rheumatol 37(11):1181–1187.

6

MECHANISMS THAT GENERATE AND MAINTAIN BONE CANCER PAIN

Juan Miguel Jimenez-Andrade and Monica Herrera

Department of Pharmacology, College of Medicine, University of Arizona, 1656 East Mabel, Tucson, Arizona 85724, USA

Patrick W. Mantyh

Department of Pharmacology, College of Medicine, University of Arizona, 1656 East Mabel, Tucson, Arizona 85724, USA and Research Service VA Medical Center, Minneapolis, Minnesota 55417, USA

INTRODUCTION

Currently, more than 10 million people are diagnosed with cancer every year and by 2020 it is estimated that 20 million new cases will be diagnosed each year.[1,2] In 2005, cancer caused 7.6 million deaths world wide.[3] In the United States, cancer is a major health problem, being the second leading cause of death. Currently, 25% of U.S. deaths are cancer related.[4]

Cancer-associated pain can be present at any time during the course of the disease, but the frequency and intensity of cancer pain tend to increase with advancing stages of cancer. In patients with advanced cancer, 62–86%

Pain in Osteoarthritis, Edited by David T. Felson and Hans-Georg Schaible
Copyright © 2009 Wiley-Blackwell.

experience significant pain that is described as moderate to severe in approximately 40–50% and as very severe in 25–30%.[5] Bone cancer pain is the most common pain in patients with advanced cancer as two-thirds of patients with metastatic bone disease experience severe pain.[6,7] Most common tumors including breast, prostate, thyroid, kidney, and lung have a remarkable affinity to metastasize to bone.[7]

Currently, the factors that drive bone cancer pain are poorly understood; however, several recently introduced models of bone cancer pain are not only providing insight into the mechanisms that drive bone cancer pain but are guiding the development of novel mechanism-based therapies to treat the pain and skeletal remodeling that accompany metastatic bone cancer.

THE CHALLENGE OF BONE CANCER PAIN

Although bone is not a vital organ, most common tumors have a strong predilection for bone metastasis. Tumor metastases to the skeleton are major contributors to morbidity and mortality in metastatic cancer. Tumor growth in bone results in pain, hypercalcemia, anemia, increased susceptibility to infection, skeletal fractures, compression of the spinal cord, spinal instability, and decreased mobility; all of which compromise the patient's survival and quality of life.[7,8] Once tumor cells have metastasized to the skeleton, tumor-induced bone pain is usually described as dull in character, constant in presentation, and gradually increasing in intensity with time.[9] As bone remodeling progresses, severe spontaneous pain frequently occurs[9] and given that the onset of this pain is both acute and unpredictable, this component of bone cancer pain can be particularly debilitating to the patient's functional status and quality of life.[8,9] Breakthrough pain, which is an intermittent episode of extreme pain, can occur spontaneously or more commonly is induced by movement of or weight-bearing on the tumor-bearing bone(s).[10]

Currently, the treatment of pain from bone metastases involves the use of multiple complementary approaches, including radiotherapy, surgery, chemotherapy, bisphosphonates, calcitonin, and analgesics.[6,9] However, bone cancer pain is one of the most difficult of all persistent pains to fully control,[9] as the metastases are generally not limited to a single site and the analgesics that are most commonly used to treat bone cancer pain. Nonsteroidal anti-inflammatory drug(s) (NSAID)[9] and opioids,[9,11–13] are limited by significant adverse side effects.[14,15]

The onset of clinically apparent bone metastases marks a crucial moment in the natural history of cancer, sharply decreasing expected survival (on average, 12 months for prostate cancer patients after the diagnosis of bone metastasis).[16] However, the length of survival continues to increase for cancer patients,[17] so to maintain the patient's quality of life and functional status, it is essential that new therapies be developed that can be administered over several years to control bone pain without the side effects commonly encountered with the currently available analgesics.

In the last decade, the first animal models of bone cancer pain were developed. These models, in terms of tumor growth, bone remodeling, and bone pain, appear to mirror several aspects of human bone cancer pain.[18–22] In the present chapter, we examine the similarities and differences between a primarily osteolytic sarcoma tumor versus a primarily osteoblastic prostate tumor in terms of bone destruction, bone formation, tumor growth, macrophage infiltration, osteoclast and osteoblast number and type, and severity of bone cancer-related pain. Additionally, we discuss the remodeling of the sensory innervation of bone in osteolytic and osteoblastic bone cancer models.

PAIN TRANSMISSION

Primary afferent sensory neurons are the gateway by which sensory information from peripheral tissues is transmitted to the spinal cord and brain and these sensory neurons innervate every organ of the body with the exception of the brain. The cell bodies of sensory fibers that innervate the head and body are housed in the trigeminal and dorsal root ganglia, respectively. Anatomically, there are three broad groups of sensory nerve fibers: large diameter myelinated A fibers, finely myelinated A fibers, and small diameter unmyelinated C fibers.

Large diameter myelinated A beta fibers originating in skin, joints, and muscles normally conduct non noxious stimuli including fine touch, vibration, and proprioception. In contrast, most small diameter sensory fibers are specialized sensory neurons known as nociceptors. These unmyelinated C fibers and finely myelinated A sensory neurons are involved in generating the chronic pain that accompanies many cancers.

TUMOR GROWTH, SKELETAL REMODELING, AND PAIN INDUCED BY PRIMARILY OSTEOLYTIC OR OSTEOBLASTIC TUMORS

When primarily osteolytic 2472 murine osteosarcoma tumor cells are injected and confined to the intramedullary space of the femur, these tumor cells grow in a highly reproducible fashion as they proliferate, replacing the hematopoietic cells in the bone marrow.[20–22] Eventually, the entire marrow space is homogeneously filled with tumor cells and tumor-associated inflammatory/immune cells. In contrast, following injection and confinement of the primarily osteoblastic ACE-1 prostate cells into the mouse femur, the tumor cells are present in small clonal colonies throughout the marrow space of the femur and these small colonies of osteoblastic tumor cells are separated from each other by extensive matrices of newly formed woven bone (Fig. 6.1).

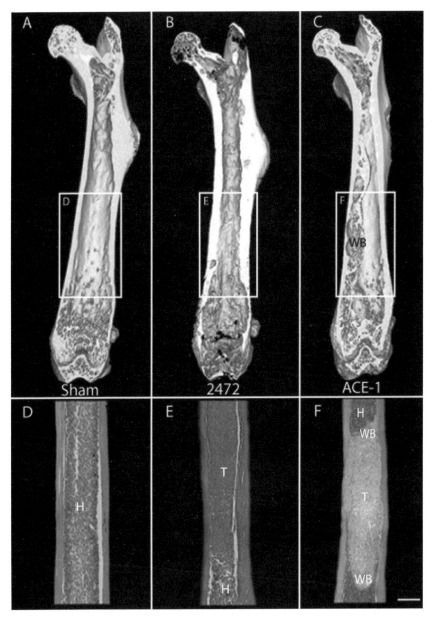

Figure 6.1. Bone remodeling and tumor growth in the 2472 sarcoma and ACE-1 prostate carcinoma-injected femurs exhibit different characteristics depending on the osteolytic or osteoblastic component of the tumor cells as assessed by μCT imaging and hematoxylin and eosin (H&E) staining. Sham-injected femurs present relative absence of bone formation or bone destruction (A, D). The 2472 sarcoma-injected femurs display a primarily osteolytic appearance, visible as regions absent of trabecular bone at the proximal and distal heads (B) as well as replacement of normal hematopoietic cells by

In regards to bone remodeling, injection of osteosarcoma cells into the femur induces predominant bone destruction, along the entire bone, including proximal and distal heads as well as the diaphysis. In sharp contrast, prostate tumor cells induce significant formation of new woven bone in the proximal and distal head of the femur as well as the diaphysis of the bone (Fig. 6.1). The marked bone formation induced by prostate cancer cells is also accompanied by bone destruction, giving the tumor-bearing femur a unique scalloped appearance when assessed by μCT or with traditional histological methodology, which is similar in appearance to that observed in human patients with prostate tumor metastases.[23]

The concurrent bone destruction and formation in the prostate cancer model is quite distinct from that observed in tumors such as sarcoma[21,24] or breast[25], where the tumor was primarily osteolytic as bone destruction predominates.[21,24] This mixed bone remodeling in the prostate tumor-bearing femurs is characterized by an increase in (1) the number of osteoclasts throughout the intramedullary space, which drives osteolytic bone remodeling, and (2) the number of macrophages scattered throughout the tumor and remaining hematopoietic spaces in the bone. In the sarcoma bone cancer pain model, there is an upregulation in the number of osteoclasts and macrophages (two-fold greater increase in macrophages than in the prostate cancer line). However, it is the increase in the number of osteoblasts found throughout the tumor-bearing intramedullary space that ultimately separates the prostate tumor from the primarily osteolytic bone tumors in which few osteoblasts are observed and little or no bone formation occurs.

In these developed models, baseline spontaneous and evoked pain behaviors in the hind limb following tumor cell injection into the intramedullary space of the femur were assessed. Ongoing and movement-evoked pain-related behaviors increased in severity with time. These pain behaviors correlate with the progressive tumor-induced bone destruction or bone formation that ensues and appears to mimic the condition in patients with primary or metastatic bone cancer.

NEUROPATHIC COMPONENT OF BONE CANCER PAIN

Numerous studies have demonstrated that the periosteum is densely innervated by both sensory and sympathetic fibers[26–28] and that it receives the greatest

---

tumor cells (E). The ACE-1 prostate carcinoma-injected femurs mainly present an osteoblastic appearance, which is characterized by pathologic bone formation in the intramedullary space (C) surrounding pockets of tumor cells that generate diaphyseal bridging structures (F). (A–F): Scale bar, 0.5 mm; T, tumor; H, normal hematopoietic cells; WB, ACE-1-induced woven bone formation.

density of nerve fibers per area.[29] Using a combination of minimal decalcification techniques and antigen amplification techniques, it has also been demonstrated that the bone marrow, mineralized bone, and periosteum all receive a significant innervation by both sensory and sympathetic nerve fibers (Fig. 6.2).[30–32] Since sensory and sympathetic neurons are present within the bone marrow, mineralized bone, and periosteum and all aspects of the bone are ultimately impacted by fractures, ischemia, or the presence of tumor cells, sensory fibers in any of these compartments may play a role in the generation and maintenance of bone cancer pain.

In examining the changes in the sensory innervation of bone induced by the primarily osteolytic sarcoma cells, sensory fibers were observed at and within the

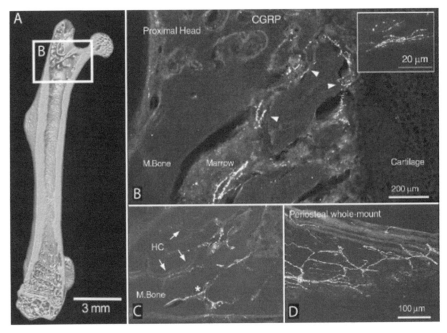

Figure 6.2. Sensory innervation of the mouse bone. (A) A μCT three-dimensional image of a mouse femur illustrating the areas used for analysis of bone innervation. (B) Confocal photomicrograph showing CGRP in the mouse femur. Low power photomicrograph is of the proximal head of the mouse femur where the CGRP-positive (+) fibers are bright white and are present in the marrow and surround the trabeculae (white arrowhead). The inset in the top right of (B) shows the average diameter of individual fibers in a bundle of CGRP fibers found in the marrow. High power photomicrographs of CGRP expressing fiber (C) in the marrow and (D) in the periosteum. Note that the CGRP+ nerve fibers are in close proximity to blood vessels within the Haversian canal (HC) system, while in the periosteum CGRP+ nerve fibers form a dense net-like meshwork. (With permission from Ref. 29.)

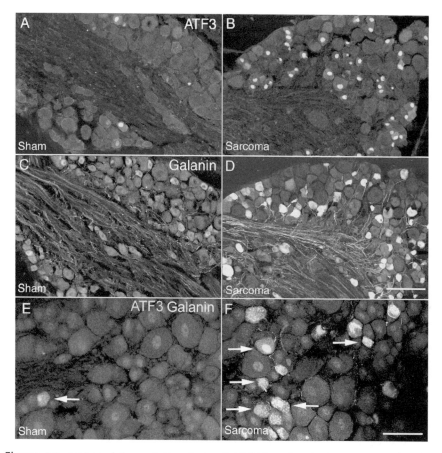

Figure 6.3. Activated transcription factor-3 (ATF-3) and galanin are upregulated in primary sensory neurons that innervate the tumor-bearing femur 14 days following injection of osteolytic sarcoma cells into intramedullary space of the femur. Neurons in the sham-vehicle L2 dorsal root ganglia express low levels of both (A) ATF-3 or (C) the neuropeptide galanin, whereas 14 days following injection and confinement of sarcoma cells to the marrow space there is a marked upregulation of both (B) ATF-3 and (D) galanin in sensory neurons in the L2 dorsal root ganglia ipsilateral to the tumor-bearing bone. Many sensory neurons that show an upregulation of galanin in response to tumor-induced injury of sensory fibers in the bone also show an upregulation of ATF-3 in their nucleus (compare part E vs. F, arrows). These data suggest tumor cells invading the bone injure the sensory nerve fibers that normally innervate the tumor-bearing bone. Scale bar = 200 µm (A–D); scale bar = 100 µm (E,F). (With permission from Ref. 24.)

leading edge of the tumor. Additionally, these sensory nerve fibers displayed a discontinuous and fragmented appearance, suggesting that following initial activation by the osteolytic tumor cells, the distal processes of the sensory fibers were ultimately injured by the invading tumor cells. In contrast, examination of

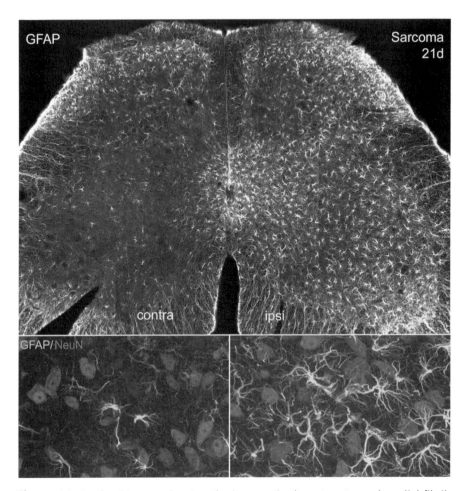

Figure 6.4. Confocal images showing the increase in the astrocyte marker glial fibril-lary acidic protein (GFAP) in a mouse with bone cancer pain in the right femur. Coronal sections of the L4 spinal cord 21 days following injection of osteolytic sarcoma cells into the intramedullary space of the femur. (A) A low power image shows that the upregulation of GFAP is almost exclusively ipsilateral to the femur with the intraosseous tumor. Higher magnification of GFAP (B) contralateral and (C) ipsilateral to the femur with cancer shows that, on the ipsilateral side, there is marked hypertrophy of astrocytes characterized by an increase in both the size of the astrocyte cell bodies and the extent of the arborization of their distal processes. Additionally, this increase in GFAP is observed without a detectable loss of neurons, as NeuN labeling remains unchanged. These images, from 60 μm thick tissue, are projected from (A) six optical sections acquired at 4 μm intervals with a 20 × lens; scale bar = 200 μm and (B,C) from 12 optical sections acquired at 0.8 μm intervals with a 60 × lens, scale bar = 30 μm. (With permission from Ref. 22.)

the sensory innervation of bone following injection of the primarily osteoblastic prostate cancer cells suggests that there is simultaneous injury and sprouting of sensory fibers in the bone.

In the sarcoma-injected animals, there was expression of activating transcription factor-3 (ATF-3) in the nucleus of sensory neurons that innervate the femur (Fig. 6.3). ATF-3 is a member of the ATF/CREB family of transcription factors, which is not expressed at detectable levels in normal sensory neurons or in sensory neurons following peripheral inflammation, but is strongly expressed in sensory neurons following injury to peripheral nerves in neuropathic pain models.[33] It is likely that the expression of ATF-3 in sensory neurons of tumor-bearing animals is a result of peripheral nerve destruction within the tumor-bearing femur.[34]

This tumor-induced injury of sensory nerve fibers in the sarcoma model was also accompanied by an increase in ongoing and movement-evoked pain behaviors, an up regulation of galanin by sensory neurons that innervate the tumor-bearing femur, an up regulation of glial fibrillary acidic protein (GFAP) (Fig. 6.4), and hypertrophy of satellite cells surrounding sensory neuron cell bodies within the ipsilateral dorsal root ganglia (DRG), and macrophage infiltration of the DRG ipsilateral to the tumor-bearing femur.[24,35,36] Similar neurochemical changes have been described following peripheral nerve injury and in other non cancerous neuropathic pain states.[37] Chronic treatment with gabapentin in the sarcoma model also did not influence tumor growth, tumor-induced bone destruction, or tumor-induced neurochemical reorganization that occurs in sensory neurons or the spinal cord, but did attenuate both ongoing and movement-evoked bone cancer-related pain behaviors.[24] These results suggest that, even when the tumor is confined within the bone, a component of bone cancer pain is due to tumor-induced injury to primary afferent nerve fibers that normally innervate the tumor-bearing bone.

SKELETAL REMODELING AND ACIDOSIS IN BONE CANCER PAIN

Recent experiments in a murine model of bone cancer pain have reported that osteoclasts play an essential role in cancer-induced bone loss and that osteoclasts contribute to the etiology of bone cancer pain.[21,38] Osteoclasts are terminally differentiated, multinucleated, monocyte lineage cells that resorb bone by maintaining an extracellular microenvironment of acidic pH (4.0–5.0) at the osteoclast–mineralized bone interface.[39] Tumor-induced release of protons and acidosis may be particularly important in the generation of bone cancer pain. Both osteolytic (bone destroying) and osteoblastic (bone forming) cancers are characterized by osteoclast proliferation and hypertrophy.[40]

Bisphosphonates, a class of antiresorptive compounds that induce osteoclast apoptosis, have also been reported to reduce pain in patients with osteoclast-induced skeletal metastases.[41–43] In a recent study of the bisphosphonate alendronate in the sarcoma model, a reduction in the number of osteoclasts and osteoclast activity was noted, as evidenced by the reduction in tumor-induced bone resorption and a reduction in the number of osteoclasts displaying the clear zone at the basal bone resorbing surface that is characteristic of highly active osteoclasts.[44] In this model, alendronate also attenuates ongoing and movement-evoked bone cancer pain, and the neurochemical reorganization of the peripheral and central nervous system, while at the same time promoting both tumor growth and tumor necrosis. The present results suggest that, in bone cancer, alendronate can simultaneously modulate pain, bone destruction, tumor growth, and tumor necrosis.

Osteoprotegerin (OPG) is a secreted soluble receptor that is a member of the tumor necrosis factor receptor (TNFR) family.[45] This decoy receptor prevents the activation and proliferation of osteoclasts by binding to and sequestering OPG ligand (OPGL; also known as receptor for activator of NFκB ligand, RANKL).[45–48] OPG has been shown to decrease pain behaviors in the sarcoma model of bone cancer.[38] These results suggest that a substantial part of the action of OPG seems to result from inhibition of tumor-induced bone destruction via a reduction in osteoclast function. This reduction of osteoclast function in turn inhibits the neurochemical changes in the spinal cord that are thought to be involved in the generation and maintenance of cancer pain, which demonstrates that excessive tumor-induced bone destruction is involved in the generation of bone cancer pain.

The finding that sensory neurons can be excited directly by protons or acid originating from cells like osteoclasts in bone has generated intense clinical interest in pain research.[49,50] Studies have shown that subsets of sensory neurons express different acid-sensing ion channels.[51,52] The two major classes of acid-sensing ion channels expressed by nociceptors are TRPV1[53,54] and the acid-sensing ion channel-3 (ASIC-3).[49,51,55] Both of these channels are sensitized and excited by a decrease in pH. Tumor stroma[56] and areas of ischemic necrosis,[57] such as that observed in the 2472 or ACE-1 prostate bone cancer model, typically exhibit lower extracellular pH than surrounding normal tissues. As inflammatory cells invade tumor stroma, they release protons that generate local acidosis. The large amount of apoptosis that occurs in the tumor environment may also contribute to the acidotic environment.

It has been shown that TRPV1 is present on a subset of sensory neuron fibers and on those that innervate the mouse femur (Fig. 6.5). TRPV1 antagonist or disruption of the TRPV1 gene results in a significant attenuation of both ongoing and movement-evoked nocifensive behaviors in a model of bone cancer pain.[36] In addition, previous studies have also shown, in the 2472 model, that administration of a TRPV1 antagonist retains its efficacy at early, middle, and late stages of tumor growth.[36] The ability of a TRPV1 antagonist to maintain its analgesic potency with disease progression is probably influenced by the fact that sensory nerve fibers innervating the tumor-bearing mouse femur maintain and upregulate the expression of TRPV1 even as tumor growth and tumor-induced bone destruction progresses.[58] Altogether these results

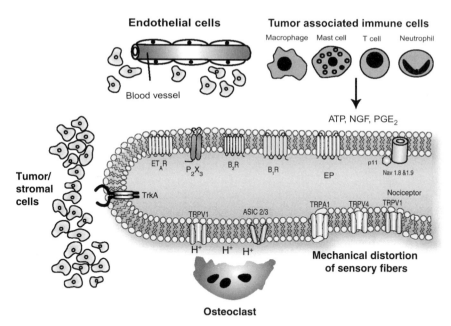

Figure 6.5. Peripheral terminal of a nociceptive nerve fiber in a tumor-bearing bone. Nociceptors use several different types of receptors to detect and transmit signals about noxious stimuli that are produced by cancer cells, tumor associated immune cells, or other aspects of the tumor microenvironment. There are multiple factors that may contribute to the pain associated with cancer. The transient receptor potential vanilloid receptor-1 (TRPV1) and acid-sensing ion channels (ASICs) detect extracellular protons produced by tumor-induced tissue damage or abnormal osteoclast-mediated bone resorption. Several mechanosensitive ion channels may be involved in detecting high threshold mechanical stimuli that occur when distal aspects of sensory nerve fiber are distended from mechanical pressure due to the growing tumor or as a result of destabilization or fracture of bone. Tumor cells and associated inflammatory (immune) cells produce a variety of chemical mediators including prostaglandins (PGE$_2$), nerve growth factor (NGF), endothelins, bradykinin, and extracellular ATP. Several of these proinflammatory mediators have receptors on peripheral terminals and can directly activate or sensitize nociceptors.

suggest that the TRPV1 channel plays a role in the integration of nociceptive signaling in a severe pain state.

TUMOR-DERIVED PRODUCTS IN GENERATION OF BONE CANCER PAIN

The tumor stroma is made up of many different cell types apart from cancer cells, including immune cells such as macrophages, neutrophils, and T lymphocytes. They secrete a variety of factors that have been shown to sensitize or directly excite primary afferent neurons, such as prostaglandins,[59,60] tumor necrosis factor α,[61-64] endothelins,[65,66] interleukin-1 (TI-1) and IL–6,[61,67,68] epidermal growth factor,[69] transforming growth factor-β,[70,71] and platelet-derived growth factor.[72-74] Receptors for many of these factors are expressed by primary afferent neurons.

Prostaglandins

Cancer cells and tumor-associated macrophages have both been shown to express high levels of cyclooxygenase (COX) isoenzymes, leading to high levels of prostaglandins.[75-79] Prostaglandins are lipid-derived eicosanoids that are synthesized from arachidonic acid by COX isoenzymes COX-1 and COX-2. Prostaglandins have been shown to be involved in the sensitization and/or direct excitation of nociceptors by binding to several prostanoid receptors expressed by nociceptors[80] (Fig. 6.5).

Studies have shown in the sarcoma model of bone cancer pain, that chronic inhibition of COX-2 activity with selective COX-2 inhibitors resulted in significant attenuation of bone cancer pain behaviors as well as many of the neurochemical changes suggestive of both peripheral and central sensitization.[21] In addition, prostaglandins have been shown to be involved in tumor growth, cell survival, and angiogenesis[81-87]; therefore, as well as having the ability to block cancer pain, COX-2 inhibitors are also capable of retarding tumor growth within bone.[21] Chronic administration of a selective COX-2 inhibitor significantly reduced tumor burden in sarcoma-bearing bones, which may, in turn, reduce factors released by tumor cells capable of exciting primary afferent fibers.[65] Acute or chronic administration of a selective COX-2 inhibitor significantly attenuated both ongoing and movement-evoked pain. Whereas acute administration of a COX-2 inhibitor presumably reduces prostaglandins capable of activating sensory or spinal cord neurons, chronic inhibition of COX-2 also appears to simultaneously reduce osteoclastogenesis, bone resorption, and tumor burden. Together, suppression of prostaglandin synthesis and release at multiple sites by selective inhibition of COX-2 may synergistically improve the survival and quality of life of patients with bone cancer pain.

Endothelins

Endothelins (endothelin-1, -2, and -3) are a family of vasoactive peptides that are expressed at high levels by several types of tumors, including those that arise from the prostate.[66] Clinical studies have shown a correlation between the severity of the pain and plasma levels of endothelins in prostate cancer patients.[88] Endothelins could contribute to cancer pain by directly sensitizing or exciting nociceptors, some primary afferent neurons express endothelin A receptors[89] (Fig. 6.5). Furthermore, direct application of endothelin to peripheral nerves induces activation of primary afferent fibers and an induction of pain-related behaviors.[90]

In the sarcoma model, acute or chronic administration of the endothelin A receptor (ET_AR) selective antagonist ABT-627 significantly attenuated ongoing and movement-evoked bone cancer pain. Chronic administration of ABT-627 also reduced several neurochemical indices of peripheral and central sensitization without influencing tumor growth or bone destruction.[91]

Kinins

Previous studies have shown that bradykinin and related kinins are released in response to tissue injury and these kinins play a significant role in driving the acute and chronic inflammatory pain.[92] The action of bradykinin is mediated by two receptors termed B_1 and B_2. Whereas the B_2 receptor is constitutively expressed at high levels by sensory neurons, the B_1 receptor is normally expressed at low but detectable levels by sensory neurons and these B_1 receptors are significantly upregulated following peripheral inflammation and/or tissue injury.[93] Tumor metastases to the skeleton induce significant bone remodeling with accompanying tissue injury, which presumably induces the release of bradykinin. It has been demonstrated that both bone cancer-induced ongoing and movement-evoked nocifensive behaviors were reduced following the pharmacologic blockade of the B_1 receptor.[94]

Nerve Growth Factor

One important concept that has emerged over the past decade is that in addition to nerve growth factor (NGF) being able to directly activate sensory neurons that express the trkA receptor, NGF modulates expression and function of a wide variety of molecules and proteins expressed by sensory neurons that express the trkA or p75 receptor. Some of these molecules and proteins include neurotransmitters (substance P and CGRP), receptors (bradykinin R), channels (P2X3, TRPV 1, ASIC-3, and sodium channels), transcription factors (ATF-3), and structural molecules (neurofilaments and the sodium channel anchoring molecule p11)[95,96] (Fig. 6.5). Additionally, NGF has been shown to modulate the trafficking and insertion of sodium channels such as Nav 1.8[97] and TRPV1[98] in the sensory neurons as well as modulating the expression profile of supporting cells in the dorsal root ganglia (DRG) and peripheral nerve, such as non myelinating Schwann cells and macrophages.[99] Therefore anti-NGF antibody therapy may be particularly effective in blocking bone cancer pain, as NGF appears to be integrally involved in the upregulation, sensitization, and disinhibition of multiple neurotransmitters, ion channels, and receptors in the primary afferent nerve and DRG fibers that synergistically increase nociceptive signals originating from the tumor-bearing bone.

In two recent studies, where the same analgesic therapy was used in the primarily osteolytic 2472 sarcoma and the primarily osteoblastic ACE-1 prostate bone cancer model, it was demonstrated that administration of an anti-NGF antibody was not only highly efficacious in reducing both early and late stage bone cancer pain-related behaviors but that this reduction in pain-related behaviors was greater than that achieved with acute administration of 10 or 30 mg/kg of morphine sulfate.[19,35] In light of these findings, the mechanisms that contribute to the efficacy of anti-NGF in blocking sarcoma or prostate tumor-induced bone pain remains a critical matter that requires further investigation.

CONCLUSION

For the first time, animal models of cancer pain are now available and effectively mirror the clinical picture observed in humans with bone cancer pain. Information generated from these models has begun to provide insight into the mechanisms that generate and maintain bone cancer pain and helped target potential mechanism-based therapies to treat this chronic pain state. It is noteworthy that, in these models, analgesics such as a bisphosphonate, osteoprotegerin, and a cyclooxygenase-2 inhibitor appear to influence disease progression in the tumor-bearing bone. Together these and other studies using models of bone cancer suggest that it may be possible to develop novel mechanism-based therapies that not only reduce tumor-induced bone pain but may provide added benefit in synergistically reducing disease progression. Successful development and clinical use of these therapies has the potential to not only positively impact survival, but also to improve the cancer patient's quality of life.

ACKNOWLEDGMENTS

This work is supported by National Institutes of Health (NS23970, NS048021) and a Merit Review from the Veterans Administration.

REFERENCES

1. Stewart B, Kleihues P. (2003). *World Cancer Report*. Geneva: World Health Organization.
2. Brennan F, Carr DB, Cousins M. (2007). Pain management: a fundamental human right. Anesth Analg 105(1):205–221.

3. WHO. (2006). *Cancer Control.* Geneva: World Health Organization.

4. Jemal A, Siegel R, Ward E, Murray T, Xu J, Thun MJ. (2007). Cancer statistics, 2007. CA Cancer J Clin 57(1):43–66.

5. van den Beuken-van Everdingen M, de Rijke J, Kessels A, Schouten H, van Kleef M, Patijn J. (2007). Prevalence of pain in patients with cancer: a systematic review of the past 40 years. Ann Oncol 18(9):1437–1449.

6. Mercadante S, Fulfaro F. (2007). Management of painful bone metastases. Curr Opin Oncol 19(4):308–314.

7. Coleman RE. (2006). Clinical features of metastatic bone disease and risk of skeletal morbidity. Clin Cancer Res 12(20 Pt 2):6243s–6249s.

8. Coleman RE. (1997). Skeletal complications of malignancy. Cancer 80 (8 Suppl):1588–1594.

9. Mercadante S. (1997). Malignant bone pain: pathophysiology and treatment. Pain 69(1-2):1–18.

10. Mercadante S, Arcuri E. (1998). Breakthrough pain in cancer patients: pathophysiology and treatment. Cancer Treat Rev 24(6):425–432.

11. Cherny N. (2000). New strategies in opioid therapy for cancer pain. J Oncol Manage 9(1):8–15.

12. Hanks GW, Conno F, Cherny N, Hanna M, Kalso E, McQuay HJ, et al. (2001). Morphine and alternative opioids in cancer pain: the EAPC recommendations. Br J Cancer 84(5):587–593.

13. Portenoy RK, Lesage P. (1999). Management of cancer pain. Lancet 353(9165): 1695–1700.

14. Foley KM. (1995). Misconceptions and controversies regarding the use of opioids in cancer pain. Anti-Cancer Drugs 6(Suppl 3):4–13.

15. Weber M, Huber C. (1999). Documentation of severe pain, opioid doses, and opioid-related side effects in outpatients with cancer: a retrospective study. J Pain Symptom Manage 17(1):49–54.

16. Storey JA, Torti FM. (2007). Bone metastases in prostate cancer: a targeted approach. Curr Opin Oncol 19(3):254–258.

17. Jemal A, Murray T, Ward E, Samuels A, Tiwari RC, Ghafoor A, et al. (2005). Cancer statistics, 2005. CA Cancer J Clin 55(1):10–30.

18. Guise TA. (1997). Parathyroid hormone-related protein and bone metastases. Cancer 80(8 Suppl S):1572–1580.

19. Halvorson KG, Kubota K, Sevcik MA, Lindsay TH, Sotillo JE, Ghilardi JR, et al. (2005). A blocking antibody to nerve growth factor attenuates skeletal pain induced by prostate tumor cells growing in bone. Cancer Res 65(20):9426–9435.

20. Honore P, Rogers SD, Schwei MJ, Salak-Johnson JL, Luger NM, Sabino MC, et al. (2000). Murine models of inflammatory, neuropathic and cancer pain each generates a unique set of neurochemical changes in the spinal cord and sensory neurons. Neuroscience 98(3):585–598.

21. Sabino MA, Ghilardi JR, Jongen JL, Keyser CP, Luger NM, Mach DB, et al. (2002). Simultaneous reduction in cancer pain, bone destruction, and tumor growth by selective inhibition of cyclooxygenase-2. Cancer Res 62(24):7343–7349.

22. Schwei MJ, Honore P, Rogers SD, Salak-Johnson JL, Finke MP, Ramnaraine ML, et al. (1999). Neurochemical and cellular reorganization of the spinal cord in a murine model of bone cancer pain. J Neurosci 19(24):10886–10897.

23. Body JJ. (1992). Metastatic bone disease: clinical and therapeutic aspects. Bone 13(Suppl 1):S57–S62.

24. Peters CM, Ghilardi JR, Keyser CP, Kubota K, Lindsay TH, Luger NM, et al. (2005). Tumor induced injury of primary afferent sensory nerve fibers in bone cancer pain. Exp Neurol 193(1):85–100.

25. Boyce BF, Yoneda T, Guise TA. (1999). Factors regulating the growth of metastatic cancer in bone. Endocrine-Related Cancer 6(3):333–347.

26. Asmus SE, Parsons S, Landis SC. (2000). Developmental changes in the transmitter properties of sympathetic neurons that innervate the periosteum. Neurosci 20(4):1495–1504.

27. Bjurholm A. (1991). Neuroendocrine peptides in bone. Int Orthop 15(4):325–329.

28. Hukkanen M, Konttinen YT, Rees RG, Gibson SJ, Santavirta S, Polak JM. (1992). Innervation of bone from healthy and arthritic rats by substance P and calcitonin gene related peptide containing sensory fibers. J Rheumatol 19:1252–1259.

29. Mach DB, Rogers SD, Sabino MC, Luger NM, Schwei MJ, Pomonis JD, et al. (2002). Origins of skeletal pain: sensory and sympathetic innervation of the mouse femur. Neuroscience 113(1):155–166.

30. Bjurholm A, Kreicbergs A, Brodin E, Schultzberg M. (1988). Substance P- and CGRP-immunoreactive nerves in bone. Peptides 9(1):165–171.

31. Bjurholm A, Kreicbergs A, Terenius L, Goldstein M, Schultzberg M. (1988). Neuropeptide Y-, tyrosine hydroxylase- and vasoactive intestinal polypeptide-immunoreactive nerves in bone and surrounding tissues. J Auton Nerv Syst 25 (2-3):119–125.

32. Tabarowski Z, Gibson-Berry K, Felten SY. (1996). Noradrenergic and peptidergic innervation of the mouse femur bone marrow. Acta Histochem 98(4):453–457.

33. Tsujino H, Kondo E, Fukuoka T, Dai Y, Tokunaga A, Miki K, et al. (2000). Activating transcription factor 3 (ATF3) induction by axotomy in sensory and motoneurons: a novel neuronal marker of nerve injury. Mol Cell Neurosci 15(2):170–182.

34. Honore P, Luger N, Sabino M, Schwei M, Rogers S, Mach D, et al. (2000). Osteoprotegerin blocks bone cancer-induced skeletal destruction, skeletal pain and pain-related neurochemcial reorganization of the spinal cord. Nat Med 6(5):521–528.

35. Sevcik MA, Ghilardi JR, Peters CM, Lindsay TH, Halvorson KG, Jonas BM, et al. (2005). Anti NGF therapy profoundly reduces bone cancer pain and the accompanying increase in markers of peripheral and central sensitization. Pain 115 (1-2):128–141.

36. Ghilardi JR, Rohrich H, Lindsay TH, Sevcik MA, Schwei MJ, Kubota K, et al. (2005). Selective blockade of the capsaicin receptor TRPV1 attenuates bone cancer pain. J Neurosci 25(12):3126–3131.

37. Obata K, Yamanaka H, Fukuoka T, Yi D, Tokunaga A, Hashimoto N, et al. (2003). Contribution of injured and uninjured dorsal root ganglion neurons to pain

behavior and the changes in gene expression following chronic constriction injury of the sciatic nerve in rats. Pain 101(1–2):65–77.

38. Luger NM, Honore P, Sabino MA, Schwei MJ, Rogers SD, Mach DB, et al. (2001). Osteoprotegerin diminishes advanced bone cancer pain. Cancer Res 61(10): 4038–4047.

39. Delaisse JM, Vaes G. (1992). Mechanism of mineral solubilization and matrix degradation in osteoclastic bone resorption. In Rifkin BR and Gay CV (eds.). *Biology and Physiology of the Osteoclast*. Ann Arbor, MI: CRC Press, pp. 289–314.

40. Clohisy DR, Perkins SL, Ramnaraine ML. (2000). Review of cellular mechanisms of tumor osteolysis. Clin Orthop Rel Res 373:104–114.

41. Berenson JR, Rosen LS, Howell A, Porter L, Coleman RE, Morley W, et al. (2001). Zoledronic acid reduces skeletal-related events in patients with osteolytic metastases. Cancer 91(7):1191–1200.

42. Fulfaro F, Casuccio A, Ticozzi C, Ripamonti C. (1998). The role of bisphosphonates in the treatment of painful metastatic bone disease: a review of phase III trials. Pain 78(3):157–169.

43. Major PP, Lipton A, Berenson J, Hortobagyi G. (2000). Oral bisphosphonates: a review of clinical use in patients with bone metastases. Cancer 88(1):6–14.

44. Horton A, Nesbitt S, Bennett J, Stenbeck G. (2002). Integrins and other cell surface attachment molecules of bone cells. In Bilezikian JP, Raisz LG, and Rodan GA (eds.). *Principles of Bone Biology*. San Diego, CA: Academic Press, pp. 265–286.

45. Simonet WS, Lacey DL, Dunstan CR, Kelley M, Chang MS, Luthy R, et al. (1997). Osteoprotegerin—a novel secreted protein involved in the regulation of bone density. Cell 89(2):309–319.

46. Anderson DM, Maraskovsky E, Billingsley WL, Dougall WC, Tometsko ME, Roux ER, et al. (1997). A homologue of the Tnf receptor and its ligand enhance T-cell growth and dendritic-cell function. Nature 390(6656):175–179.

47. Yasuda H, Shima N, Nakagawa N, Yamaguchi K, Kinosaki M, Mochizuki S, et al. (1998). Osteoclast differentiation factor is a ligand for osteoprotegerin/osteoclastogenesis-inhibitory factor and is identical to TRANCE/RANKL. Proc Nat Acad Sci USA 95(7):3597–3602.

48. Rodan GA, Martin TJ. (2000). Therapeutic approaches to bone diseases. Science 289(5484):1508–1514.

49. Sutherland S, Cook S, McCleskey EW. (2000). Chemical mediators of pain due to tissue damage and ischemia. Prog Brain Res 129:21–38.

50. Woolf CJ. (2004). American College of Physicians, American Physiological Society. Pain: moving from symptom control toward mechanism-specific pharmacologic management. Ann Intern Med 140(6):441–451.

51. Olson TH, Riedl MS, Vulchanova L, Ortiz-Gonzalez XR, Elde R. (1998). An acid sensing ion channel (ASIC) localizes to small primary afferent neurons in rats. Neuroreport 9(6):1109–1113.

52. Julius D, Basbaum AI. (2001). Molecular mechanisms of nociception [Review]. Nature 413(6852):203–210.

53. Caterina MJ, Schumacher MA, Tominaga M, Rosen TA, Levine JD, Julius D. (1997). The capsaicin receptor: a heat-activated ion channel in the pain pathway. Nature 389(6653):816–824.

54. Tominaga M, Caterina MJ, Malmberg AB, Rosen TA, Gilbert H, Skinner K, et al. (1998). The cloned capsaicin receptor integrates multiple pain-producing stimuli. Neuron 21(3):531–543.

55. Bassilana F, Champigny G, Waldmann R, de Weille JR, Heurteaux C, Lazdunski M. (1997). The acid-sensitive ionic channel subunit ASIC and the mammalian degenerin MDEG form a heteromultimeric H^+-gated Na^+ channel with novel properties. J Biol Chem 272(46):28819–28822.

56. Griffiths JR. (1991). Are cancer cells acidic? Br J Cancer 64:425–427.

57. Deigner HP, Kinscherf R. (1999). Modulating apoptosis: current applications and prospects for future drug development. Curr Med Chem 6(5):399–414.

58. Niiyama Y, Kawamata T, Yamamoto J, Omote K, Namiki A. (2007). Bone cancer increases transient receptor potential vanilloid subfamily 1 expression within distinct subpopulations of dorsal root ganglion neurons. Neuroscience 148(2):560–572.

59. Galasko CS. (1995). Diagnosis of skeletal metastases and assessment of response to treatment. Clin Orthop Relat Res 312:64–75.

60. Nielsen OS, Munro AJ, Tannock IF. (1991). Bone metastases: pathophysiology and management policy. J Clin Oncol 9(3):509–524.

61. DeLeo JA, Yezierski RP. (2001). The role of neuroinflammation and neuroimmune activation in persistent pain. Pain 90:1–6.

62. Watkins LR, Maier SF, Goehler LE. (1995). Immune activation: the role of pro-inflammatory cytokines in inflammation, illness responses and pathological pain states. Pain 63(3):289–302.

63. Watkins LR, Maier SF. (1999). Implications of immune-to-brain communication for sickness and pain. Proc Nati Acad Sci U S A 96(14):7710–7713.

64. Nadler RB, Koch AE, Calhoun EA, Campbell PL, Pruden DL, Bennett CL, et al. (2000). IL-1beta and TNF-alpha in prostatic secretions are indicators in the evaluation of men with chronic prostatitis. J Urol 164(1):214–218.

65. Davar G. (2001). Endothelin-1 and metastatic cancer pain. Pain Med 2(1):24–27.

66. Nelson JB, Carducci MA. (2000). The role of endothelin-1 and endothelin receptor antagonists in prostate cancer. BJU Int 85(Suppl 2):45–48.

67. Opree A, Kress M. (2000). Involvement of the proinflammatory cytokines tumor necrosis factor alpha, IL-1 beta, and IL-6 but not IL-8 in the development of heat hyperalgesia: effects on heat evoked calcitonin gene-related peptide release from rat skin. J Neurosci 20(16):6289–6293.

68. Watkins LR, Goehler LE, Relton J, Brewer MT, Maier SF. (1995). Mechanisms of tumor necrosis factor-alpha (TNF-alpha) hyperalgesia. Brain Res 692(1-2):244–250.

69. Stoscheck CM, King LE Jr. (1986). Role of epidermal growth factor in carcinogenesis. Cancer Res 46(3):1030–1037.

70. Poon RT, Fan ST, Wong J. (2001). Clinical implications of circulating angiogenic factors in cancer patients. J Clin Oncol 19(4):1207–1225.

71. Roman C, Saha D, Beauchamp R. (2001). TGF-beta and colorectal carcinogenesis. Microsc Res Tech 52(4):450–457.

72. Silver BJ. (1992). Platelet-derived growth factor in human malignancy. Biofactors 3(4):217–227.

73. Daughaday WH, Deuel TF. (1991). Tumor secretion of growth factors. Endocrinol Metab Clin North Am 20(3):539–563.

74. Radinsky R. (1991). Growth factors and their receptors in metastasis. Semin Cancer Biol 2(3):169–177.

75. Shappell SB, Manning S, Boeglin WE, Guan YF, Roberts RL, Davis L, et al. (2001). Alterations in lipoxygenase and cyclooxygenase-2 catalytic activity and mRNA expression in prostate carcinoma. Neoplasia 3(4):287–303.

76. Kundu N, Yang QY, Dorsey R, Fulton AM. (2001). Increased cyclooxygenase-2 (COX-2) expression and activity in a murine model of metastatic breast cancer. Int J Cancer 93(5):681–686.

77. Ohno R, Yoshinaga K, Fujita T, Hasegawa K, Iseki H, Tsunozaki H, et al. (2001). Depth of invasion parallels increased cyclooxygenase-2 levels in patients with gastric carcinoma. Cancer 91(10):1876–1881.

78. Molina MA, Sitja-Arnau M, Lemoine MG, Frazier ML, Sinicrope FA. (1999). Increased cyclooxygenase-2 expression in human pancreatic carcinomas and cell lines: Growth inhibition by nonsteroidal anti-inflammatory drugs. Cancer Res 59(17):4356–4362.

79. Dubois RN, Radhika A, Reddy BS, Entingh AJ. (1996). Increased cyclooxygenase-2 levels in carcinogen-induced rat colonic tumors. Gastroenterology 110(4): 1259–1262.

80. Vasko MR. (1995). Prostaglandin-induced neuropeptide release from spinal cord. Prog Brain Res 104:367–380.

81. Sonoshita M, Takaku K, Sasaki N, Sugimoto Y, Ushikubi F, Narumiya S, et al. (2001). Acceleration of intestinal polyposis through prostaglandin receptor EP2 in Apc(Delta 716) knockout mice. Nat Med 7(9):1048–1051.

82. Sheng H, Shao J, Kirkland SC, Isakson P, Coffey RJ, Morrow J, et al. (1997). Inhibition of human colon cancer cell growth by selective inhibition of cyclooxygenase-2. J Clini Invest 99(9):2254–2259.

83. Williams CS, Tsujii M, Reese J, Dey SK, DuBois RN. (2000). Host cyclooxygenase-2 modulates carcinoma growth. J Clini Invest 105(11):1589–1594.

84. Masferrer JL, Leahy KM, Koki AT, Zweifel BS, Settle SL, Woerner BM, et al. (2000). Antiangiogenic and antitumor activities of cyclooxygenase-2 inhibitors. Cancer Res 60(5):1306–1311.

85. Harris RE, Alshafie GA, Abou-Issa H, Seibert K. (2000). Chemoprevention of breast cancer in rats by celecoxib, a cyclooxygenase 2 inhibitor. Cancer Res 60(8):2101–2103.

86. Reddy BS, Hirose Y, Lubet R, Steele V, Kelloff G, Paulson S, et al. (2000). Chemoprevention of colon cancer by specific cyclooxygenase-2 inhibitor, celecoxib, administered during different stages of carcinogenesis. Cancer Res 60(2):293–297.

87. Lal G, Ash C, Hay K, Redston M, Kwong E, Hancock B, et al. (2001). Suppression of intestinal polyps in Msh2-deficient and non-Msh2-deficient multiple intestinal neoplasia mice by a specific cyclooxygenase-2 inhibitor and by a dual cyclooxygenase-1/2 inhibitor. Cancer Res 61(16):6131–6136.

88. Nelson JB, Hedican SP, George DJ, Reddi AH, Piantadosi S, Eisenberger MA, et al. (1995). Identification of endothelin-1 in the pathophysiology of metastatic adenocarcinoma of the prostate. Nat Med 1(9):944–949.

89. Pomonis JD, Rogers SD, Peters CM, Ghilardhi JR, Mantyh PW. (2001). Expression and localization of endothelin receptors: implication for the involvement of peripheral glia in nociception. Neurosci 21(3):999–1006.

90. Davar G, Hans G, Fareed MU, Sinnott C, Strichartz G. (1998). Behavioral signs of acute pain produced by application of endothelin-1 to rat sciatic nerve. Neuroreport 9(10):2279–2283.

91. Peters CM, Lindsay TH, Pomonis JD, Luger NM, Ghilardi JR, Sevcik MA, et al. (2004). Endothelin and the tumorigenic component of bone cancer pain. Neuroscience 126(4):1043–1052.

92. Couture R, Harrisson M, Vianna RM, Cloutier F. (2001). Kinin receptors in pain and inflammation. Eur J Pharmacol 429(1-3):161–176.

93. Fox A, Wotherspoon G, McNair K, Hudson L, Patel S, Gentry C, et al. (2003). Regulation and function of spinal and peripheral neuronal B1 bradykinin receptors in inflammatory mechanical hyperalgesia. Pain 104(3):683–691.

94. Sevcik MA, Ghilardi JR, Halvorson KG, Lindsay TH, Kubota K, Mantyh PW. (2005). Analgesic efficacy of bradykinin B1 antagonists in a murine bone cancer pain model. J Pain 6(11):771–775.

95. Hefti FF, Rosenthal A, Walicke PA, Wyatt S, Vergara G, Shelton DL, et al. (2006). Novel class of pain drugs based on antagonism of NGF. Trends Pharmacol Sci 27(2):85–91.

96. Pezet S, McMahon SB. (2006). Neurotrophins: mediators and modulators of pain. Annu Rev Neurosci 29:507–538.

97. Gould HJ 3rd, Gould TN, England JD, Paul D, Liu ZP, Levinson SR. (2000). A possible role for nerve growth factor in the augmentation of sodium channels in models of chronic pain. Brain Res 854(1-2):19–29.

98. Ji RR, Samad TA, Jin SX, Schmoll R, Woolf CJ. (2002). p38 MAPK activation by NGF in primary sensory neurons after inflammation increases TRPV1 levels and maintains heat hyperalgesia. Neuron 36(1):57–68.

99. Heumann R, Korsching S, Bandtlow C, Thoenen H. (1987). Changes of nerve growth factor synthesis in nonneuronal cells in response to sciatic nerve transection. J Cell Biol 104(6):1623–1631.

7

SYMMETRY, T-CELLS, AND NEUROGENIC ARTHRITIS

Nicholas G. Shenker

Department of Rheumatology, Addenbrooke's Hospital, Cambridge University NHS Foundation Trust, Cambridge CB2 2QQ, United Kingdom

David R. Blake and Candida S. McCabe

The Royal National Hospital for Rheumatic Diseases, Bath BA1 1RL, United Kingdom and School for Health, University of Bath, Claverton Down BA2 7AY, United Kingdom

Richard C. Haigh

Department of Rheumatology, Royal Devon & Exeter Hospital (Wonford), Exeter EX2 5DW, United Kingdom

Paul I. Mapp

Academic Department of Rheumatology, University of Nottingham, City Hospital, Nottingham NG5 1PB, United Kingdom

SYMMETRY IN CLINICAL DISEASE

Symmetry in clinical disease is common and can be seen in a wide spectrum of conditions. Symmetrical diseases are found within the realms of rheumatology, dermatology, ophthalmology, and neurology, as might be expected given the anatomical duplicity of the systems with which these specialities deal. The consistency of the presence of this clinical finding points to an underlying mechanism.

Bilateral expression of a unilateral stimulus has best been studied in the neurosciences and Koltzenburg et al.[1] reviewed this phenomenon in 1999. They summarized the work of several teams who had independently described symmetrical, topographically precise, time-dependent changes in response to specific local neurological insults. Neural connections between left and right sides of the spinal cord are hypothesized to account for these changes (Fig. 7.1).

Detailed histological examination in the spinal cords of primates and other vertebrates[2,3] demonstrates posterior decussation of significant numbers of neurons at all levels of the spinal cord. These fibers terminate in the contralateral substantia gelatinosa (Rexed's laminae I–II) as well as in the deeper layers (laminae III–IV) and their function has yet to be described.

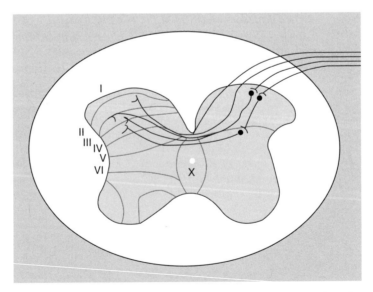

Figure 7.1. Scheme demonstrating routes identified from histological studies of sensory fibres decussating via the dorsal commissure without significant cranio-caudal transmission.

The implication that bilateral neurally mediated pathways exist and determine symmetrical disease patterns is important because conditions that exhibit symmetry are common and their etiology largely unknown. Skin psoriasis, for example, is much more symmetrical than expected by chance.[4] Other dermatological symmetrical conditions include vitiligo and pityriasis rosacea. The classic inflammatory example seen in ophthalmology is sympathetic ophthalmia. This is a bilateral uveitis complicating a unilateral perforating wound. Interestingly, acute demyelinating plaques seen in the brains of patients with multiple sclerosis are associated with subtle contralateral changes seen on diffusion MRI.[5] Glomerulonephritis and pulmonary fibrosis never occur unilaterally and this is noteworthy in itself.

SYMMETRY IN DEGENERATIVE ARTHRITIS

With respect to the musculoskeletal system, both degenerative and inflammatory arthritides are symmetrical. The Heberden's nodes of osteoarthritis (OA), the commonest arthritis of them all, are symmetrical. This is emphasized by a recent epidemiological survey from the Framingham population,[6] which demonstrated that symptomatic OA is remarkably symmetrical, especially in women. Proprioceptive feedback is abnormal in a radiologically normal knee that is contralateral to an osteoarthritic knee. This contralateral sensory deficit is more abnormal than expected when compared to age-matched patients who have no OA.[7,8] These observations suggest that neural deficits exist before the symmetrical expression of OA occurs. Further evidence that the neural supply to the joint is fundamental to the expression of this disease is that neural disruption prevents the development of Heberden's nodes (Table 7.1).

TABLE 7.1   Reports in the Literature of the Development of Arthritic Diseases in Partially Paralysed Patients[a]

Disease	Neural Injury	Outcome Suppressed
OA	Hemiplegia	Heberden's nodes
OA	Hemiplegia	Heberden's nodes
OA	Hemiplegia	Heberden's nodes
OA	Poliomyelitis	OA knee and hip
OA	Nerve injury	OA and Heberden's nodes
RA	Hemiplegia	Digital vasculitis, RA and RA nodules
RA	Hemiplegia	Arthritis
RA	Hand dominance	Radiological changes of arthritis
RA	Hand dominance	Radiological changes of arthritis
RA	Poliomyelitis	Arthritis
Gout	Hemiplegia	Arthritis and tophi deposits

[a]Modified from Dixon[40].

SYMMETRY IN INFLAMMATORY ARTHRITIS

A symmetrical pattern of involvement is clinically so important in rheumatoid arthritis that it is a feature of its diagnostic criteria.[9] There have been recent publications noting that inflammatory arthritis is symmetrical irrespective of rheumatoid factor[10] and that some of the seronegative arthritides, such as psoriatic,[11] are more symmetrical than would be expected by chance.

The pathophysiology of inflammatory arthritis currently centers on T- and B-lymphocyte dominated autoimmune processes. Yet, how could the immune system, effected by blood-borne agents, manifest clinically symmetrical disease? This chapter supports a neurogenic hypothesis to explain disease symmetry, and with reference to immune mediated disease, presents possible mechanisms for the interface between some neuropeptides and the immune system.

ROLE OF THE NEUROPEPTIDES SUBSTANCE P AND CGRP IN ARTHRITIS

Hench's classical report of symmetrical palindromic rheumatism dates more than 50 years and in it he describes wheals and flares occurring over affected joints. The similarity between this observation and Lewis's triple flare–wheal response was quickly made. The flare–wheal response is dependent on an intact nerve supply and, more specifically, on the release of the colocalized neuropeptides substance P (SP) and calcitonin gene-related peptide (CGRP) contained within populations of unmyelinated neurons. These are the commonest neuropeptides found in small diameter nerve fibers. It is now known that some of the unmyelinated fibers that innervate joint structures also have sprouting peripheral terminals that project into the surrounding skin. The skin changes that Hench described could well be attributed to the vasodilatory effects, known to be caused by the release of SP and CGRP, via an antidromic route. The role of these neuropeptides in the inflammatory processes of arthritis is therefore of interest.

Experimental work on a variety of animal species utilizing a number of insults to generate mono- and systemic arthritides have demonstrated that there is a release of SP in response to an arthritic insult.[12,13] There is a corresponding increase in the production of SP and CGRP in the nerve cell bodies located in the rat dorsal root ganglion.[14,15] The finding that joints "primed" with substance P demonstrate a more severe subsequent arthritis[16] supports the importance of the role of substance P in inflammatory arthritis. Furthermore, it can be shown that the depletion of these neuropeptides through denervation[17] or exposure to capsaicin[18] attenuates the progression and severity of an acute polyarthritis. Thus the presence of SP worsens, and its absence improves, experimental arthritis.

There is a persistent increase in SP in the synovial fluid of patients with RA compared with normal controls.[19] This is a consistent finding reported by several groups independently and SP levels are raised in the synovial fluid from patients with inflammatory arthritis when compared to both plasma concentrations and patients with noninflammatory arthritis.[12] Histochemical studies support the release of neuropeptides from arthritic synovium by finding a reduction in the presence of neural SP.[12] Interestingly, both CGRP and SP are produced by peripheral lymphocytes and this route may also contribute to the presence of neuropeptide release in the inflamed synovial joint.[20,21]

INFLUENCE OF NEUROPEPTIDES ON T CELLS

Neuropeptide-containing nerves are in contact with immune cells throughout the lifespan of T cells and intimate connections have been demonstrated in the thymus, lymph node, and spleen. There is a rich neuropeptide innervation to the blood vessels within lymph nodes in which there appears to be an especially strong anatomical link to the T cells rather than to the B cells.[22] Indeed, although B cells have recently been given significant attention following the successful introduction of anti-CD20 antibodies for active rheumatoid arthritis, it is still the T cell that has received more attention when neuropeptide–immune interactions are reviewed.

SP and CGRP are located perivascularly in the synovium.[12] CGRP has powerful vasodilatory effects[23] and will therefore increase synovial circulation significantly. These neuropeptides are also important in the migration of lymphocytes from the circulation to the joint. Capsaicin, an SP- and CGRP-depleting agent, reduces the influx of T cells into the acutely arthritic joint of guinea pigs.[24] This is a specific effect on these T cells because macrophage influx was unaffected in the same model.

Substance P binds to a particular subset of T lymphocytes via specific receptors and causes proliferation of these lymphocytes.[25] Furthermore, Levite's work suggests that neuropeptides can cause T lymphocytes to produce a rather different and distinctive pattern that is described as "forbidden." T_H0 cells are driven by antigenic stimulation to induce rather fixed patterns of cytokine secretion characterized by the "proinflammatory" T_H1 (e.g., IL-2, IFN-γ) and the "proantibody" T_H2 (e.g., IL-4, IL-10) cytokine profiles. The "forbidden" pattern that is induced by some neuropeptides combines both the characteristic T_H1 responses with the additional secretion of IL-4 and IL-10, and the characteristic T_H2 responses with the additional secretion of IL-2 and IFN-γ.[26] These *in vitro* studies need confirmation *in vivo*. Neuropeptide mediated T-helper responses, however, obviate the need for antigen and may well contribute to the immune dysregulation seen in rheumatoid arthritis.

Neuropeptides have an important role in both the trafficking and the subsequent immunomodulation of T cells in inflammatory arthritis. This has been illustrated by the demonstration that GnRH I and II, neuropeptides mainly produced in the brain, have effects on the endothelial binding of T cells and their localization in specific organs.[27] Vasoactive intestinal peptide (VIP) alters the T-lymphocyte response by reducing the costimulatory capacity of antigen presenting cells; preferentially inducing T_H2-type responses; and by generating antigen-specific regulatory T cells (T_{reg}) through the induction of tolerogenic dendritic cells.[28–30] Neuropeptide Y (NPY) also has a role in controlling T cells via the Y1 receptor. It can do this through both the antigen presenting cells, where it has been demonstrated that Y1−/− (NPY receptor 1) knockout mice have functionally defective antigen presenting dendritic cells, as well as the Y1 receptor located on T lymphocytes, which is a strong negative regulator.[31] αMSH, derived from proopiomelanocortin, also has pleiotropic effects on the immunoinflammatory response and has at least two receptors (MC1R and MC5R) identified on T cells. Broadly, αMSH appears to have regulatory functions and inhibits T-cell replication.[30,32]

The exact role of neuropeptides in inflammatory arthritis is not known. Substance P, CGRP, VIP, NPY, and GnRH I and II as well as other neuropeptides are anatomically, physiologically, and pharmacologically relevant to the mechanisms seen in the pathological processes of inflammatory arthritis.

THE NERVOUS SYSTEM IN ARTHRITIS

The role that the nervous system has in rheumatoid arthritis in humans is well documented. There are numerous examples of both lower motor and upper motor neuron lesions ameliorating the progression of this deforming joint disease. Denervation also prevents deformities caused by osteoarthritis, gout, and seronegative arthritides. Table 7.1 summarizes some of the identified case reports. The presence of an intact nervous system is important to allow the full expression of these arthritides.

A putative mechanism can be proposed whereby an inflammatory insult, such as a monoarthritis, triggers changes in the ipsilateral neural network, which are then mirrored to the contralateral side either through the spinal cord or via higher brain centers, to predispose this side to a similar inflammatory state. This is an example of an autoregulatory loop and this hypothesis is testable.

CONTRALATERAL INFLUENCES OF NEUROINFLAMMATORY INSULTS

Rotshenker and Tal[33] reported in both frogs and mice that sprouting in the contralateral neuromuscular junction followed nerve section and degeneration of the ipsilateral neuromuscular junctions. These contralateral fine extra sprouts were first seen 5 days after the sciatic nerve was proximally sectioned and this sprouting occurred much more frequently than in control rats.

Associated contralateral increases in GAP43, neuropeptide mRNA and expression, and proliferation of microglia were also seen.[1]

An inflammatory lesion induced in a rat knee using latex spheres resulted in a thickening bilaterally of the synovial intimal layer and this was accompanied by a bilateral cellular infiltrate.[34] No changes were detectable in any of the other joints. There were also contralateral changes in bradykinin-induced extravasation from the knee joint, as measured using Evans blue, which followed the course of this latex monoarthritis. This somatotopic distant response to a local inflammatory insult can only be mediated through the neural network. Systemic circulatory factors cannot display such topographical precision and biomechanical influences fail to explain the lack of response in other load-bearing joints. In further support of a neurogenic mechanism, the expression of substance P in the dorsal root ganglion was increased within 3 days *bilaterally* in this monoarthritis model.

There exists a body of published evidence to corroborate the findings that a unilateral insult induces contralateral topographically precise changes associated with appropriately located changes at the spinal level. This literature has been reviewed and updated and is summarized in Table 7.2.

It is important to note that although contralateral changes in the periphery can be seen from these models, the earliest changes on the contralateral side occur within the spinal cord. These are seen at the cellular level with changes in neuropeptide expression in the contralateral nerve cell bodies.[34]

It has been documented that unilateral capsaicin injections, the pungent extract of chili that induces the release of SP and CGRP, alters contralateral depolarization thresholds and reflexes.[35] We were able to demonstrate contralateral central pain responses in humans by detecting contralateral allodynia and hyperalgesia within 30 minutes following a unilateral intradermal injection of capsaicin (Fig. 7.2). In a group of 20 normal control subjects, 9 (45%) demonstrated contralateral sensory changes that were between 5% and 50% of the hypersensitive area induced by the capsaicin injection. In a group of 21 subjects with rheumatoid arthritis, 11/21 (52%) demonstrated contralateral sensory changes. This is the first demonstration of contralateral sensitization occurring in humans and allows a clinical model for examining the physiology of this in more detail.

The prior development of changes within the central nervous system implies that this is driving any contralateral peripheral change. This physiological loop may well be important in conferring survival benefit, as will be discussed later, but "physiology begets pathology". It is therefore possible that the nervous system not only underlies the symmetry of some diseases but may be principal in their etiopathogenesis as well.

Charcot was the first to note the possible role of the nervous system in arthritis and his name has become synonymous with the neuroarthropathic joint. It is therefore no coincidence that the clinical history of these joints reflects the surmised role that neuropeptides have in their etiology.

TABLE 7.2   The Contralateral Effects of Localised Unilateral Inflammation[a]

Lesions Inducing Arthritis	Contralateral Effect
CFA (1 μg) in knee	Decrease in anabolism of cartilage for 6–72 h
Freund's adjuvant in knee (0.05 ml of 1 mg/ml)	Increase in SP, CGRP and NPY in knee for 2–24 h
	Increase in NK-A in knee at 2 h and at 24 h
Carrageenan 2% (0.05 ml) in knee	Increase in CGRP and NPY for 2–24 h
	Increase in SP at 2 h and at 24 h; and NK-A at 24 h
Human recombinant IL-1 (0.05 ml of 1 mg/ml) in knee	Increase in CGRP and NPY for 2–24 h
	Increase in NK-A at 2–6 h and SP at 2 h
SP (0.05 ml of 10^{-5} M) in knee	Increase in SP for 2–24 h, CGRP for 6–24 h and NPY for 2–6 h
	No increase in NK-A
SP in knee (0.2, 1, 2, 10, 20 μg in 50 μl)	Decrease in anabolism of cartilage for 6–72 h
500 μl of mBSA in knee of rats preimmunised with 1 ml CFA/2 mg MTb	Histopathological and biochemical evidence of joint destruction up to 80 d
500 μg (50 μl) mBSA in knee of pre-sensitized rats	Increased proteoglycan loss and mechanical hyperalgesia up to 9 d
CFA (250 μg/100 μl) in knee	Antidromic action potentials increased in contralateral saphenous nerve measured compared to control
	Evans blue extravasation increased in knee compared to control
100 μl of 1% latex spheres in knee	Bradykinin-induced plasma extravasation enhanced between 10–21 d
	Macrophage infiltration noted between 3–10 d

TABLE 7.2. (Continued)

Lesions Inducing Hindpaw Oedema	Contralateral Effect
CFA (100 µl)	TNF-alpha levels elevated up to 120 h
Carrageenan (0.1 ml of 2%)	CGRP levels increase in hindpaw perfusate at 3–4 h
	Thermal and mechanical withdrawal latencies reduced at 3–4 h
Carrageenan 100 µl of 2%	Mechanical hyperalgesia between 3–5 d
Formaldehyde 50 µl (0.1%, 5%, 10%)	Licking responses occur at 10–60 min
Bee venom 100 µl (0.2 mg)	Heat (not mechanical) withdrawal latency reduced for 2–48 h
Repeated saline injection 150 µl on 3 consecutive days	Reduction in mechanical withdrawal latencies for 3–5 h
	Increase in paw thickness for 3–5 h
Urate, pyrophosphate and oxalate crystals (3 mg in 150 µl)	Swelling observed, maximal at 5 h
CGRP 100 µl (300 pmol)	Oedema induced at 5–24 h
NGF injections (3 d of 4 µg/d) in hindpaw or ear or forepaw.	Increased expression of preprotachykinin and preproCGRP mRNA in nerve (sciatic; trigeminal; or brachial plexus)
IL-1beta (10 ng)	B1 receptor-mediated mechanical hyperalgesia for 1–6 h
Thermal stimuli (55C for 15 s)	Thermal foot withdrawal latencies reduced at 24 h
Thermal stimuli (55C for 15–20 s)	Thermal foot withdrawal latencies reduced at 24 h
Thermal stimuli to decerebrate rat (75C for 60 s)	Reduction in the flexor reflex threshold to mechanical and thermal stimuli at 1 h

[a]All of these studies were performed in rats, unless otherwise indicated.

Key: CFA – complete Freund's adjuvant; SP – substance P; NPY – neuropeptide Y; CGRP – calcitonin gene related peptide; NK-A – neurokinin A; IL-1 – interleukin 1; MBSA – methylated bovine serum albumin; MTb – *mycobacterium tuberculosis*; TNF – tumour necrosis factor; NGF – nerve growth factor; RNA – ribonucleic acid.

Sella and Barrette[36] were able to identify five stages of neuroarthropathy in the feet of diabetics from the careful evaluation of clinical histories and radiological tests. In stage 0 the patient presents with a locally swollen, warm, and often painful foot. It is this stage that is often missed clinically as patients tend to present later. Radiographs are negative whereas a technetium 99 bone scan is markedly positive. In addition to these clinical findings, there are also periarticular cysts, erosions, and localized osteopenia radiologically in stage 1. Stages 2–4 demonstrate the progressive joint subluxations, dislocations,

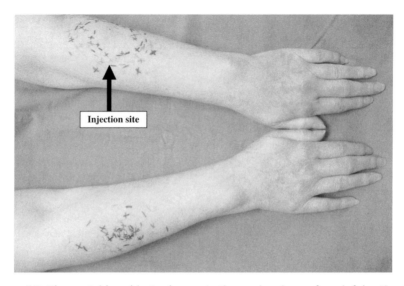

Figure 7.2. Rheumatoid subject demonstrating mirroring of painful stimulus. Ipsilateral capsaicin injection in the left forearm. Using Semmes Weinstein filaments, the sensory changes are then mapped using different colors to represent 10–minute intervals between 10–60 minutes. Changes in allodynia are marked with an 'x'. Changes to mechanical hyperalgesia are marked with '-'. Note the development of both allodynia and hyperalgesia in a topographically-precise contralateral region.

and destruction of the joints in the diabetic foot. Clinically in these stages, there is no temperature gradient between the two feet. Radiologically, there is bony trabeculation across joint spaces indicative of mature fusion.

Histological examination of Charcot joints has been difficult because tissue from early disease is rare to find and most samples have been removed from destroyed joints that are late in the disease process. Most of these specimens show nonspecific changes consistent with an inflammatory process, but there are isolated reports that show scattered lymphocytes.[37]

As can be seen from the experimental evidence presented above, neuropeptides from damaged nerve terminals increase both the synovial blood supply and the influx of activated macrophages and lymphocytes into the joint. These cells alter the complex neurochemical intra-articular matrix substantially to lead to massive rapid destruction of the joint. Later in the disease, however, neural damage has sufficiently depleted neuropeptides so that their vasodilatory effects are negligible. Interestingly, Charcot joints are not uncommonly bilateral.[38]

SURVIVAL HYPOTHESIS OF AN AUTO-NEUROINFLAMMATORY LOOP

There is evolutionary pressure for rapid appropriate responses to be available as part of an organism's defense against noxious environs.[39] Bilaterality has evolved so that there is functional capacity should one part be irreparably damaged. It is therefore vitally important that the contralaterally homonymous area should be protected following focal damage. A neuroinflammatory loop, whereby protective responses are contralaterally rapidly upregulated, would therefore be a useful addition to any symmetrical organism's protection and long-term survival. The advantage that this precise response has over any systemic mechanism is that it is economic with the energy expended and limits widespread self-damage caused by inappropriate inflammation. Similarly, pain withdrawal reflexes are primed through previously documented electrophysiological changes in the spinal cord so that the contralateral limb can be withdrawn more quickly. There is more chance of damage limitation from a dangerous environment if such responses existed and it is argued that survival is enhanced through the use of such pathways.

As our control over the environment has reduced the risk of noxious exposure in modern society, these pathways may now unfortunately be more associated with disease states. There is insufficient evolutionary pressure to downregulate these pathways because these diseases have a limited effect on reproductive capacity as their peak onset is after childbearing years.

CONCLUSION

Chronic inflammatory disease is symmetrical where possible. This symmetry is mediated neurogenically through neuropeptide mechanisms that define a neuroinflammatory loop that is insult specific and topographically precise. The immune system can fundamentally be affected by the release of such neuropeptides through their effects on T cells. This interaction may be important not only in the expression of symmetry in disease but also in their etiopathogenesis.

REFERENCES

1. Koltzenburg M, Wall PD, McMahon SB. (1999). Does the right side know what the left side is doing? TINS 22:122–127.
2. Light AR, Perl ER. (1979). Reexamination of the dorsal root projection to the spinal dorsal horn including observation of the differential termination of coarse and fine fibres. J Comp Neurol 186:117–132.
3. Culberson JL, Haines DE, Kimmel DL, Brown PB. (1979). Contralateral projection of primary afferent fibres to mammalian spinal cord. Expl Neurol 64:83–97.
4. Farber EM, Nickoloff BJ, Recht B, Fraki JE. (1986). Stress, symmetry and psoriasis: possible role of neuropeptides. J Am Acad Dermatol 14:305–311.
5. Werring DJ, Brassat D, Droogan AG, et al. (2000). The pathogenesis of lesions and normal-appearing white matter changes in multiple sclerosis: a serial diffusion MRI study. Brain 123:1667–1676.

6. Niu J, Zhang Y, LaValley M, Chaisson CE, Aliabadi P, Felson DT. (2003). Symmetry and clustering of symptomatic hand osteoarthritis in elderly men and women: the Framingham study. Rheumatology 42:343–348.

7. Garsden LR, Bullock-Saxton JE. (1999). Joint reposition sense in subjects with unilateral osteoarthritis of the knee. Clin Rehabil 13:148–155.

8. Sharma L, Pai YC, Holtkamp K, Rymer WZ. (1997). Is knee joint proprioception worse in the arthritic knee versus the unaffected knee in unilateral knee osteoarthritis? Arthritis Rheum 40:1518–1525.

9. Arnett FC, Edworthy SM, Bloch DA, et al. (1988). The American Rheumatism Association 1987 revised criteria for the classification of rheumatoid arthritis. Arthritis Rheum 31:315–324.

10. Bukhari M, Lunt M, Harrison BJ, Scott DG, Symmons DP, Silman AJ. (2002). Erosions in inflammatory polyarthritis are symmetrical regardless of rheumatoid factor status: results from a primary care-based inception cohort of patients. Rheumatology (Oxford) 41:246–252.

11. Helliwell PS, Hetthen J, Sokoll K, Green M, Marchesoni A, Lubrano E, Veale D, Emery P. (2000). Joint symmetry in early and late rheumatoid and psoriatic arthritis. Arthritis Rheum 43:865–871.

12. Garrett NE, Mapp PI, Cruwys SC, Kidd BL, Blake DR. (1992). Role of substance P in inflammatory arthritis. Ann Rheum Dis 51:1014–1018.

13. Holzer P. (1988). Local effector functions of capsaicin-sensitive sensory nerve endings: involvement of tachykinins, calcitonin gene-related peptide and other neuropeptides. Neuroscience 24:739–768.

14. Hanesch U, Blecher F, Stiller RU, Emson PC, Schaible HG, Heppelmann B. (1995). The effect of a unilateral inflammation at the rat's ankle joint on the expression of preprotachykinin-A mRNA and preprosomatostatin mRNA in dorsal root ganglion cells—a study using non-radioactive in situ hybridization. Brain Res 700:279–284.

15. Mapp PI, Terenghi G, Walsh DA, Chen ST, Cruwys SC, Garrett N, Kidd BL, Polak JM, Blake DR. (1993). Monoarthritis in the rat knee induces bilateral and time-dependent changes in substance P and calcitonin gene-related peptide immunoreactivity in the spinal cord. Neuroscience 57:1091–1096.

16. Levine JD, Clark R, Devor M, Helms C, Moskowitz MA, Basbaum AI. (1984). Intraneuronal substance P contributes to the severity of experimental arthritis. Science 226:547–549.

17. Levine JD, Dardick SJ, Basbaum AI, Scipio E. (1985). Reflex neurogenic inflammation. I. Contribution of the peripheral nervous system to spatially remote inflammatory responses that follow injury. J Neurosci 5:1380–1386.

18. Donaldson LF, McQueen DS, Seckl JR. (1995). Neuropeptide gene expression and capsaicin-sensitive primary afferents: maintenance and spread of adjuvant arthritis in the rat. J Physiol 486:473–482.

19. Westermark T, Rantapaa-Dahlqvist S, Wallberg-Jonsson S, Kjorell U, Forsgren S. (2001). Increased content of bombesin/GRP in human synovial fluid in early arthritis: different pattern compared with substance P. Clin Exp Rheumatol 19:715–720.

20. Qian BF, Zhou GQ, Hammarstrom ML, Danielsson A. (2001). Both substance P and its receptor are expressed in mouse intestinal T lymphocytes. Neuroendocrinology 73:358–368.

21. Wang H, Xing L, Li W, Hou L, Guo J, Wang X. (2002). Production and secretion of calcitonin gene-related peptide from human lymphocytes. J Neuroimmunol 130:155–162.

22. Weihe E, Krekel J. (1991). The neuroimmune connection in human tonsils. Brain Behav Immun 5:41–54.

23. Brain SD, Williams TJ, Tippins JR, Morris HR, MacIntyre I. (1985). Calcitonin gene-related peptide is a potent vasodilator. Nature 313:54–56.

24. Hood VC, Cruwys SC, Urban L, Kidd BL. (2001). The neurogenic contribution to synovial leucocyte infiltration and other outcome measures in a guinea pig model of arthritis. Neurosci Lett 299:201–204.

25. McGillis JP, Mitsuhashi M, Payan DG. (1990). Immunomodulation by tachykinin neuropeptides. Ann NY Acad Sci 594:85–94.

26. Levite M. (2001). Nervous immunity: neurotransmitters, extracellular potassium and T-cell function. Trends Immunol 22:2–5.

27. Chen A, Ganor Y, Rahimipour S, Ben-Aroya N, Koch Y, Levite M. (2002). The neuropeptides GnRH-II and GnRH-I are produced by human T cells and trigger laminin receptor gene expression, adhesion, chemotaxis and homing to specific organs. Nat Med 8:1421–1426.

28. Delgado M, Abad C, Martinez C, Leceta J, Gomariz RP. (2001). Vasoactive intestinal peptide prevents experimental arthritis by downregulating both autoimmune and inflammatory components of the disease. Nat Med 7:563–568.

29. Ganea D, Gonzalez-Rey E, Delgado M. (2006). A novel mechanism for immunosuppression: from neuropeptides to regulatory T cells. J Neuroimmune Pharmacol 1:400–409.

30. Gonzalez-Rey E, Chorny A, Delgado M. (2007). Regulation of immune tolerance by anti-inflammatory neuropeptides. Nat Rev Immunol 7:52–63.

31. Wheway J, Mackay CR, Newton RA, Sainsbury A, Boey D, Herzog H, Mackay F. (2005). A fundamental bimodal role for neuropeptide Y1 receptor in the immune system. J Exp Med 202:1527–1538.

32. Steinman L. (2004). Elaborate interactions between the immune and nervous systems. Nat Immunol 5:575–581.

33. Rotshenker S, Tal M. (1985). The transneuronal induction of sprouting and synapse formation in intact mouse muscles. J Physiol 360:387–396.

34. Kidd BL, Cruwys SC, Garrett NE, Mapp PI, Jolliffe VA, Blake DR. (1995). Neurogenic influences on contralateral responses during experimental rat monoarthritis. Brain Res 688:72–76.

35. Gjerstad J, Tjolsen A, Svendsen F, Hole K. (2000). Inhibition of spinal nociceptive responses after intramuscular injection of capsaicin involves activation of noradrenergic and opioid systems. Brain Res 859:132–136.

36. Sella EJ, Barrette C. (1999). Staging of Charcot neuroarthropathy along the medial column of the foot in the diabetic patient. J Foot Ankle Surg 38:34–40.

37. Clement GB, Grizzard K, Vasey FB, Germain BF, Espinoza LR. (1984). Neuro-pathic arthropathy (Charcot joints) due to cervical osteolysis: a complication of progressive systemic sclerosis. J Rheumatol 11:545–548.

38. Armstrong DG, Todd WF, Lavery LA, Harkless LB, Bushman TR. (1997). The natural history of acute Charcot's arthropathy in a diabetic foot speciality clinic. Diab Med 14:357.

39. Kidd BL, Mapp PI, Gibson SJ, Polak JM, O'Higgins F, Buckland-Wright JC, Blake DR. (1989). A neurogenic mechanism for symmetrical arthritis. Lancet 8762:1128–1129.

40. Dixon A. (1989). Hemiplegia, hand dominance and asymmetry of expression of arthritis in relation to intra-articular pressure. In Dixon A and Hawkins C (eds.). *Raised Intra-Articular Pressure—Clinical Consequences*. Bath: Bath Institute for Rheumatic Diseases. p. 65.

PART II

OSTEOARTHRITIS AND PAIN

8

JOINT MECHANICS IN OSTEOARTHRITIS

Walter Herzog

Faculties of Kinesiology, Engineering, and Medicine, University of Calgary, 2500 University Drive NW, Calgary AB T2N 1N4, Canada

Douglas Bourne and Aliaa Rehan Youssef

Faculty of Kinesiology, University of Calgary, 2500 University Drive NW, Calgary AB T2N 1N4, Canada

INTRODUCTION

The primary goal of our research is to quantify the in vivo loading of normal and osteoarthritic joints, and to determine the pathways linking joint loading to the onset and progression of osteoarthritis (OA). Much of the biomechanics of OA has been focused on articular cartilage and its changing properties measured using explant tissue preparations. We feel that, although critically important to our understanding of cartilage mechanics and biology, these experiments may not be directly transferable to interpreting the in vivo joint mechanics and to elucidate the detailed mechanisms of onset and progression of OA. Therefore we have attempted to measure the loading of the intact knee in

Pain in Osteoarthritis, Edited by David T. Felson and Hans-Georg Schaible
Copyright © 2009 Wiley-Blackwell.

feline and lapine models of OA. We have found that, upon anterior cruciate ligament (ACL) transection in the cat, knee joints are more flexed during locomotion, muscle forces are decreased, normal muscle coordination patterns are changed, and muscles atrophy. In the initial stage of this OA model (0–6 months following ACL transection), articular cartilage initially becomes thicker, softer, and more permeable, resulting in generally increased joint contact areas, and decreased peak pressures compared to control values. In the midstage of OA (6 months to about 12 years), normal muscle coordination patterns and locomotion biomechanics are recovered in the cat, and although there are clinical signs of OA, there is no pain. In the final stages of the cat ACL transection model of OA (>12 years post ACL transection), cartilage becomes thinner, there is complete erosion of articular cartilage from specific areas of the joint, there are joint "mice," the subchondral bone has lost some integrity, and the animals start limping because of joint pain. In this phase, joint contact areas become smaller and peak pressures increase. Based on these results, we propose that altered joint mechanics with a concomitant unloading of the joint causes the knee to degenerate following ACL transection, and that this degeneration leading to OA cannot be stopped even when recovering normal joint biomechanics. The onset of joint pain in the cat model seems to be associated with the complete erosion of cartilage from specific areas of the joint, and from ∼ 1 mm diameter, spherical, hard, cartilaginous inclusions in the joint (joint mice).

DEFINITIONS

Biomechanics is the science that deals with the external and internal forces acting on biological systems, and the effects produced by these forces. For the purpose of this chapter, the system under consideration is the joint. The external forces may be represented by gravitational, inertial, and contact forces; and the internal forces are the forces acting on and within joint structures, such as the articular cartilage, ligaments, muscles, tendons, and menisci.

A joint is the junction between two or more bones. Joints are classified as fibrous, cartilaginous, and synovial, and it is the latter that is of particular interest in this context. Joints permit movement between segments and transfer forces from one bone to the next. When performing biomechanical analyses in the context of joint OA, ideally, we would like to know the instantaneous internal forces acting on all structures in and around the joint, specifically the variable pressure distribution acting on the articular cartilages.

The joint equipollence equations relate the internal (muscular, ligamentous, and bony contact forces) to the resultant joint forces and moments. The resultant joint forces and moments can be obtained readily for most situations using the so-called inverse dynamics approach.[1] However, calculating the associated internal forces is typically much more complex because of the redundant nature of human and animal joints. Typically, a joint has many more internal force unknowns than the system has degrees of freedom; thus there is an infinite number of possible solution for the internal forces.[2] For example, the human knee has at least ten independent muscles, four major ligamentous and two primary bony articulating forces (Fig. 8.1), whereas the joint has merely six degrees of freedom (and thus six independent scalar equations). Mathematical optimization has frequently been used to solve for the internal forces, as it has been argued, with some merit, that muscles may be recruited during normal locomotion in such a way that metabolic cost or

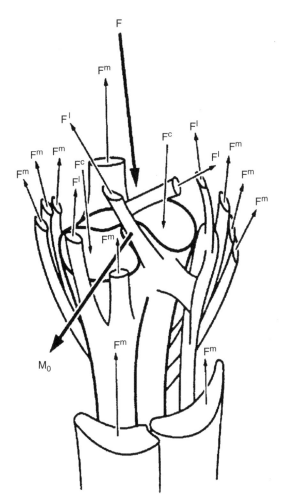

Figure 8.1. Force distribution in the knee and its equipollent replacement by a resultant external force (F) and a resultant external joint moment (M_0) (From Ref. 2 with permission.)

fatigue is minimized or endurance is maximized. Independent of the precise nature of these approaches and the function to be optimized, the validity of such optimization approaches has been questioned,[3] and rigorous validation is missing despite the availability of general solutions for the most widely used optimization techniques.[4] Therefore determination of internal forces in joints must be done using experiments, as theoretical approaches are too crude at present and cannot provide more than rough estimates of the internal force distributions in and around joints.

Osteoarthritis (OA) is a joint disease of primarily unknown origin. Its end stage is defined by complete cartilage erosion from all, or parts, of the articular surfaces. As such, it is often considered a disease of the articular cartilage. However, we would like to define it in much broader terms. OA is a joint disease associated with damage to the articular surfaces, accompanied by osteophyte formation, with changes in the subchondral bone structure, the ligaments, menisci, the synovial fluid, and so on.

It has typically been assumed that OA is associated, in one way or another, with joint loading. However, this has not been proved with absolute certainty. Nevertheless, we will adopt the notion that joint loading, which can be quantified through the in vivo joint mechanics, triggers the onset of OA, and once triggered, the disease continues and, at present, cannot be stopped or reversed. This progression of the disease, typically over years, may also be associated with altered joint loading, as some animal models of OA would suggest.[5] However, this notion is much more tentative and does not receive support from a recently completed study on ACL transection in cats that were followed for more than 12 years post intervention (unpublished observations).

If we adopt the premise that a certain type of joint loading produces joint degeneration leading to OA, the following basic questions emerge:

1. What is the type of loading that is harmful to the joint in terms of magnitude, rate of application, frequency, and other mechanical descriptors?
2. What is the biological response to these loading conditions that produces the osteoarthritic response?
3. And probably most importantly, what are the pathways (or mechanisms) linking the load to the degenerative response?

In order to answer the first two questions, it seems imperative that the normal in vivo joint loading is quantified and compared to situations that are known to produce end-stage OA, and that the biological responses to such in vivo loading are measured. Theoretically, such experiments should be straightforward, but little progress has been made toward these goals, probably because the work involved is extremely time consuming, and such long-term experiments are expensive. The third question is arguably the most interesting and important but also the most elusive to date. Impressive research aimed at relating "mechanical loading" to biological responses has been made in studies using articular cartilage explants that are exposed to well-defined loading conditions in a laboratory setting.[6-9] However, the boundary conditions of explants under these artificial loading conditions are far removed from real in vivo joint loading. Therefore the results from these studies, although interesting from a materials property point of view, may bear little relevance to physiologically occurring joint loading and the associated pathogenesis of human OA. Of course, there exists the possibility that articular cartilage cylinders with perfectly flat-shaved surfaces subjected to confined, or unconfined, in vitro loading conditions between two metal plates may behave similarly to the naturally rounded cartilage surfaces attached to their native bone that are exposed to the gliding and compression loading from their adjacent cartilage surfaces. However, if so, this must be demonstrated. Here, we will not discuss the vast number of excellent studies on articular cartilage explants, partly because of a lack of relevance in the current context, and partly because those studies have received much attention and are summarized in a series of excellent reviews.[10-13]

Instead, we will focus on studies aimed at quantifying the internal and external forces occurring in diarthrodial joints of experimental models of bona fide end-stage OA. This will be done by presenting research on the ground reaction forces and kinematic patterns of the ACL transected cat, by discussing work on the corresponding muscle forces and activation patterns, and by showing results of the associated degenerative responses. Following this discussion, we would like to present work on the biological response of articular cartilage to controlled in vivo loading of joints, and on an experimental model of muscle weakness. We have evidence that physiological loading of joints produces biosynthetic responses from the articular cartilage that are often conceptually different from those obtained using comparable loading conditions in cartilage/bone explants. These differences might contain crucial clues as to the relationship between joint loading and onset of OA. The muscle weakness work is motivated by the clinical observations that OA is associated with altered muscle coordination patterns, muscle inhibition, weakness, and atrophy. It has been suggested that muscle weakness might be an independent risk factor for OA, rather than just an associated occurrence, but although there is ample anecdotal observation and clinical support,[14,15] there is little quantitative and systematic evidence in support of this suggestion.

METHODS, TECHNIQUES, AND APPROACHES

The Cat Model of Osteoarthritis

There are only a few experimental animal models of OA that have been followed longitudinally over years. Two such models are the anterior cruciate ligament (ACL) transected dog[16] and cat.[17] Both these models have been found to present a history of onset and progression of OA similar to the human disease and have led to complete erosion of articular cartilage from specific areas of the articular surfaces. We chose ACL transection of the cat as our model for in vivo investigation for two primary reasons: (1) the cat hind limb is arguably the best known mammalian system in terms of muscular anatomy, in vivo force production, and neurophysiological movement control; and (2) the cat knee does not suffer from naturally occurring OA; therefore degenerative changes in joint structure, control, and movement can be associated directly with targeted interventions, even when animals are followed over years where age effects might play a role in other experimental models, such as the dog. The detailed approach to arthroscopic and open joint ACL transection surgery has been described previously.[18,19]

External Forces and Kinematics

The external ground reaction forces for walking animals, before and after experimental intervention, were measured using a pair of animal-sized (10×15 cm) force platforms (AMTI, Amherst, USA) embedded in a specifically designed walkway.[17,20] These platforms measure the three-dimensional forces and moments acting from the ground on the animal's paws, and simultaneously provide the location of the center of pressure of the resultant ground reaction force. Hind limb kinematics were measured using a high speed video system (Motion Analysis, Santa Rosa, CA, 200 Hz), with a correction algorithm to account for skin marker movement.[21]

Muscle Forces and Activation Patterns

Forces in selected ankle extensor muscles were measured using E-shaped, external tendon force transducers (Fig. 8.2) based on a strain-gauged design.[22]

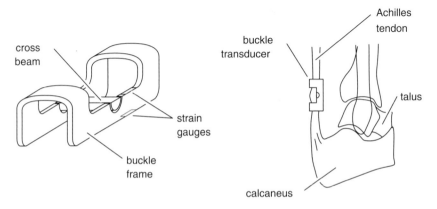

Figure 8.2. Schematic illustration of a buckle tendon force transducer (left) and a possible arrangement on an Achilles tendon (right).

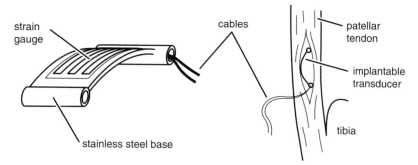

Figure 8.3. Schematic illustration of an implantable force transducer (left) and a possible arrangement in a patellar tendon (right). (From Ref. 23 with permission.)

Forces in the knee extensors (patellar tendon) were quantified using an omega-shaped, implantable force transducer based on the design of Xu et al.[23] and tested and adapted by Herzog et al.[24] and Hasler et al.[25] (Fig. 8.3). Activation patterns of selected knee and ankle extensor and flexor muscles were measured using indwelling, Teflon coated, bipolar, fine wire electrodes embedded into the midbelly of the target muscles with an approximate interelectrode distance of 5 mm, and aligned in the approximate direction of the muscle fibers.[26]

Joint Pressure Distribution

In situ joint pressure distributions in normal and ACL transected knees were measured using Fuji low and medium grade, pressure sensitive films.[27] Films were packaged in 12×120 mm strips for multiple measurements and were sealed in polyethylene adhesive layers for moisture proofing.[28] Film strips were inserted into the joint space through a lateral opening (approximately 20 mm). Once inserted, controlled knee extensor activation was produced by stimulating the femoral nerve via a bipolar cuff electrode and a Grass (S88) stimulator. Knee extensor force was measured using a specifically designed tibial restraining bar, and the force was adjusted by changing the voltage and frequency of stimulation. Fuji film calibration and analysis were performed as outlined in detail by Clark et al.[29]

RESULTS AND DISCUSSION

Osteoarthritis

Transection of the cat ACL causes increases in thickness, softness, and permeability of the articular cartilage and produces osteophyte formation, increases in thickness and mass of the medial collateral ligament and medial

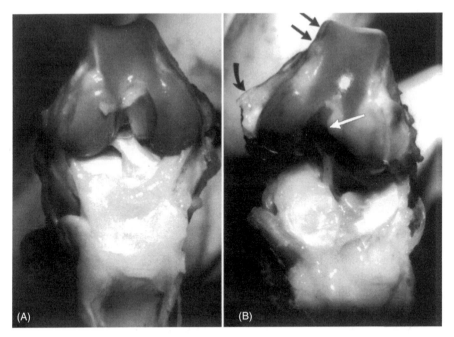

Figure 8.4. (A) Intact cat knee and (B) anterior cruciate ligament transected knee 16 weeks postintervention. Note the missing ACL, the enlarged medial capsule (curved arrow), and the osteophytes at the joint margins (straight arrows).

joint capsule, and atrophy of the hind limb musculature within weeks (Fig. 8.4).[18] Over time, site-specific articular surfaces are eroded away, cartilages become soft and lose internal structure, the joint space becomes narrower, and osteophytes increase in number and size (Fig. 8.5).

Mechanics

Mechanically, ACL transection is associated with an immediate instability of the knee that results in an excessive anterior translation and internal rotation of the tibia relative to the femur for a given amount of force or moment, respectively.[19,30] Muscle forces, external ground reaction forces, and knee angles decrease immediately following ACL transection,[17,25] and activation patterns of the knee extensor and flexor musculature show two distinct features: (1) a burst-like (rather than the normal, continuous) firing pattern of the knee extensors; and (2) an additional phase of activation of the knee flexors (semitendinosus) to compensate for the loss of mechanical function associated with ACL transection (Fig. 8.6).

Within approximately 4 months of ACL transection, joint stability in the anterior and internal rotation direction are fully reestablished.[30] This result is in

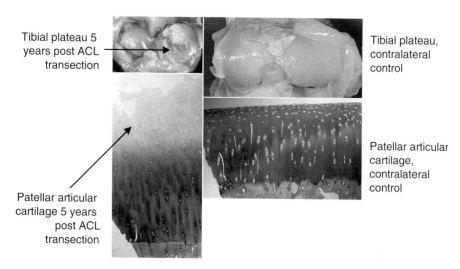

Tibial plateau 5 years post ACL transection

Tibial plateau, contralateral control

Patellar articular cartilage, contralateral control

Patellar articular cartilage 5 years post ACL transection

Figure 8.5. Tibial plateau and retropatellar articular cartilage samples from an anterior cruciate ligament deficient cat, 5 years postintervention. Left panel: experimental side; right panel: contralateral side. Note the complete erosion of articular cartilage from the medial tibial plateau of the experimental hind limb (arrow), and the loss of structure and fissuring in the surface zone (arrow) of the experimental articular cartilage. The contralateral tibial plateau and articular cartilage (right panel) look relatively normal.

contrast to the notion that continuing joint instability, particularly the pronounced anterior shift of the tibia relative to the femur in many animal species[31] and humans, is responsible, at least in part, for the progression of joint degeneration. Despite attempts to accurately measure the relative movements of tibia and femur using sonomicrometry (Sonometrics Corp., London, ON, Canada) with a 16 µm spatial resolution, we have not been able to detect the anterior tibial shift typically observed in ACL deficient humans, dogs, and sheep at the instant of foot contact during locomotion.[31,32] We speculate that the activation of the semitendinosus just prior to paw contact in the cat (Fig. 8.6, third row figure, arrows) might prevent the anterior shift of the tibia relative to the femur. If so, one could argue that proper neuromuscular adaptation offsets the mechanical loss of function associated with ACL deficiency. However, the crucial clinical question of whether semitendinosus firing is a meaningful adaptation of muscle coordination that slows down joint degeneration has not been addressed. It does not prevent final stage, symptomatic OA, as will be discussed later.

The detailed adaptations responsible for the quick reestablishment of knee stability following ACL transection in the cat are not known. We speculate that the initial increase in articular cartilage thickness, the strengthening of the medial capsule, the increase in mass of the medial collateral ligament, and the appearance of osteophytes at the joint margins might contribute to the observed increase in joint stability.[33] However, despite the apparent lack of anterior

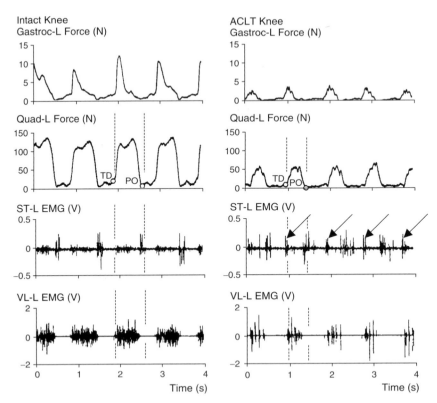

Figure 8.6. Gastrocnemius (Gastroc) and knee extensor (Quad) forces, as well as semitendinosus (ST) and vastus lateralis (VL) EMG before (Intact knee) and 10 days after anterior cruciate ligament transection (ACLT knee). The values shown are for slow walking (0.4 m/s) on a motor driven treadmill. Observe the decrease in muscle force and the change in EMG patterns and continuity from before to after ACL transection. Vertical line TD shows the touch down of the hind limb during the step cycle; the corresponding vertical line PO indicates the instant of paw off.

translation of the tibia during locomotion, and the reduction of anterior translation and medial rotation to normal values within 4 months of ACL transection, the cat knee continues to degenerate. Therefore joint instability might be a factor contributing to the onset and progression of OA, but it does not appear to be a necessary condition for the progression of OA.

The ground reaction forces decrease immediately following ACL transection. However, similar to the observations on knee instability, the ground reaction force patterns recover to normal values within about 16 weeks for static (quiet standing) tasks, and within about 6 months for dynamic (straight walking and running) tasks (Fig. 8.7). These results are of interest, as in the ACL transected dog, neither the ground reaction forces nor knee stability appear to recover following ACL transection, not even after 54 months.[16]

Fz
(% of body weight)

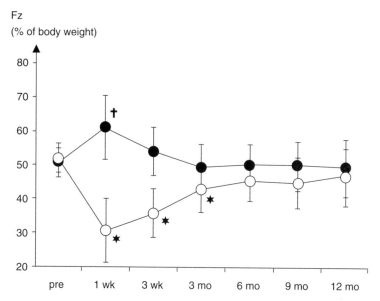

Figure 8.7. Peak vertical ground reaction forces (means $\pm$ 1 SD, $n = 7$) as a percentage of body weight for the ACL transected (open symbols) and the corresponding contralateral, intact hind limb (solid symbols) during cat walking and running before (pre) and at various time periods after unilateral ACL transection (1 week to 12 months). Note that the forces differ statistically at 1 week, 3 weeks, and 3 months post intervention, but not for the other time points. A minimum of 10 step cycles for both hind limbs was used at each time point and each animal to calculate the mean values shown.

Therefore we have two models of experimentally induced OA whose pathogenesis is very similar[18,34] but the long-term external mechanics are completely different. In the dog, the ACL transected joint remains unstable over years, while in the cat, such instability is never observed during walking, and in anterior or medial rotation displacement tests, the initial instability is abolished within 4 months following ACL transection. Similarly, the ACL transected dog shows reduced vertical ground reaction forces over years, while such force reductions are all but gone in the cat after 4–6 months.

Although the interpretation of the pathogenesis of these two animal models of OA, in consideration of the directly measured joint mechanics, is wide open, the following scenario appears the most obvious, and although by no means proved, might stimulate discussion about how altered joint mechanics may produce OA. First, one has to acknowledge that the mechanical changes to the joint are similar in the cat and dog in the early stages following intervention, and the pathogenesis is similar too. Second one has to consider that, after approximately 4–6 months, the mechanics start to differ substantially, but the progression of the disease remains similar. This scenario suggests that ACL transection in the cat and dog disrupts the mechanics of the knee, and that this event is responsible for triggering events leading to degeneration and OA of the joint. We are not sure what these events are, but, in general, the muscular forces, contact pressures, and external ground reaction forces are decreased substantially, thus leading to the hypothesis that there is an initial "unloading" of the joint. Therefore unloading of the joint, rather than the commonly believed "overloading," might trigger degenerative events in the knee.

Furthermore, once these degenerative processes have been initiated, the stabilization of the joint, and the normalization of its mechanics, does not affect the end result (bona fide OA development), suggesting that once degenerative processes are initiated, the disease progresses to end stage, although the rate of progression might vary. While the ACL transected dog is unloading its affected hind limb, presumably because of pain, the cat does not until approximately 12 years following intervention, when the knee becomes painful and the cat starts limping again as it did immediately following ACL transection. These results imply that rehabilitation strategies aimed at establishing normal movement patterns and joint loading would be most successful early in the rehabilitation process; that is, as soon as possible following a traumatic event that might pose a risk for OA. Furthermore, if we accept the notion that the cat progresses to "symptomatic OA" much slower than the dog, it would appear that rehabilitation strategies based on restoring normal joint mechanics would likely not prevent OA if initiated late in the rehabilitation process, but might slow down joint degeneration leading to symptomatic OA. This is a tragic conclusion insofar as most degenerative joint diseases are typically diagnosed at an advanced state only, when, according to our interpretation of the results, any mechanical or neuromuscular intervention is too late to prevent OA. Therefore diagnosing the possibility for joint degeneration needs to be done immediately upon an insult or trauma, and people at risk should be identified at an early age, as preventative measures might be much more powerful prior to the onset of OA compared to once a joint is painful. Therefore the identification of people at risk and the very early detection of joint degeneration and OA are likely of prime importance for the successful fight against this disease.

Muscle Forces and EMG

As indicated earlier (Fig. 8.6), ankle and knee extensor forces are dramatically reduced in the first few weeks following ACL transection in the cat. No muscle force measurements are available from any other experimental model of OA, nor have there been measurements months or years after intervention. However, it is trivial to show that a given direction and magnitude of the ground reaction force is associated with specific muscle force patterns,[35] assuming that there is no substantial amount of cocontraction. Therefore, since the external ground reaction forces and moments are, on average, back to normal at about 6 months following ACL transection in the cat, we may assume that the individual muscle forces are also similar prior to and about 6 months following

ACL transection. Electromyographical patterns of eight muscles in the cat hind limb are indistinguishable in terms of timing relative to the step cycle, the magnitude and the frequency content, 6 months following ACL transection compared to normal (unpublished observations).

One result concerning muscle forces and EMGs deserves further attention. In Fig. 8.6, it can be seen that gastrocnemius and quadriceps forces are reduced following ACL transection. But not only are the muscle forces reduced, they are also "jerky" rather than "smooth." When comparing the EMG patterns in the vastus lateralis (VL—one of the quadriceps muscles) before and after intervention, it is apparent that the continuous EMG during the stance phase prior to intervention changes to a 3–5 burst pattern during stance following intervention. This result suggests that the "jerkyness" of the knee extensor forces following intervention is caused by this burst-like (rather than the normal continuous) firing pattern. We assume that these individual bursts during stance represent a fight between an excitatory mechanism aimed at preventing the knee from collapsing and an inhibitory mechanism of unknown origin, possibly associated with the instability of the knee in the early phase following intervention. We further speculate that this perturbed activation pattern, which results in poorly coordinated muscle actions, and thus presumably poorly controlled fine mechanics of joint movement, might be the mechanism for triggering some of the degenerative responses that are seen quickly following joint perturbation. Again, this is an unproven idea but has some appeal in that it is well known that we lose fine muscle control with advanced age because of a diminishing number of motor units per muscle.[36] Thus one might speculate that OA in old age is not necessarily caused by the natural aging process of the articular cartilage, but is associated with the loss of fine motor control and thus presumably loss of smooth joint loading. This idea can readily be tested in an animal model of "smooth" versus "jerky" joint loading and, if our hypothesis is correct, would provide a novel way to treat joint degeneration in the elderly.

Joint Contact Pressure Distribution Patterns

In the most perfect world, joint loading would be described accurately by the instantaneous and time-evolving stress and strain states of all the individual tissues that make up a joint. However, that is not possible. An acceptable compromise to this perfect scenario would be the instantaneous and time-evolving pressure distribution patterns on the articular joint surfaces during normal movements. However, even such measurements have not been made to date, although pressure distributions and contact forces have been measured in artificial joints of select patients with instrumented joint prostheses.[37,38] We have measured the joint surface pressure distributions in the cat knee using Fuji pressure sensitive film for a variety of knee angles and knee extensor forces representing those observed during normal locomotion,[27,39] in normal and ACL deficient knees.

Among the many results, arguably the most important was that pressure distribution changed dramatically from pre to post ACL transection. In 38 measurements of joint contact patterns in five cats, we found that the contact areas in the patellofemoral joint increased by 22% ($\pm 37\%$), and the corresponding peak pressure decreased by 55% ($\pm 21\%$) at 16 weeks post ACL transection compared to the normal, contralateral joint (Fig. 8.8). This result demonstrated for the first time that joint contact loading changes quickly following ACL transection, and that a given resultant joint loading produces completely different pressure distribution patterns on the articular surfaces as joint degeneration proceeds.

The increase in contact area and the decrease in peak pressure observed in this study with the progression of disease could readily be explained by the increased thickness and decreased stiffness of the articular cartilage at 16 weeks post ACL transection.[27] This result illustrates two important points. First, measurement of ground reaction forces, and even muscular forces, says little about the local loading (stress–strain states) of the articular cartilage. However,

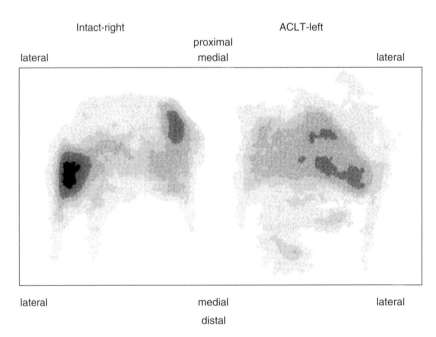

Figure 8.8. Pressure distribution in the patellofemoral joint of a cat 16 weeks post ACL transection. The contact area in the intact joint (Intact–right) is smaller, and the peak pressure (gray scale) is greater compared to the ACL transected joint (ACLT–left) for the same force across the joint. These results were statistically significant across measurements in five different cats (38 measurements total)

it is likely that local loading conditions are responsible for the differential joint degeneration observed experimentally; therefore understanding them is essential and should be a top priority for future research. Second, local loading conditions change continuously in a degenerating joint; thus the biological responses for a given load are likely changing too. The possibility that identical loading conditions in a normal and a diseased joint might produce completely different biological responses has not been investigated systematically but might contain important clues about how to slow down, stop, or even reverse joint degeneration.

Physiological Joint Loading and Biological Response

In order to elucidate the detailed mechanisms underlying joint degeneration leading to OA, it is essential that the in vivo local loading of the target joint is known. Aside from the standard measurements in humans and animal models of OA involving gait analysis, measurement of the external ground reaction forces, and possibly EMG, quantification of the muscle forces and pressure distribution patterns is possible and can provide much needed insight into the joint mechanics.

One of the properties associated with articular cartilage is that of damping impact forces. However, cartilage surface layers tend to be thin, a few millimeters at most in big mammalian joints, such as the human knee, but merely a fraction of a millimeter in most joints of midsized animals such as rabbits and cats. Therefore damping of impact forces is limited by the thickness of cartilage. When measuring the contact areas, peak pressures, and mean pressures in the cat patellofemoral joint for knee extensor forces ranging from normal everyday loading experienced during locomotion (50–200 N) to the maximal force that can be produced by nerve stimulation (about 500 N), we discovered that patellofemoral contact areas increased nonlinearly with knee extensor forces (Fig. 8.9A). Specifically, for physiologically relevant loading conditions (50–200 N), contact area increased with increasing loads by a factor of 5–10, while mean and peak pressures only increased by 25% and 71%, respectively.[29] This result suggests that one of the primary functions of cartilage may be to help increase contact area for increasing muscular loads to keep pressures low (Fig. 8.9B). When loading of the patellofemoral joint was maintained for either 2 s or 5 min, contact area increased by up to 33% for the 5 min loading condition, indicating that the viscoelastic properties of cartilage enable it to distribute loads over ever increasing surface areas to accommodate long-term joint loading by reducing local strains and pressures.[29]

The crucial question, however, remains: What are the biological responses of a joint to physiological or damaging loading conditions? In order to answer this question, we developed methods for artificial electrical nerve stimulation that allow for precisely controlled application of muscular forces to a joint.

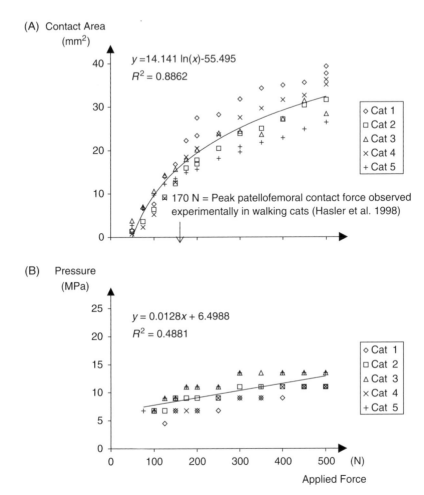

Figure 8.9. (A) Contact area as a function of applied force for five subjects under short duration load. Values calculated from low-grade Fuji pressure sensitive film. (B) Mean pressure as a function of applied force for five subjects under short duration load. Values are calculated from medium-grade film and plotted as the median value of the pressure range.

Specifically, we tested this approach in rabbit knee joints and stimulation of the knee extensor musculature through the femoral nerve.[40] In addition, we also developed an impact loading system in which the flexed rabbit patellofemoral joint can be impacted with any load in approximately 2 ms. This approach is similar to that described in the literature.[41,42]

Intermittent muscular loading of the patellofemoral joint over a 1 hour period (2 s of knee extensor stimulation every 30 s at about 50% of the total maximal isometric force) produced significant changes in mRNA expression of key proteins and proteinases.[40] Specifically, mRNA expression of TIMP-1 and MMP-3 (Fig. 8.10) was increased immediately following load application while bFGF was decreased compared to unloaded control specimens. Furthermore, these genes also exhibited a location-specific response (femur vs. patella). Similarly, biglycan, decorin, and aggrecan mRNA levels in response to long-term muscular joint loading were found to vary as a function of bone (femur vs. patella), indicating that not only loading but also the location of the articular cartilage within the joint played a significant role in the biological responses. We concluded from these results that not only the local loading changed within a joint but so did the biosynthetic responses of the cartilage, indicating that the relationship between joint loading and adaptive/degenerative changes in the joint is complex and needs careful investigation.

One of the proposed mechanisms for OA initiation and progression is the idea that joint loading causes cell death, and since the turnover time for chondrocytes is long, there might be insufficient active cells to maintain a healthy and strong cartilage matrix. In order to test cell viability following joint loading, we exposed rabbit patellofemoral joints to maximal muscular loading and impact loading of similar peak contact pressures. Maximal muscle loading was not associated with increased cell death while impact loading was, despite the similarity in load magnitudes (Fig. 8.11). However, the impact load was applied within about 2 ms, while muscular loading induced by supramaximal stimulation of the femoral nerve takes about 250 ms for full force development. Furthermore, impact loading on rabbit patellofemoral joints at 4 weeks post ACL transection (Impact loading ACLT—Fig. 8.11) resulted in increased cell death compared to the same impact load on normal knees, as did a 1 hour

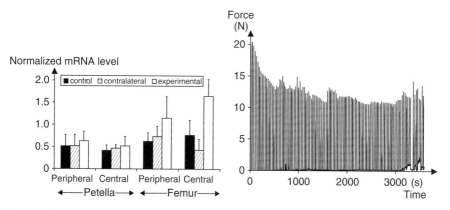

Figure 8.10. Normalized mRNA levels of metalloproteinase 3 (MMP3) from articular cartilage of central and peripheral regions of patella and femoral groove. The experimental samples were loaded in vivo for 1 hour as shown in the right panel. The contralateral knees and control knees from normal animals were used as unloaded controls.

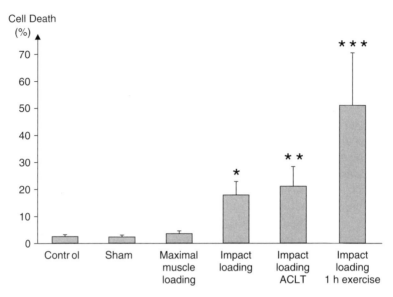

Figure 8.11. Percent cell death in the rabbit knee for control (control) animals, sham treated animals (sham), animals subjected to a 10 s maximal knee extensor contraction produced by supramaximal stimulation of the femoral nerve (maximal muscle loading), animals subjected to an impact load of 5 J energy applied to the intact, hyperflexed knee (impact loading), and animals subjected to impact loading at 4 weeks following anterior cruciate ligament transection (impact loading ACLT) and following a 1 hour, 20% of maximal voluntary contraction exercise bout (impact loading 1 h exercise).

exercise bout preceding impact loading (Fig. 8.11). We concluded from these results that the speed of load application (impact vs. muscular loading) plays a much more important role than the peak contact pressure. Furthermore, we concluded that cartilage that is in the initial phase of joint degeneration (4 weeks post ACL transection) is more vulnerable to cell death than cartilage in healthy control joints, and cartilage subjected to impact loading following exhaustive exercise is highly vulnerable to cell death.

Muscle Weakness

In the first part of this chapter, we described the important role of muscles in joint loading and provided evidence that neuromuscular malfunctioning produces conditions that may cause the onset of OA. Muscular atrophy has been an acknowledged factor associated with OA, and people with muscle weakness have been implicated as being at higher risk for OA than people with normal strength.[14,15] However, there is no direct evidence linking muscle weakness to joint degeneration.

Recently, we developed a first model of experimental muscle weakness aimed at investigating if muscle weakness indeed is an independent risk factor for the development of OA.[43] Rabbit knee extensor muscles were injected with botulinum toxin type-A (BTX-A). BTX-A inhibits acetylcholine release at the neuromuscular junction and thus inhibits muscle contraction in the presence of voluntary activation. A single injection of BTX-A of approximately 3.5 units per kilogram body mass resulted in muscle atrophy (Fig. 8.12), and a decrease in muscle strength of 70% that lasted for a 4 week period, and monthly repeat injections maintained muscle weakness for the 6 month experimental period (Fig. 8.13).[44] This muscle weakness model also resulted in decreased functional capacity as described by a reduction in the vertical ground reaction push off forces during rabbit hopping (Fig. 8.14).

The crucial question now remained if this model of muscle weakness was also associated with signs of joint degeneration. In order to test this hypothesis, we randomly assigned ten rabbits to a control ($n = 4$) or an experimental group ($n = 6$). The experimental group animals received a unilateral injection

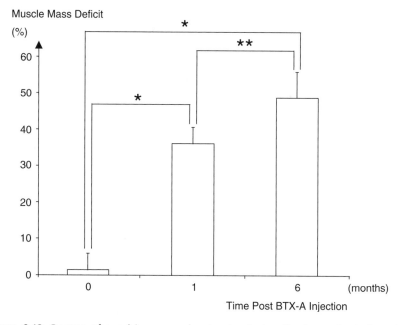

Figure 8.12. Degree of quadriceps muscle atrophy during the 6 month study period: percent muscle mass between the experimental and the corresponding contralateral control hind limb. Group means and standard deviations are shown. The 1 month and 6 month post BTX-A injections group had a significantly greater muscle mass deficit than that found between the hind limbs of control rabbits (*$p < 0.01$). Muscle mass deficit was significantly greater 6 months post BTX-A injections versus 1 month post injection (*$p < 0.02$).

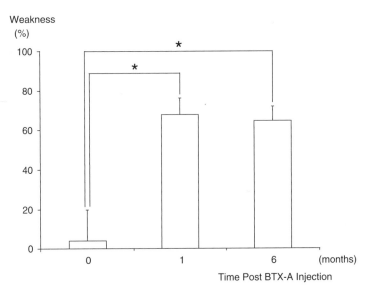

Figure 8.13. Percent muscle weakness during the 6 month study period. Percent weakness reflects the relative decrease in torque between experimental and contralateral hind limb. Group means and standard deviations are shown. The 1 month and 6 month post BTX-A injections groups had significantly greater muscle weakness than the control group (*$p < 0.01$).

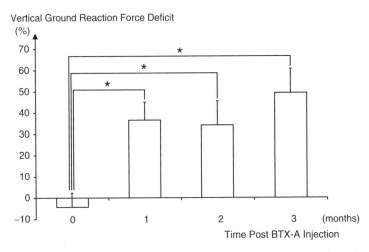

Figure 8.14. Vertical ground reaction force deficits during the 6 month study period. Percent force deficit reflects the relative decreases in vertical ground reaction force between the experimental and the corresponding contralateral control hind limb at push-off. Group means and standard deviations are shown. Significantly greater deficits in vertical ground reaction forces were found at 1 month, 3 month, and 6 month post BTX-A injections when compared to controls (*$p < 0.01$).

of BTX-A into the quadriceps musculature as described previously. The control animals received a unilateral injection of physiological saline of equal volume. Four weeks following BTX-A injections, muscle atrophy and weakness were present as shown earlier.[43] But in addition, histological evaluation of the retropatellar surface cartilage using a modified Mankin scoring system revealed significantly increased degeneration in the experimental compared to the control group animals. We conclude from these results that muscle weakness is an independent risk factor for the onset of joint degeneration leading to OA. However, we cannot distinguish if this result was obtained because of the functional changes in hind limb use associated with muscle weakness or because of the muscle weakness itself.

CONCLUSION

Osteoarthritis is associated with joint loading. However, little is known about the local loading of intact joints under physiologically relevant conditions, such as locomotion and other everyday movement conditions. Therefore it is of utmost importance for biomechanics researchers to develop approaches for the accurate measurement or theoretical determination of local loading conditions in joints. Once these mechanical conditions are known, they can be related to clinical or scientific measures of onset and progression of joint degeneration leading to OA. Such results might hold the key to understanding the intricate and changing relationship between mechanical loading of joints and the associated biological (adaptive and degenerative) responses.

REFERENCES

1. Andrews JG. (1974). Biomechanical analysis of human motion. Kinesiology 4: 32–42.
2. Crowninshield RD, Brand RA. (1981). The prediction of forces in joint structures: distribution of intersegmental resultants. Exerc Sport Sci Rev 159–181.
3. Herzog W. (1996). Force-sharing among synergistic muscles: theoretical considerations and experimental approaches. In Holloszy JO (ed.). *Exercise and Sport Sciences Reviews*. Baltimore: Williams & Wilkins, pp. 173–202.
4. Ait-Haddou R, Jinha A, Herzog W, Binding P. (2004). Analysis of the force-sharing problem using an optimization model. Math Biosci 191:111–122.
5. Brandt KD, Myers SL, Burr D, Albrecht M. (1991). Osteoarthritic changes in canine articular cartilage, subchondral bone, and synovium fifty-four months after transection of the anterior cruciate ligament. Arthritis Rheum 34:1560–1570.

6. Burton-Wurster N, Vernier-Singer M, Farquhar T, Lust G. (1993). Effect of compressive loading and unloading on the synthesis of total protein, proteoglycan, and fibronectin by canine cartilage explants. J Orthop Res 11:717–729.

7. Quinn TM, Grodzinsky AJ, Buschmann MD, Kim YJ, Hunziker EB. (1998). Mechanical compression alters proteoglycan deposition and matrix deformation around individual cells in cartilage explants. J Cell Sci 111:573–583.

8. Sah RL, Kim YL, Doong J-YH, Grodzinsky AJ, Plaas AHK, Sandy JD. (1989). Biosynthetic response of cartilage explants to dynamic compression. J Orthop Res 7:619–636.

9. Torzilli PA, Grigiene R, Huang C, Friedman SM, Doty SB, Boskey AL, Lust G. (1997). Characterization of cartilage metabolic response to static and dynamic stress using a mechanical explant test system. J Biomech 30:1–9.

10. Guilak F, Sah RL, Setton LA. (1997). Physical regulation of cartilage metabolism. In Mow VC and Hayes WC (eds.). *Basic Orthopaedics Biomechanics*. Philadelphia: Lippincott-Raven Publishers, pp. 179–207.

11. Hasler EM, Herzog W, Wu JZ, Muller W, Wyss U. (1999). Articular cartilage biomechanics: theoretical models, material properties, and biosynthetic response. Crit Rev Biomed Eng 27(6):415–488.

12. Mow VC, Bachrach NM, Setton LA, Guilak F. (1994). Stress, strain, pressure and flow fields in articular cartilage and chondrocytes. In Mow VC, Guilak F, Tran-Son-Tray R, and Hochmuth RM (eds.). *Cell Mechanics and Cellular Engineering*. New York: Springer Verlag, pp. 345–379.

13. Sah RL, Grodzinsky AJ, Plaas AHK, Sandy JD. (1992). Effects of static and dynamic compression on matrix metabolism in cartilage explants. In Kuettner K, Peyron JG, Schleyerbach R, and Hascall VC (eds.). *Articular Cartilage and Osteoarthritis*. New York: Raven Press, pp. 373–392.

14. Slemenda C, Brandt KD, Heilman DK, Mazzuca S, Braunstein EM, Katz BP, Wolinsky FD. (1997). Quadriceps weakness and osteoarthritis of the knee. Ann Intern Med 127:97–104.

15. Slemenda C, Heilman DK, Brandt KD, Katz BP, Mazzuca S, Braunstein EM, Byrd D. (1998). Reduced quadriceps strength relative to body weight. A risk factor for knee osteoarthritis in women? Arthritis Rheum 41:1951–1959.

16. Brandt KD, Braunstein EM, Visco DM, O'Connor B, Heck D, Albrecht M. (1991). Anterior (cranial) cruciate ligament transection in the dog: a bona fide model of osteoarthritis, not merely of cartilage injury and repair. J Rheumatol 18: 436–446.

17. Suter E, Herzog W, Leonard TR, Nguyen H. (1998). One-year changes in hindlimb kinematics, ground reaction forces and knee stability in an experimental model of osteoarthritis. J Biomech 31:511–517.

18. Herzog W, Adams ME, Matyas JR, Brooks JG. (1993). A preliminary study of hindlimb loading, morphology and biochemistry of articular cartilage in the ACL-deficient cat knee. Osteoarthritis Cart 1:243–251.

19. Maitland ME, Leonard TR, Frank CB, Shrive NG, Herzog W. (1998). Method to assess in vivo knee stability longitudinally in an animal model of ligament injury. J Orthop Res 16:441–447.

20. Kaya M, Leonard TR, Herzog W. (2008). Premature deactivation of soleus during the propulsive phase of cat jumping. J R Soc Interface 5:415–426. DOI: 10.1098/rsif.2007.1158.

21. Goslow GE, Reinking RM, Stuart DG. (1973). The cat step cycle: hind limb joint angles and muscle lengths during unrestrained locomotion. J Morphol 141:1–42.

22. Walmsley B, Hodgson JA, Burke RE. (1978). Forces produced by medial gastrocnemius and soleus muscles during locomotion in freely moving cats. J Neurophysiol 41:1203–1215.

23. Xu WS, Butler DL, Stouffer DC, Grood ES, Glos DL. (1992). Theoretical analysis of an implantable force transducer for tendon and ligament structures. J Biomech Eng 114:170–177.

24. Herzog W, Hasler EM, Leonard TR. (1996). In-situ calibration of the implantable force transducer. J Biomech 29:1649–1652.

25. Hasler EM, Herzog W, Leonard TR, Stano A, Nguyen H. (1998). In-vivo knee joint loading and kinematics before and after ACL transection in an animal model. J Biomech 31:253–262.

26. Guimaraes ACS, Herzog W, Allinger TL, Zhang YT. (1995). The EMG–force relationship of the cat soleus muscle and its association with contractile conditions during locomotion. J Exp Biol 198:975–987.

27. Herzog W, Diet S, Suter E, Mayzus P, Leonard TR, Muller C, Wu JZ, Epstein M. (1998). Material and functional properties of articular cartilage and patellofemoral contact mechanics in an experimental model of osteoarthritis. J Biomech 31:1137–1145.

28. Liggins AB, Hardie WR, Finlay JB. (1995). The spatial and pressure resolution of Fuji pressure-sensitive film. Exp Mech 35:166–173.

29. Clark AL, Herzog W, Leonard TR. (2002). Contact area distribution in the feline patellofemoral joint under physiologically meaningful loading conditions. J Biomech 35:53–60.

30. Maitland ME, Leonard TR, Frank CB, Shrive NG, Herzog W. (1998). Longitudinal measurement of tibial motion relative to the femur during passive displacements and femoral nerve stimulation in the ACL-deficient cat model of osteoarthritis. J Orthop Res 16:448–454.

31. Tashman S, DuPré K, Goitz H, Lock T, Kolowich P, Flynn M. (1995). A digital radiographic system for determining 3D joint kinematics during movement. Am Soc Biomech 249–250.

32. Korvick DL, Pijanowski GJ, Schaeffer DJ. (1994). Three-dimensional kinematics of the intact and cranial cruciate ligament-deficient stifle of dogs. J Biomech 27:77–87.

33. Maitland ME. (1996). Longitudinal measurement of tibial motion relative to the femur during passive displacements and femoral nerve stimulation in the ACL-deficient cat model of osteoarthritis. University of Calgary, Calgary, AB, Canada.

34. Adams ME. (1989). Cartilage hypertrophy following canine anterior cruciate ligament transection differs among different areas of the joint. J Rheumatol 16:818–824.

35. Kaya M, Leonard TR, Herzog W. (2006). Control of ground reaction forces by hindlimb muscles during cat locomotion. J Biomech 39:2752–2766.

36. McComas AJ. (1996). *Skeletal Muscle: Form and Function*. Champaign, IL: Human Kinetics.

37. Bergmann G, Graichen F, Rohlmann A. (1993). Hip joint loading during walking and running, measured in two patients. J Biomech 26(8):969–990.

38. Krebs DE, Elbaum L, Riley PO, Hodge WA, Mann RW. (1991). Exercise and gait effects on in vivo hip contact pressures. Phys Ther 71:301–309.

39. Herzog W, Hasler EM, Leonard TR. (2000). Experimental determination of in vivo pressure distribution in biologic joints. J Musculoskel Res 4(1):1–7.

40. Clark A, Mills L, Hart DA, Herzog W. (2004). Muscle-induced patellofemoral joint loading rapidly affects cartilage mRNA levels in a site specific manner. J Musculoskel Res 8(1):1–12.

41. Ewers BJ, Newberry WN, Haut RC. (2000). Chronic softening of cartilage without thickening of underlying bone in a joint trauma model. J Biomech 33:1689–1694.

42. Haut RC, Ide TM, De Camp CE. (1995). Mechanical responses of the rabbit patello-femoral joint to blunt impact. J Biomech Eng 117:402–408.

43. Longino D, Frank CB, Leonard TR, Herzog W. (2005). Proposed model of botulinum toxin-induced muscle weakness in the rabbit. J Orthop Res 23: 1411–1418.

44. Longino D, Frank C, Herzog W. (2005). Acute botulinum toxin-induced muscle weakness in the anterior cruciate ligament-deficient rabbit. J Orthop Res 23: 1404–1410.

9

NEUROMUSCULAR ASPECTS OF OSTEOARTHRITIS

Kenneth D. Brandt

Kansas University Medical Center, 5755 Windsor Drive, Fairway, Kansas 66205, USA

INTRODUCTION

In contrast to other types of arthritis, osteoarthritis (OA) is a mechanically induced disease that occurs when the level of mechanical stress exceeds the capacity of the shock-absorbing mechanisms of the joint. For the clinician, the overriding neuromuscular problem associated with OA is joint *pain;* if it were not painful, OA would receive little attention. Epidemiologic data suggest that reduction of excessive mechanical stress (e.g., by prevention of obesity and traumatic injury and by modification of workplace ergonomics) would significantly reduce the incidence of OA of the hip and knee. In clinical trials, nonpharmacologic interventions that modulate stress on the OA joint and improve joint physiology have been shown to relieve OA pain.

In patients with OA, proprioceptive acuity may be impaired as a result of local joint pathology, but diminished proprioception may also be the result of

Pain in Osteoarthritis, Edited by David T. Felson and Hans-Georg Schaible
Copyright © 2009 Wiley-Blackwell.

157

an underlying generalized neurologic deficit, which, by impairing protective muscular reflexes, increases the mechanical stress on joints.

Similarly, quadriceps weakness often develops as a consequence of painful knee OA but because the muscle is an important stabilizer of the knee joint and the major antigravity muscle in the lower extremity, by increasing impulsive loading of the knee during gait, quadriceps weakness may also be a risk factor for incident knee OA.

Current pharmacologic treatment of OA pain with analgesics and nonsteroidal anti-inflammatory drugs is often unsatisfactory because of lack of efficacy and adverse effects. Despite treatment with therapeutic doses of such drugs, many patients still have OA pain, raising the question of whether an element of their pain is neurogenic in origin, with peripheral and central sensitization. This has led to the investigation of new mechanism-based therapeutic approaches for OA pain, such as intra-articular injection of botulinum toxin.

This chapter is a sequel to one that was published in the proceedings of a 2003 Novartis Foundation Symposium on OA pain.[1] However, although it notes some of the recent basic and clinical research that is relevant to the neuromuscular aspects of OA, it differs considerably from its predecessor insofar as it reflects the views of a physician who has treated patients with OA for many years.

For the clinician, the overriding neuromuscular problem associated with OA is joint *pain*. If OA were not painful, it would receive little attention. Liang[2] succinctly framed the issue: "X-rays don't weep." Patients weep.

As pointed out by Hadler,[3] at all ages more people suffer knee pain than exhibit radiographic evidence of OA. Although it is somewhat more likely that those with more severe X-ray changes will have difficulty with mobility, the radiographic progression of OA is usually slow and the course unpredictable. Symptoms of knee OA wax and wane independent of radiographic progression.[4] Among subjects with far advanced X-ray changes of hip OA, nearly 50% may not have hip pain.[5,6] Still, the prevalence of radiographic OA is very high: the Framingham study suggested that radiographic OA occurred in 33% of people who were age 63 and older.[7] Even if joint pain occurs in only a minority, it presents a major public health problem with enormous medicoeconomic and socioeconomic costs. Biochemists and molecular biologists studying cartilage or bone from OA joints, radiologists imaging OA joints, and researchers assaying biologic fluids for molecules derived from OA joints have yet to explain why some are painful and others painless. Anxiety, depression, and quadriceps weakness may be better predictors of pain in subjects with knee OA than the severity of radiographic changes.[8]

Unlike the therapeutic successes we have achieved with disease-modifying drugs (DMARDs) and biologicals for rheumatoid arthritis, efforts to develop disease-modifying OA drugs (DMOADs, formerly called chondroprotective drugs and now called also structure-modifying OA drugs (SMOADs)) that can interrupt or reverse the pathogenetic processes underlying OA have not been unambiguously successful.[9,10] We have contended that the reason for this lack of success is our failure to appreciate sufficiently that garden-variety OA, from its earliest stages and in whichever joint it occurs, is a *mechanically induced disease.*[10]

Normally, articular cartilage is protected from excessive loads by the periarticular muscle and underlying subchondral bone, which serve as active and passive shock absorbers, respectively. The mechanical factors that cause OA and result in its progression can be developmental or genetic in origin or can arise as the result of previous trauma or joint infection. Regardless of the basis, if the stress (force/unit area) on the joint exceeds the physiologic limits (e.g., with obesity, varus–valgus malalignment, or meniscus damage) and overwhelms the protective mechanisms, OA will develop. Idiopathic, garden-variety OA resembles OA that results from, for example, obesity, joint instability, or an inadequately treated staphylococcal infection of the joint.

Most of the stress on joints is generated by contraction of the muscles that span the joint, not by body weight. Because the thickness of the articular cartilage and subchondral bone in an interphalangeal joint is small, contraction of the powerful finger flexor muscles may produce stresses on it that are as great as, or greater than, those in a knee or hip.[11] This may be a factor in the development of Heberden's nodes, especially if the collateral ligaments are damaged.[12]

In OA, an abnormal concentration of stress on habitually loaded areas of the joint provokes biochemically mediated local joint damage by stimulating the synthesis and release of tissue-degrading enzymes and toxic oxygen radicals by chondrocytes and other cells. Although the most obvious pathologic changes in an OA joint are usually seen in the articular cartilage, all of the tissues of the joint are involved, including bone, synovium, muscles, nerves, and ligaments. The site of origin of OA pain, however, may vary from patient to patient and, within the same patient, from visit to visit (Table 9.1).

The likelihood that a drug that inhibits a specific enzyme or cytokine in the pathways of cartilage breakdown or further stimulates the already active synthesis of cartilage matrix molecules will solve the problem of painful OA is, in our view, small.[10,13] Because cartilage repair cannot deal with the

TABLE 9.1 Origins of Joint Pain in Patients with OA

Tissue	Mechanism(s) of Pain
Subchondral bone	Medullary hypertension, microfractures
Osteophytes	Stretching of nerve endings in periosteum
Ligaments	Stretch
Entheses	Inflammation
Joint capsule	Distension, inflammation
Periarticular muscle	Spasm
Synovium	Inflammation
Articular cartilage(?)	Mechanical stress (?)

underlying mechanical abnormality, it cannot solve the problem of OA. Remodeling of the subchondral bone may mitigate the underlying mechanical abnormality but, in doing so, may cause joint pain.

Unless the abnormal stresses on the joint are corrected, it is unlikely that the progression of damage will be interrupted or reversed pharmacologically. Indeed, if they *are* corrected, pharmacologic intervention may be superfluous. Regardless of the potential to generate new cartilage or to inhibit further breakdown of OA cartilage that a drug may exhibit in vitro or in relatively short-term preclinical studies in vivo, in the patient, the joint will continue to exist in the adverse mechanical environment that got it into trouble in the first place.[13] Furthermore, there is no assurance that a drug that slowed the progression of structural damage in an OA joint would have a beneficial effect on the patient's symptoms.

A decade ago, considering risk factors for OA from an epidemiologic perspective and strategies for prevention of OA in the hip or knee, Felson[14] reckoned that elimination of obesity, prevention of knee injury, and elimination of jobs requiring knee bending and carrying heavy loads—each of which can cause increased stress on the joints under consideration—would decrease the incidence of OA in those joints. We contend that such considerations are important not only for the prevention of incident OA but also in the treatment of established OA. Given the current interest in development of SMOADs, consider the following selected examples of pain relief in OA by mechanical (i.e., physiologic) rather than pharmacologic interventions.

Patients with knee OA who undergo valgus osteotomy—a *nonpharmacologic* approach to alter the mechanical stresses across the joint—report relief of knee pain on follow-up exam. Clinical improvement is unrelated to whether the hyaline articular cartilage remains unchanged from baseline, shows worsening of OA pathology, or is replaced with fibrocartilage.[15] As further evidence that OA is not a cartilage disease,[13] consider the slide in the 1972 Arthritis Foundation Clinical Teaching Collection[16] of a histologic section through a Heberden's node from a patient with nodal OA. Bony hypertrophy (osteophyte) is apparent at the articular margin of the distal phalanx but the thicknesses of the articular cartilages on both sides of the joint space are normal and the cartilage surfaces are intact (Fig. 9.1).

A recent systematic review and meta-analysis of patellar taping for patellofemoral OA provides a further example of successful treatment of painful OA with a mechanical intervention.[17] In three studies, taping of patients with symptomatic radiographic patellofemoral OA, to exert a medially directed force on the patella, decreased chronic knee pain in comparison with no taping or sham taping (in both cases, $p \leq 0.001$). The results are consistent with evidence that anterior knee pain in patients with patellofemoral OA is due to lateral displacement of the patella, relative to the trochlear groove, with increased loading of the lateral facet of the patella.[18]

In subjects with relatively mild structural changes of knee OA, those with knee pain had significantly higher medial compartment loads than those who

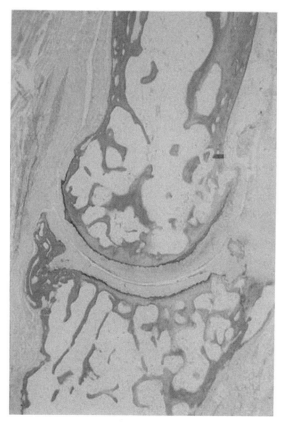

Figure 9.1. Section through a distal interphalangeal joint of a patient with nodal OA, showing a prominent dorsal osteophyte. Note the normal thickness and intact surface of the articular cartilage on both sides of the joint space. (Used with permission of the American College of Rheumatology.)

were asymptomatic, whereas medial compartment loads in those who were asymptomatic were no different from those in normal controls. The results suggest that, at this stage of structural damage, individuals with symptomatic OA differ biomechanically from those with asymptomatic disease.[19]

Interest has focused on the importance in knee OA of the peak adduction moment, which is considered to be a proxy for the dynamic load on the tibiofemoral joint.[20] Cross-sectional studies have shown that the peak adductor moment is significantly greater in patients with medial compartment knee OA than in controls and in patients with more severe OA than in those with less severe disease.[21,22] Longitudinal studies suggest that the peak adductor moment strongly predicts radiographic progression in patients with medial compartment OA[23] and the development of knee pain in asymptomatic older subjects.[24]

PROPRIOCEPTION

Awareness by the central nervous system (CNS) of the position of a joint in space generates muscle activity that results in the control of movement and stability of the joint and protects it from injury. Periarticular muscle is not only an effector organ that is essential for movement of a joint, but is also an important sensory organ by virtue of its content of highly specialized sensory nerve endings (muscle spindles). The afferent fibers of muscle spindles, like receptors in tendons, joint capsule, ligaments, horns of the menisci, and skin, provide proprioceptive input that contributes to protective muscular reflexes and to voluntary muscle activity. Proprioceptive impulses are transmitted through the dorsal root ganglion into the spinal cord, where reflexes are established whose efferent arm is a motor nerve to periarticular muscle.

Proprioceptive activity diminishes with age, and in subjects with unilateral knee OA, proprioception is less accurate—even in the apparently normal contralateral knee—than in nonarthritic controls. In patients who, on clinical and radiographic grounds, were considered to have unilateral knee OA, reduction in proprioception has been shown to be present bilaterally.[25] Furthermore, impairment of proprioception at the knee of patients with knee OA has been shown to be present also at the elbows,[26] raising the possibility that a subclinical neurological defect is of etiological importance in some subjects with idiopathic knee OA, as had been suggested previously.[27]

Recently, it was shown that poor knee joint proprioception in patients with knee OA was related to limitation of function (walking time, $r = 0.30$; Get Up and Go time, $r = 0.30$; WOMAC physical function subscale, $r = 0.26$, $p < 0.05$ for each).[28] Although the strength of the association between impairment of function and impairment of proprioception in patients with OA was only modest, among OA patients with poor proprioception, reduction of lower extremity muscle strength increased the severity of the functional impairment.

Although proprioception may be improved with elastic bandages, knee sleeves, orthoses, and exercise, whether improving proprioception has beneficial effects on joint pain, function, or progression of structural damage in OA is unclear. Experimental evidence indicates that normal joints are protected from damage even after they have been deprived of ipsilateral sensory input, suggesting that reprogramming of the central nervous system may occur after joint damage.[29]

The rate of impulsive loading of the knee, and not only the magnitude of the load, appears to be important in causing joint damage.[30] Proprioception involves neural pathways that originate peripherally in articular or periarticular structures, with afferent impulses traveling through the dorsal root ganglia and ascending via the dorsal columns of the spinal cord to the cerebellum and sensory cortex. In contrast, central pattern generators (CPGs), which can coordinate locomotor movements in the absence of movement-related afferent feedback, can be activated much more rapidly.[31] Johansson and Sjölander[32] concluded that the time required for a nerve impulse from a mechanoreceptor in a joint to travel proximally to activate a protective contraction of periarticular muscle was too long to prevent the potentially damaging movement. The importance of neural protective mechanisms other than proprioception in protecting normal and arthritic joints from damage awaits further elucidation.

QUADRICEPS WEAKNESS

Periarticular Muscle as a Shock Absorber for the Knee Joint

The bodys active shock-absorbing mechanisms for joints are associated with the use of muscles and joint motion in "negative work". Although contraction of muscles can move a joint, muscles can also act as large rubber bands. When a slightly stretched muscle is subjected to greater stretch as a result of movement of a joint, it can absorb a large amount of energy. Most of the muscle activity generated during activity is not used to propel the body forward but to absorb energy to decelerate the body.

For example, when we jump off a ledge or table, we normally land on our toes, come down on our heels, and straighten our flexed knees and hips. During this smooth action our muscles perform negative work, that is, they absorb energy. As we dorsiflex our ankles, we stretch our calf muscles; as we straighten our knees, we flex our quadriceps muscle; as we straighten our hips, we stretch our hamstrings. The amount of energy absorbed by this is enormous.[33] The energy produced by normal walking is sufficient to tear all the ligaments of the knee; that this does not occur routinely attests to the importance and effectiveness of this active energy absorption mechanism in the muscles that surround our joints and cushion them from mechanical stress.

Small, unexpected loads for which we are unprepared are much more damaging to joints than large ones that we have anticipated. Consider what happens when we come down stairs, misjudge a step, and abruptly slip a couple of steps. Because our muscles are not prepared to accommodate the load, we feel a sharp jolt. To prepare a neuromuscular reflex to handle an impact load requires approximately 75 ms. Therefore a fall of very brief duration (e.g., of only about 1 inch) does not afford sufficient time to bring protective muscular reflexes into play. Under such conditions, the load is transmitted to the cartilage and bone. In contrast, during a fall from a greater height, sufficient time is available for activation of the appropriate reflexes so that the energy of impact is absorbed by the lengthening of the muscles surrounding the joint and movement of the joint, and the articular cartilage is protected.[34]

As indicated previously, not only the magnitude but also the *rate* of loading of a joint is important with respect to the possibility of damage. Experimentally, repetitive acute (e.g., 50 ms, onset to peak) impulsive loading results in damage to articular cartilage and subchondral bone of the knee, whereas loads of greater magnitude, if applied more gradually (500 ms, onset to peak), are not detrimental.[30] Rapid delivery of load does not permit sufficient time for activation of the muscles surrounding the joint, which are the major shock absorbers protecting the joint.

Implications for Osteoarthritis

Muscle weakness, due to disuse atrophy or reflex inhibition,[35] both of which may occur in association with OA, or an increase in the latent period of the reflex (which may occur with peripheral neuropathy due to aging or other causes) will reduce the effectiveness of this shock-absorbing mechanism.

The quadriceps muscle protects the knee from mechanical damage by virtue of the fact that it is the major antigravity muscle of the lower extremity and serves as a brake on the pendular action of the lower limb during ambulation, thereby minimizing the forces generated with heelstrike. In addition, it is important in stabilizing the knee joint. After a femoral nerve block (to temporarily paralyze the quadriceps), the load rate in normal subjects who had no force-transient profile during gait increased more than twofold—to approximately $150 \times$ body weight/second,[36] suggesting that a force transient can be caused by failure to decelerate the lower extremity prior to heelstrike. In normal individuals, minor incoordination in muscle recruitment, resulting in failure to decelerate the leg, may generate impulsive forces at the knee with heelstrike that are as high as $65 \times$ body weight/second. Whether this micro-incoordination of neuromuscular control, which has been called "microklutzi-ness,"[36] is a risk factor for knee OA remains to be established.

While the periarticular muscles serve a primary motor function, Hurley[37] has emphasized the importance of the *sensory* function of muscle and the proprio-ceptive impulses that originate in muscle and are transmitted to the central nervous system. Data suggest that muscle weakness due either to disuse atrophy or reflex inhibition of muscle contraction because of intra-articular pathology could result in joint degeneration.

In patients with knee OA, quadriceps weakness is common. Often, atrophy of the muscle is obvious from the concave appearance of the anterior thigh. The general view is that the atrophy is due to disuse that is the result of painful arthritis, which has led the patient to avoid loadbearing on the extremity in order to avoid discomfort. However, in a study of older individuals living in communities in central Indiana who had not seen the need to seek medical care for knee pain, felt they were doing as well as, or better than, their peers, and had normal knee X-rays, we found that decreased quadriceps strength in women, but not in men, was associated with development of radiographic knee OA: that is, weakness was a risk factor for, rather than the result of, knee OA.[38] It has been shown that a weak quadriceps results in an increase in the stress transient at the knee during heelstrike,[39] immediately prior to which quadriceps action decelerates the pendulum action of the lower extremity.

In contrast to the evidence that quadriceps weakness is a risk factor for incident radiographic OA of the knee in women, it did not increase the risk of X-ray progression among women with established radiographic OA.[40] Sharma et al.[41] found, similarly, that quadriceps weakness was not generally associated with radiographic progression of OA. However, among subjects with knee OA who had varus–valgus malalignment or knee laxity, the investigators found that greater quadriceps strength was associated with an *increased* rate of radiographic progression.

In a cross-sectional study of nearly 2500 subjects at least 60 years old who were enrolled in the Beijing Osteoarthritis Study, isometric quadriceps weakness was related to tibiofemoral and patellofemoral OA, with the strongest association occurring in subjects with mixed tibiofemoral and patellofemoral X-ray changes.[42] Pain may have contributed to some of the weakness, but even after the exclusion of subjects with knee pain, the relationship between muscle weakness and mixed tibiofemoral and patellofemoral OA remained significant.

Among patients with knee OA who had high degrees of varus–valgus laxity, van der Esch et al.[43] found that the relationship between lower extremity muscle strength and functional ability, as assessed by the Western Ontario and McMaster Universities Osteoarthritis Index (WOMAC) and 100 m walk time, was stronger than in those with lesser degrees of laxity. The authors concluded that among patients with knee OA who have high grade laxity, those who also have lower extremity weakness were at greatest risk of being disabled. As noted previously,[28] reduction of muscle strength increases the severity of functional impairment also among patients with knee OA who have impaired proprioception.

Knee pain in subjects with radiographic OA was shown to have a negative association with quadriceps strength, postural sway, and disability in comparison with radiographic OA in the absence of symptoms. However, in comparison with normal subjects, pain-free radiographic OA had a significant negative effect on quadriceps strength and disability.[44] In comparison with normals, all subjects with knee pain and/or radiographic OA exhibited quadriceps weakness ($p < 0.01$), but intergroup differences in weakness were not significant.

To the patient with OA, especially if elderly, quadriceps weakness poses the threat of falling, with the possible serious consequences of fracture,[45] subdural hematoma, and so on, especially if the patient is taking an anticoagulant. Li and Aspden[46] and Grynpas et al.[47] have shown that the subchondral cortical bone and cortical bone from patients with OA is less highly mineralized than that from age-matched controls. Thus, although the amount of bone is increased in OA (as reflected, e.g., by the increased density (sclerosis) of subchondral bone on the radiograph), from a material standpoint bone density is *decreased*. This may help, in part, to explain the increased fracture risk in people with knee OA. Buckling (i.e., giving way of the knee) may lead to falls, may occur in the presence or absence of knee pain, and may create functional limitations (e.g., in stair climbing) in people with knee OA.[48]

Can exercise, in addition to improving symptoms in patients with OA, improve structural joint damage? Roos and Dahlberg[49] reported that, in a randomized, placebo-controlled, 4 month clinical trial of moderate intensity neuromuscular and aerobic training in patients who had previously undergone a partial medial meniscectomy and had structurally mild knee OA, the glycosaminoglycan concentration of knee articular cartilage, based on changes in delayed gadolinium-enhanced magnetic resonance imaging (dGEMRIC), increased relative to that of the control subjects. The differences were most apparent when examined in relation to self-reported change in the physical activity level during the study. Notably, however, the exercise group and controls did not differ significantly at either baseline or after 4 months of participation with respect to aerobic capacity, quadriceps strength, or muscular performance tests, except for significantly greater improvement in one-leg jumps by the exercise group. Whether the improvement in dGEMRIC could be sustained over longer periods or the progression of structural damage in the OA joint could be delayed, and whether the increase in glycosaminoglycan concentration was accompanied by an improvement in the mechanics of the OA cartilage in load-bearing, however, remain to be shown.

NEUROGENIC ARTHRITIS

A variety of inflammatory mediators (e.g., prostaglandins, thromboxanes, leukotrienes, kinins) are present in synovial fluid from OA joints. Intra-articular injection of these mediators directly enhances the response of joint afferent fibers to pressure or mechanical stimuli.[50] Afferent nerve fibers containing neuropeptides, for example, substance P and calcitonin gene related peptide (CGRP), are common in joint tissues and evidence suggests that release of these peptides is directly involved in "neurogenic arthritis,"[51] which occurs as the result of the stimulation by these neuropeptides of chemotaxis, neutrophil activation, mast cell degranulation, and fibroblast proliferation, that is, features of the inflammatory response. The severity of experimentally induced acute synovitis was reduced significantly in animals that were pre-treated with capsaicin, which depletes substance P from nerve endings, or with a substance P antagonist.[52]

Peripheral and Central Sensitization in Osteoarthritis Pain

Neuropeptides sensitize nociceptive terminals within the joint (peripheral sensitization), increasing joint pain in response to chemical and mechanical stimuli.[50] Under these conditions, stimuli that are not normally painful cause pain (allodynia), those that are normally painful become more painful than usual (hyperalgesia), and sensory stimuli may be perceived in an exaggerated fashion (hyperesthesia). Although the importance of substance P in the pathogenesis of joint inflammation in OA is not clear, it plays an important role in mediating joint pain in this disease OA and its pharmacologic inhibition may be useful in palliating OA pain.

Central sensitization has been suggested as a basis for the residual joint pain experienced by patients with OA whose joint pain is not adequately relieved by NSAIDs and simple analgesics. The concept of central sensitization relates to sustained pain that is present despite only mild tissue damage and appears to depend on persistent transmission from local nociceptors to the dorsal horn of the spinal cord.[53] With central sensitization, sustained sensory input from C and A-δ afferents originating in the periphery (e.g., joint) depolarizes dorsal horn neurons so that Mg^{2+} is released from N-methyl-D-aspartate (NMDA)-linked ion channels. Release of Mg^{2+} is followed by an influx of extracellular Ca^{2+} and generation of nitric oxide (NO), which promotes the exaggerated release of excitatory amino acids and substance P from the termini of presynaptic afferent neurons, causing hyperexcitability of the dorsal horn neurons.

In addition, glial cells in the spinal cord may become activated and release proinflammatory cytokines, excitatory amino acids, and CGRP, all of which increase the depolarization of NMDA receptor sites in the dorsal horn.[54] As a consequence, neurons in the cord that project to the brain become hyperexcitable; that is, their threshold for firing is lowered and their receptor fields are enlarged so that stimuli of modest intensity now produce greatly augmented transmission of nociceptive impulses to the brain, resulting in enhanced pain sensitivity from stimuli arising at the site of original injury (the joint), and also more generally. For example, patients with painful unilateral hip OA may exhibit a diminished threshold to a painful stimulus in the area around the normal contralateral hip.[55]

Some unexpected results obtained in the acetaminophen (ACET) control arm of a small uncontrolled study, whose purpose was to assess the sensitivity of quantitative MRI in evaluating synovial changes in response to NSAID treatment of painful knee OA, may provide some insight into neurogenic inflammation in OA.[56] We found that therapeutic doses of acetaminophen (ACET) reduced the total synovial effusion volume and synovial tissue volume to a degree comparable to that seen in patients treated with a variety of NSAIDs. Severity of the flare of joint pain after drug washout was similar in both groups and reinstitution of the patient's previous treatment resulted in a substantial (50%) decrease in pain in both treatment groups. The mean total effusion volume measured during the flare of knee pain was similar in the two groups (approx. 16–17 mL) and similar decreases in effusion volume were observed after reinstitution of either ACET or NSAID (approx. 4 mL, respectively, p = not significant).

These findings suggested that ACET had a significant anti-inflammatory action in these patients with knee OA, leading us to speculate that it may have suppressed neurogenic inflammation. The results are consistent with the reduction of jaw swelling after administration of ACET in placebo-controlled trials of dental patients after third molar extraction.[57,58]

ACET has been shown to interfere with nociception-associated spinal activation of NMDA receptors through inhibition of spinal nitric oxide (NO) mechanisms.[59,60] Like substance P, NO has been implicated as an inflammatory mediator in OA and inhibition of inducible NO synthase ameliorated the severity of joint damage in a canine cruciate-deficiency model of OA.[61] However, whether therapeutic doses of ACET reduce the levels of substance P and/or NO in the OA joint is unknown.

Intraarticular Injection of Botulinum Neurotoxin

An experimental approach that is currently under evaluation as a treatment for OA pain is the intraarticular injection of botulinum toxin type A (BTX-A), a zinc-dependent endopeptidase that is comprised of a 100 kD chain that is involved in binding and membrane translocation and a 50 kD chain that contains the catalytic site. As elucidated by studies of the mechanism underlying the inhibition by botulinum neurotoxins of acetylcholine release at the neuromuscular junction, which accounts for their ability to reduce local muscle contractions (e.g., in dystonias), the various BTX serotypes cleave one or more of the synaptosomal regulatory proteins (SNAREs, soluble N-ethyl maleimide-sensitive factor [NSF] attachment protein receptor) that are required for vesicle docking and, as a consequence, the release of acetylcholine from the motor neuron.[62] When injected into a muscle, BTX-A binds irreversibly to specific receptors in nerve terminal membranes and is internalized as an endosome in the cytosol of the nerve ending, where it interrupts release of acetylcholine by cleaving one of the SNAREs, the 25 kD synaptosome-associated protein (SNAP-25), which is involved in the docking of the synaptic vesicle and fusion of the vesicle to the plasma membrane for subsequent release of neurotransmitter.[63] Proteolysis of SNAP-25 by BTX-A inhibits release of acetylcholine when the nerve is depolarized, blocking neurotransmission at the endplate of the alpha motoneuron.

Germane to its possible utility in ameliorating OA pain, BTX inhibits release from the termini of peripheral afferent nerves of mediators involved in nociception (e.g., substance P, CGRP, glutamate).[64] Effects of BTX-A have been studied in the rat formalin pain model, in which botulinum neurotoxins inhibited release of substance P from embryonic rat dorsal root ganglia neurons.[65] Pretreatment with BTX-A was found to reduce inflammation and levels of inflammatory mediators in the limb, and also reduced central sensitization in the spinal cord.[66,67] Similarly, in the rat carageenan model of inflammation, pretreatment of the hind paw with BTX-A resulted in significant reduction in paw edema, suggesting that the neurotoxin had an effect on neurogenic inflammation. In summary, the results in these animal models suggested that under conditions of inflammation and sustained pain, BTX-A exerted antinociceptive effects by inhibiting the release of vesicle-mediated mediators, substance P, CGRP, and glutamate, from peripheral afferent terminals, thereby indirectly inhibiting the local release of other inflammatory mediators, such as bradykinin, prostaglandins, and serotonin, which are involved in neurogenic inflammation. Aoki[64] proposed that this reduction in pain and peripheral sensitization led to decreased transmission of nociceptive impulses to the spinal cord, inhibiting the release of substance P and glutamate in the cord and reducing central sensitization.

In a small uncontrolled study, BTX-A was shown to provide long-lasting pain relief following injection into human OA joints.[63] Subsequently, a preliminary 3 month analysis of a randomized placebo-controlled trial of BTX-A injection into moderately to severely painful knees of patients with OA ($n = 37$) or rheumatoid arthritis ($n = 5$) also reports positive results, due to a much greater effect than placebo in those with severe knee pain.[68] Although imaging (e.g., ultrasound, fluoroscopy) was not used to guide needle placement in the above studies, problems due to injection of the drug into a periarticular site or to diffusion of BTX-A out of the joint space into periarticular muscle were not reported. Further studies are needed.

REFERENCES

1. Brandt KD. (2004). Neuromuscular aspects of osteoarthritis: a perspective. In *Osteoarthritic Joint Pain*. Novartis Foundation Symposium 260. London: Wiley, pp. 49–63.

2. Liang MH. (2004). Pushing the limits of patient-oriented outcome measurements in the search for disease modifying treatments for osteoarthritis. J Rheum 31: 61–65.

3. Hadler NM. (1992). Knee pain is the malady—not osteoarthritis. Ann Int Med 116:598–599.

4. Massardo L, Watt I, Cushnaghan J, et al. (1989). Osteoarthritis of the knee joint: an eight year prospective study. Ann Rheum Dis 48:893–897.

5. Lawrence JS, Bremmer JM, Bier F. (1966). Osteo-arthrosis. Prevalence in the population and relationship between symptoms and X-ray changes. Ann Rheum Dis 25:1–24.

6. Lawrence JS. (1977). Osteoarthrosis. In *Rheumatism in Populations*. Bristol: JW Arrowsmith Ltd., pp. 98–155.

7. Felson DT, Naimark A, Anderson J, et al. (1987). The prevalence of knee osteoarthritis in the elderly. Arthritis Rheum 30:914–918.

8. O'Reilly SC, Muir KR, Doherty M. (1998). Knee pain and disability in the Nottingham community: association with poor health status and psychological distress. Br J Rheumatol 57:588–594.

9. Felson DT, Kim Y. (2007). The futility of current approaches to chondroprotection. Arthritis Rheum 56:1378–1383.

10. Brandt KD, Radin EL, Dieppe PA, et al. (2007). Letter. The futility of current approaches to chondroprotection—a different perspective: comment on the special article by Felson and Kim. Arthritis Rheum 56:3873–3874.

11. Radin EL, Parker HG, Paul IL. (1971). Pattern of degenerative arthritis. Preferential involvement of distal finger joints. Lancet 1:377–379.

12. Tan AL, Toumi H, Benjamin M, et al. (2006). Combined high-resolution magnetic resonance imaging and histology to explore the role of ligaments and tendons in the phenotypic expression of early hand osteoarthritis. Ann Rheum Dis 65:1267–1272.

13. Brandt KD, Radin EL, Dieppe PA, et al. (2006). Yet more evidence that OA is not a cartilage disease. Ann Rheum Dis 65:1261–1264.

14. Felson DT. (1998). Preventing knee and hip osteoarthritis. Bull Rheum Dis 47:1–4.

15. Bergennud H, Johnell O, Redlund-Johnell I, Lohmander LS. (1992). The articular cartilage after osteotomy for gonarthrosis: biopsies after 2 years in 19 cases. Acta Orthop Scand 63:413–416.

16. 1972-2004 American College of Rheumatology Clinical Slide Collection. American College of Rheumatology Atlanta, GA.

17. Warden SJ, Hinman RS, Watson MA Jr, et al. (2008). Patellar taping and bracing for the treatment of chronic knee pain: a systematic review and meta-analysis. Arthritis Rheum 59:73–83.

18. Niu J, Zhang YQ, Nevitt M, et al. (2005). Patellar malalignment is associated with prevalent patellofemoral osteoarthritis: the Beijing Osteoarthritis Study. Arthritis Rheum 52(Suppl 9):S456–S457.

19. Thorp LE, Sumner DR, Wimmer MA, et al. (2007). Relationship between pain and medial knee joint loading in mild radiographic knee osteoarthritis. Arthritis Rheum 57:1254–1260.

20. Birmingham TB, Hunt MA, Jones IC, Jenkyn TR, Giffin JR. (2007). Test–retest reliability of the peak knee adduction moment during walking in patients with medial compartment knee osteoarthritis. Arthritis Rheum 57:1012–1017.

21. Baliunas AJ, Hurwitz DE, Ryals AB, et al. (2002). Increased knee joint loads during walking are present in subjects with knee osteoarthritis. Osteoarthritis Cartilage 10:573–579.

22. Mundermann A, Dyrby CO, Hurwitz DE, et al. (2004). Potential strategies to reduce medial compartment loading in patients with knee osteoarthritis of varying severity: reduced walking speed. Arthritis Rheum 50:11172–11178.

23. Miyazaki T, Wada M, Kawahara H, et al. (2002). Dynamic load at baseline can predict radiographic disease progression in medial compartment knee osteoarthritis. Ann Rheum Dis 61:617–622.

24. Amin S, Luepongsak N, McGibbon CA, et al. (2004). Knee adduction moment and development of chronic knee pain in elders. Arthritis Rheum 51:371–376.

25. Sharma L, Pai Y-C, Holtkamp K, et al. (1997). Is knee joint proprioception worse in the arthritic knee versus the unaffected knee in unilateral osteoarthritis? Arthritis Rheum 40:1518–1525.

26. Lund H, Juul-Kristensen B, Christensen H, et al. (2004). Impaired proprioception of both knees and elbows in patients with knee osteoarthritis compared to healthy controls. Osteoarthritis Cartilage 12(Suppl B):S25.

27. O'Connor BL, Brandt KD. (1993). Neurogenic factors in the etiopathogenesis of osteoarthritis. Rheum Dis Clin North Am 19:581–605.

28. van der Esch M, Steultjens M, Harlaar J, Knol D, Lems W, Dekker J. (2007). Joint proprioception, muscle strength, and functional ability in patients with osteoarthritis of the knee. Arthritis Rheum 57:787–793.

29. O'Connor BL, Visco DM, Brandt KD, et al. (1993). Sensory nerves only temporarily protect the unstable canine knee joint from osteoarthritis. Arthritis Rheum 36:1154–1163.

30. Radin EL, Boyd RD, Martin RB, et al. (1985). Mechanical factors influencing cartilage damage. In Peyron JG (ed.). *Osteoarthritis: Current Clinical and Fundamental Problems*. Paris: Geigy, pp. 90–99.

31. Vilensky JA. (2003). Innervation of the joint and its role in osteoarthritis. In Brandt KD, Doherty M, and Lohmander LS (eds.). *Osteoarthritis*, 2nd ed. Oxford, UK: Oxford University Press, pp. 161–167.

32. Johansson H, Sjölander P. (1993). Neurophysiology of joints. In Wright V and Radin EL (eds.). *Mechanics of Human Joints*. New York: Marcel Dekker, pp. 243–290.

33. Hill AV. (1960). Production and absorption of work by muscle. Science 131:897–903.

34. Jones CM, Watt DG. (1971). Muscular control of landing from unexpected falls in man. J Physiol 219:729–737.

35. Stokes M, Young A. (1984). The contribution of reflex inhibition to arthrogenous muscle weakness. Clin Sci 67:7–14.

36. Radin EL, Yang KH, Riegger C, Kish VL, O'Connor JJ. (1991). Relationship between lower limb dynamics and knee joint pain. J Orthop Res 9:398–405.

37. Hurley MV. (1999). The role of muscle weakness in the pathogenesis of osteoarthritis. Rheum Dis Clin North Am 25:299–314.

38. Slemenda C, Heilman DK, Brandt KD, et al. (1998). Reduced quadriceps strength relative to body weight: a risk factor for knee osteoarthritis in women? Arthritis Rheum 41:1951–1959.

39. Jefferson RJ, Collins JJ, Whittle MW, et al. (1990). The role of the quadriceps in controlling impulsive forces around heelstrike. Proc Inst Mech Eng 204:21–28.

40. Brandt KD, Heilman DK, Slemenda C, et al. (1999). Quadriceps strength in women with radiographically progressive osteoarthritis of the knee and those with stable radiographic changes. J Rheum 26:2431–2437.

41. Sharma L, Dunlop DD, Cahue S, et al. (2003). Quadriceps strength and osteoarthritis progression in malaligned and lax knees. Ann Intern Med 38:13–19.

42. Baker KR, Xu L, Zhang Y, et al. (2004). Quadriceps weakness and its relationship to tibiofemoral and patellofemoral knee osteoarthritis in Chinese: the Beijing Osteoarthritis Study. Arthritis Rheum 50:1815–1821.

43. van der Esch M, Steultjens M, Knol DL, Dinant H, Dekker J. (2006). Joint laxity and the relationship between muscle strength and functional ability in patients with osteoarthritis of the knee. Arthritis Rheum 55:953–959.

44. Hall MC, Mockett SP, Doherty M. (2006). Relative impact of radiographic osteoarthritis and pain on quadriceps strength, proprioception, static postural sway and lower limb function. Ann Rheum Dis 65:865–870.

45. Arden NK, Nevitt MC, Lane NE, et al. (1999). Osteoarthritis and risk of falls, rates of bone loss, and osteoporotic fractures. Study of Osteoporotic Fractures Research Group. Arthritis Rheum 42:1378–1385.

46. Li B, Aspden RM. (1997). Mechanical and material properties of the subchondral bone plate from the femoral head of patients with osteoarthritis or osteoporosis. Ann Rheum Dis 56:247–254.

47. Grynpas MD, Alpert B, Katz I, et al. (1991). Subchondral bone in osteoarthritis. Calcif Tissue Int 49:20–26.

48. Fitzgerald GK, Piva SR, Irrgang JJ. (2004). Report of joint instability in knee osteoarthritis: its prevalence and relationship to physical function. Arthritis Rheum 51:941–946.

49. Roos EM, Dahlberg L. (2005). Positive effects of moderate exercise on glycosaminoglycan content in knee cartilage: a four-month randomized, controlled trial in patients at risk of osteoarthritis. Arthritis Rheum 52:3507–3514.

50. Schaible H-G, Grubb BD. (1993). Afferent and spinal mechanisms of joint pain. Pain 55:5–54.

51. Marshall KW, Chan ADM. (1993). Neurogenic contributions to degenerative and inflammatory arthroses. Curr Opin Orthop 4:48–55.

52. Lam FY, Ferrell WR. (1989). Inhibition of carrageenan induced inflammation in the rat knee joint by substance P antagonist. Ann Rheum Dis 48:928–932.

53. Bradley LA. (2004). Recent approaches to understanding osteoarthritis pain. J Rheum 31(Suppl 70):54–60.

54. Watkins LR, Milligan ED, Maier SF. (2001). Glial activation: a driving force for pathological pain. Trends Neurosci 24:450–455.

55. Kosek E, Orderberg G. (2000). Lack of pressure pain modulation by heterotopic noxious conditioning stimulation in patients with painful osteoarthritis before, but not following, surgical pain relief. Pain 88:69–78.

56. Brandt KD, Mazzuca SA, Buckwalter B. (2006). Acetaminophen, like conventional NSAIDs, may reduce synovitis in osteoarthritic knees. Rheumatology 5:1389–1394.

57. Bjornsson GA, Hannaes HR, Skoglund LA. (2003). A randomized double-blind crossover trial of paracetamol 1000 mg four times daily vs ibuprofen 600 mg: effect on swelling and other postoperative events after third molar surgery. Br J Clin Pharmacol 55:405–412.

58. Skelbred P, Lokken P, Skoglund LA. (1984). Postoperative administration of acetaminophen to reduce swelling and other inflammatory events. Curr Ther Res 35:377–385.

59. Bjorkman R, Hallman KM, Hedner J, et al. (1994). Acetaminophen blocks spinal hyperalgesia induced by NMDA and substance P. Pain 57:259–264.

60. Bjorkman R. (1995). Central anti-nociceptive effects of non-steroidal anti-inflammatory drugs and paracetamol. Experimental studies in the rat. Acta Anesthesiol Scand 103(Suppl):1–44.

61. Pelletier JP, Jovanovic D, Fernandes JC, et al. (1998). Reduced progression of experimental osteoarthritis in vivo by selective inhibition of inducible nitric oxide synthase. Arthritis Rheum 41:1275–1286.

62. Humeau Y, Doussau F, Grant NJ, et al. (2000). How botulinum and tetanus neurotoxins block neurotransmitter release. Biochimie 82:427–446.

63. Mahowald ML, Singh JA, Dykstra D. (2006). Long term effects of intra-articular botulinum toxin A for refractory joint pain. Neurotox Res 9:179–188.

64. Aoki KR. (2003). Pharmacology and immunology of botulinum toxin type A. Clin Dermatol 21:476–480.

65. Welch MJ, Purkiss JR, Foster KA. (2000). Sensitivity of embryonic rat dorsal root ganglia neurons to *Clostridium botulinum* neurotoxins. Toxicon 38:245–258.

66. Cui M, Li Z, You S, et al. (2002). Mechanisms of the antinociceptive effect of subcutaneous botox: inhibition of peripheral and central nociceptive processing. Arch Pharmacol 365(Suppl 2):R17.

67. Cui M, Khanijou S, Rubino J, et al. (2004). Subcutaneous administration of botulinum toxin A reduces formalin-induced pain. Pain 107:125–133.

68. Mahowald ML, Singh JA, Goelz E, et al. (2007). Intra-articular botulinum toxin type A (IA-BoNT/A) for refractory knee pain: randomized controlled trial in patients with rheumatoid arthritis (RA) and osteoarthritis (OA). Arthritis Rheum 6(Suppl):S662.

10

PRESSURE-DRIVEN INTRAVASATION OF OSSEOUS FAT IN THE PATHOGENESIS OF OSTEOARTHRITIC PAIN

Peter A. Simkin

*Division of Rheumatology, University of Washington,
Seattle, Washington 98195, USA*

INTRODUCTION

Intraosseous hypertension has been implicated as an important factor in osteoarthritic pain of weight-bearing human joints.[1,2] The characteristic story is one of pain that is deep, aching, exacerbated by use, often worse at night, and relieved by surgical decompression. Though not the only pattern of osteoarthritic pain, these symptoms are common and they arguably comprise the most frequent rationale for total joint replacement.

Since intraosseous pressure values are not accessible without invasive determinations, it is not surprising that the direct evidence of hypertension is meager. Most of the data are old, and I have not found useful additions within the new millennium. Instead, there has been persuasive documentation of a direct relationship between increasing articular pain and progression of "bone edema" recognized by serial magnetic resonance imaging (MRI) assessments.[3–5] If, as I believe, this finding results from pressure-driven intravasation of subchondral

Pain in Osteoarthritis, Edited by David T. Felson and Hans-Georg Schaible
Copyright © 2009 Wiley-Blackwell.

fat, the new data provide indirect evidence of intraosseous hypertension in this disease. In support of that hypothesis, I review some of the available physiology of normal and abnormal intraosseous pressure and consider how that may apply to the bone edema of osteoarthritis.

NORMAL PRESSURE

Normal human epiphyseal bone is pressurized at rest.[6] This property was recognized in the human hip by Ficat and Arlet,[7] who regularly found pressures substantially higher in the femoral head than those in midshaft, diaphyseal bone. In so doing, they confirmed the findings of Kabakele,[8] who observed striking site differentials in his large series of African subjects of all ages (Table 10.1). Ficat and Arlet pointed out that the inflow of arterial blood provides the obvious driver for intraosseous pressure and the existence of consistent regional gradients "presupposes the presence of adaptable barriers and permanent differences in neurovascular control."[7]

The putative system they envision may control either the arterial input or the venous outflow and both locations could be subject to pharmacologic manipulation. After the nutrient arteries enter long bones, they divide to yield long, slender arteriolar capillaries, which serve as the principal vessels of the immediate subchondrium. These then dive back down into the metaphysis, where they empty into the dilated, saccular sinusoids characteristic of all marrow compartments.[9,10] At the site of outflow into collecting venules, there appear to be sphincters that may control intraosseous pressure just as outflow resisters control the comparable pressures within the eye and in normal erectile tissues.

When epinephrine is infused into the nutrient artery, there is apparent constriction of the arterioles with a consequent abrupt fall in intraosseous pressure.[11,12] Conversely, bradykinin infusions appear to dilate the same vessels and to increase the intraosseous pressure.[13] In further studies, acetylcholine,

TABLE 10.1. Mean Tibial Intramedullary Pressures[a]

Area	Child[b]	Adult
Epiphysis	26.1 (24)[c]	—
Metaphysis	22.3 (69)[c]	19.9 (14)
Diaphysis	13.6 (124)[c]	11.8 (26)

Source: Reference 8.

[a]Pressures are in mmHg with the number of observations in parentheses.

[b]Children were 3–17 years old.

[c]Single, high outlying values were deleted from each of the three bony regions in children.

ephedrine, and serotonin caused variable pressure responses. In clinical practice, cyclosporine, a well-known vasoconstrictor, has been implicated as a cause of symptomatic osseous hypertension that can be relieved by vasodilators.[14,15]

The work on vascular control of intraosseous pressure was limited in scope and most of it was performed long ago. None of the most recent cytokines (not even the prostaglandins) have been characterized well, so much remains to be learned. We know only that this tissue is turgid, that both inflow and outflow may be subject to control, and that their balance will determine the epiphyseal pressure both at rest and during exercise.

All joints experience use-related loading and the manner in which they handle loading energy is of immense potential importance to students of osteoarthritis. Since the cartilage is relatively thin, most of the burden is transmitted through this layer into the underlying trabecular bone.[16] There, it encounters quite different patterns of organization in the opposing members of the joint. The concave side (such as the glenoid fossa or the acetabulum) has a relatively thick subchondral plate supported by sturdy struts and a relatively open trabecular framework. Together, these features make the surface stiff and noncompliant. Conversely, the opposing convex member (such as the humeral or femoral head) has a thin subchondral plate and a highly compartmentalized underpinning of slender trabecular walls. These aspects allow the convex joint members to be both flexible and strong.[17]

The contrasting structural features lead to important differences in mechanical behavior: (1) Under the same load, bony deflection was six times greater in the canine humeral head than in the opposing glenoid fossa.[18] (2) At the same 9 mm subchondral depth, the humeral hydraulic resistance to infused saline was ninefold greater in the canine humeral head than that within the opposing scapula.[19] (3) Reflecting both the greater deflection of its surface and the greater resistance to displacement of its fluid content, the load-induced pressure was almost three times greater at sites within the human femoral head than it was under the acetabulum with the same concurrent load.[20] Comparable findings can be anticipated when these characteristics are studied within other, normal ball-and-socket joints.

Together, these features support the concept that loading forces are hydraulically distributed throughout the convex subchondrium.[21] This system then enlists a large trabecular area to serve as a hydraulic spring that accepts loading energy while sparing both the articular cartilage and the more distal shaft. At the same time, it transiently stores energy that can then be recovered to perform useful work. Thus load-driven pressurization of the subchondral space is a normal, physiologic function.

It must be noted as well that the experiments summarized above were all carried out in dead, excised bone without the benefit of the vessel-driven pressurization that we now recognize as basic, normal physiology. Were that pressurization in force, the hydraulic spring would be enhanced just as internal pressurization amplifies the bounce of an inflated basketball or a rubber tire.

PATHOLOGIC PRESSURE AND OSTEONECROSIS

The most extensive studies of intraosseous hypertension have occurred in the context of osteonecrosis (avascular necrosis of bone).[1,7] There, current concepts focus on outflow obstruction, which may be caused by extrinsic venous compression or by intravascular obstruction. In either case, obstruction of venous outflow will cause the intraosseous pressure to rise just as the pressure rises in the lake behind a dam. The most common compressive event occurs when fat cells (the predominant component of subchondral tissue) hypertrophy in response to therapeutic corticosteroids or chronic abuse of ethanol. Other compressive, extravascular factors include Gaucher's cells and infiltration of inflammatory or malignant cells as in myeloma or acute leukemia. In any of these cases, cellular proliferation and/or hypertrophy results in compression of outflow veins since they are the most compliant component within the closed intraosseous space.

The best-studied examples of intravascular obstruction are those caused by aggregation of misshapen erythrocytes in sickle cell anemia, and by the clots

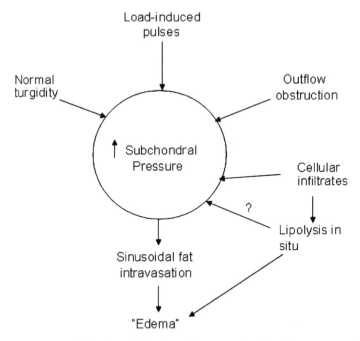

Figure 10.1. Factors in focal mobilization of osseous fat. Baseline pressures in bony epiphyses, normally akin to those of the eye, may be elevated further in osteoarthritis. Under acute loads, the baseline intraosseous pressure response is then amplified, osseous fat is driven into venous sinusoids, and the expelled fat is replaced by water and cells to yield the MRI finding of "bone edema." Comparable displacement, with similar MRI findings, occurs in other bony pathologic processes but is not discussed here.

induced when nitrogen bubbles injure the endothelium during decompression after industrial or recreational exposure to high pressure environments. More recent evidence suggests that hypercoagulability factors and perhaps antiphospholipid antibodies should be added to the list of entities that induce osseous hypertension by intravascular obstruction of venous outflow.[22]

Each of these obstructive processes will increase the pressure further within the already turgid confines of the epiphyseal subchondrium. Then, when affected individuals walk, run, jump, or fall, the load-induced response will be amplified by the higher baseline (Fig. 10.1). This is the setting where we have suggested that the interstitial pressure may exceed that of the feeding arterioles. If so, intravasated fat within the venous sinusoids may find that its egress path of least resistance lies not downstream through the obstructed venules, but upstream into the slender arteriolar capillaries. There, these retrograde emboli may lodge at bifurcations and block subsequent arteriolar inflow.[23,24] Obstructing fat emboli within the arteriolar tree have long been considered as leading contenders for the cause of tissue infarction in avascular necrosis of bone. The above hypothesis offers plausible support for that role. It suggest that infarctions ensue not from systemic embolization (for which there is no credible evidence) but from local, retrograde emboli comprised of osseous fat. Furthermore, it explains why this problem would be most likely in convex articular members (such as the femoral head) where load-induced pressurization is a prominent feature of the normal physiology. Finally, it provides a rationale for the occurrence of this problem in young, active people rather than older, less active individuals who might be on comparable does of corticosteroids.

PATHOLOGIC PRESSURE AND OSTEOARTHRITIS

Osteoarthritis is the other major entity with extensive evidence of intraosseous hypertension.[1,2] As in osteonecrosis, surgical decompression may dramatically relieve the pain of osteoarthritis and this finding suggests that sustained, pressure-induced trabecular tension may be the source of the pain, although other possible mechanisms such as ischemia must also be considered and the precise pathophysiology remains unclear.

As in osteonecrosis, the source of the hypertension lies clearly in outflow obstruction rather than in increased arteriolar input. Unlike osteonecrosis, however, the cause or causes of that obstruction remain unidentified. The most impressive evidence comes from impaired clearance both of injected isotopes and of radiopaque dyes.[25] These studies reveal striking distension of the obstructed venous sinusoids. If that distension ensues from constricted outflow sphincters, pharmacologic relaxation of those sphincters could provide crucial relief of osteoarthritic pain. This possibility offers an intriguing opportunity for medical relief of what has been thought to be a largely mechanical problem.

SINUSOIDAL INTRAVASATION

Venous sinusoids are perhaps the most conspicuous feature of the normal intraosseous vasculature. Since there is no system of lymphatic vessels, the sinusoids serve as the only route to the bloodstream for cells and any other particulates within the marrow space. This, of course, is how most of the normal cells of blood begin their useful lives. It is also the path by which osseous malignant cells, for instance, those of osteosarcoma, enter the blood.[26] Since there is no lymphatic filter, any cells or particulates picked up by the sinusoids will travel first to the heart and then to the lungs. Experimentally, 15 µm microspheres, which obstruct the arteriolar capillaries of bone after injection into the arterial stream, are cleared immediately through the sinusoids after injection into the bony interstitium.[27] More impressively, similar intraosseous injections of 100 µm particulates leads to their immediate clearance through the normal venous flow.[28] This dimension gains relevance when it is considered in view of the 55–65 µm size of normal osseous adipocytes.[29,30]

Embolization of osseous fat to the lung has been well known for years through the dreaded fat embolus syndrome that is recognized most often after major long bone fractures.[31] There, massive amounts of bone fat may embolize the pulmonary vasculature and lead ultimately to pulmonary failure and death. A similar pathogenesis may underlie the serious acute chest syndrome of patients with sickle cell anemia.[32] More recently, the syndrome has been recognized as a complication of arthroplastic surgery.

In joint replacement surgery, the recipient bone must be carved and reamed to provide a close-fitting socket for the successful implant. This process necessarily raises the intraosseous pressure and that pulse then drives intravasation of osseous fat. The resultant pulmonary embolization is predictable. It has been followed in patients by transesophageal echocardiography, which permits visualization of the fat as it passes through the heart en route to the lung.[33,34] In experiments using sheep and baboons, fat was quantified in the vena cava and its amount was found to correlate directly with the pressure induced within the reamed bone.[35,36] This work then led to modifications in equipment and technique that have reduced the pressure response and, with it, the amount of fat embolization.[37] Thus surgical necessity has led to the most conclusive evidence that raised intraosseous pressure drives intravasation of osseous fat.

IMPLICATIONS FOR OSTEOARTHRITIS

A large, blinded, crossover study of patients with painful osteoarthritis of the knee found no significant benefit from the local anesthetic Bupivacaine when it was compared to simple saline.[38] Impaired proprioception indicated that the synovium was anesthetized and the lack of symptomatic relief from that anesthesia implies that synovium is not a major contributor to the pain of this disease. The aneural cartilage seems even less likely, and this by default leaves the subchondral bone as that articular tissue most likely to be the source of major osteoarthritic pain in this disease. This should come as no surprise. Bone is the site of the sclerosis, osteophytosis, and cyst formation that together with "joint space" loss comprise the classic radiographic hallmarks of this disease. Those changes, however, correlate only moderately with the pain of these lesions. Now, extensive (and expensive) studies have employed MRI to find further that bone marrow lesions (BMLs) correlate better with pain in affected knees and that their progression corresponds to worsening of the pain.

These BMLs (still widely referred to as "bone marrow edema") represent the appearance of an aqueous MRI signal at subchondral sites normally occupied by fat. Both sides of this equation are relevant. Since the volume of this space is fixed by bony limits, zero sum principles must apply. This means that more water (whether in interstitial edema or in infiltrating cells) means less fat.

This chapter suggests that osseous fat is lost through pressure-driven intravasation at venous sinusoids. The epiphyses and metaphyses where BMLs occur are normally turgid at rest and subject to load-induced, cyclic pulses above their baseline pressure. For reasons unknown, but most probably neurovascular, that baseline is often elevated in patients with painful osteoarthritis. When such elevations are amplified by normal loading, they would seem fully capable of driving intravasation of fat with secondary "edema" as the lost fat is replaced by cells and interstitial water.

REFERENCES

1. Simkin PA. (2004). Bone pain and pressure in osteoarthritic joints. Osteoarthritic joint pain. In *Novartis Foundation Symposium 260*. East Hanover, NJ: Novartis, pp. 179–190.

2. Lemperg RK, Arnoldi CC. (1978). The significance of intraosseous pressure in normal and diseased states with special reference to the intraosseous engorgement–pain syndrome. Clin Orthop Relat Res 136:143–156.

3. Felson DT, Chaisson CE, Hill CL, Totterman SMS, Gale E, Skinner KM, Kazis L, Gale DR. (2001). The association of bone marrow lesions with pain in knee osteoarthritis. Ann Intern Med 134:541–549.

4. McQueen FM. (2007). A vital clue to deciphering bone pathology: MRI bone oedema in rheumatoid arthritis and osteoarthritis. Ann Rheum Dis 66:1549–1551.

5. Felson DT, Niu J, Guermazi A, Roemer F, Aliabadi P, Clancy M, Torner J, Lewis CE, Nevitt MC. (2007). Correlation of the development of knee pain with enlarging bone marrow lesions on magnetic resonance imaging. Arthritis Rheum 56:2986–2992.

6. Wilkes CH, Visscher MB. (1975). Some physiological aspects of bone marrow pressure. J Bone Joint Surg Am 57:49–57.

7. Ficat RP, Arlet J. (1980). *Ischemia and Necroses of Bone*. Baltimore: Williams & Wilkins.

8. Kabakele M. (1972). Contribution au diagnostic précoce de l'ostéonécrose drépanocytaire. Thèse dagrègation, Kinshasa, Zaire.

9. Obtani O, Gannon B, Obtsuka A, Mutakami T. (1982). The microvasculature of bone and especially of bone marrow as studied by scanning electron microscopy of vascular cast-a review. Scan Electron Microsc 1:427–434.

10. Kessel RG, Kardon RH. (1979). *Tissues and Organs: A Text-Atlas of Scanning Electron Microscopy*. San Francisco: WH Freeman.

11. Stein AH Jr, Morgan HC, Porras RF. (1958). The effect of pressor and depressor drugs on intramedullary bone-marrow pressure. J Bone Joint Surg Am 40:1103–1110.

12. Shim SS. (1968). Physiology of blood circulation of bone. J Bone Joint Surg Am 50:812–824.

13. Schneider T, Drescher W, Becker C, Schlack W, Sager M, Assheuer J, Ruther W. (1998). The impact of vasoactive substances on intraosseous pressure and blood flow alterations in the femoral head: a study based on magnetic resonance imaging. Arch Orthop Trauma Surg 118:45–49.

14. Barbosa LM, Gauthier VJ, Davis CL. (1995). Bone pain that responds to calcium channel blockers. A retrospective and prospective study of transplant recipients. Transplantation 59:541–544.

15. Kart-Koseoglu H, Yucel AE, Isyklar I, Turker I, Akcali Z, Haberal M. (2003). Joint pain and arthritis in renal transplant recipients, and correlation with cyclosporine therapy. Rheumatol Int 23:159–162.

16. Radin EL, Paul IL, Lowy M. (1970). A comparison of the dynamic force-transmitting properties of subchondral bone and articular cartilage. J Bone Joint Surg Am 52:444–456.

17. Simkin PA, Graney DO, Fiechtner JJ. (1980). Roman arches, human joints, and disease: differences between convex and concave sides of joints. Arthritis Rheum 23:1308–1311.

18. Simkin PA, Houglum SJ, Pickerell CC. (1985). Compliance and viscoelasticity of canine shoulders loaded in vitro. J Biomechanics 10:735–743.

19. Simkin PA, Pickerell CC, Wallis W. (1985). Hydraulic resistance in bones of the canine shoulder. J Biomechanics 18:657–663.

20. Downey DJ, Simkin PA, Taggart R. (1988). The effect of compressive loading on intraosseous pressure in the femoral head in vitro. J Bone Joint Surg 70A:871–877.

21. Simkin PA. (2004). Hydraulically loaded trabeculae may serve as springs within the normal femoral head. Arthritis Rheum 50:3068–3075.

22. Jones LC, Mont MA, Le TB, Petri M, Hungerford DS, Wang P, Glueck CJ. (2003). Procoagulants and osteonecrosis. Rheumatol 30:783–789.

23. Simkin PA, Downey DJ. (1987). Hypothesis: retrograde embolization of marrow fat may cause osteonecrosis. J Rheumatol 14:870–872.

24. Simkin PA, Gardner GC. (1994). Osteonecrosis: pathogenesis and practicalities. Hosp Pract 29:73–84.

25. Arnoldi CC, Djurhuus JC, Heerfordt J, Karle A. (1980). Intraosseous phlebography, intraosseous pressure measurements and ^{99m}Tc-polyphosphate scintigraphy in

patients with various painful conditions in the hip and knee. Acta Orthop Scan 51:19–28.

26. Jeffree GM, Price CH, Sissons HA. (1975). The metastatic patterns of osteosarcoma. Br J Cancer 32:87–107.

27. Robertson WW Jr, Janssen HF, Walker RN. (1985). Passive movement of radioactive microspheres from bone and soft tissue in an extremity. J Orthop Res 4: 405–411.

28. Janssen HF, Robertson WW, Berlin S. (1988). Venous drainage of the femur permits passage of 100-micron particles. J Orthop Res 6:671–675.

29. Rozman C, Reverter JC, Feliu E, Berga L, Rozman M, Climent C. (1990). Variations of fat tissue fraction in abnormal human bone marrow depend both on size and number of adipocytes: a stereologic study. Blood 76:892–895.

30. Allen JE, Henshaw DL, Keitch PA, Fews AP, Eatough JP. (1995). Fat cells in red bone marrow of human rib: their size and spatial distribution with respect to the radon-derived dose to the haemopoietic tissue. Int J Radiat Biol 68:669–678.

31. Mellor A, Soni N. (2001). Fat embolism. Anaesthesia 56:145–154.

32. Vichinsky E, Williams R, Das M, Earles AN, Lewis N, Adler A, McQuitty J. (1994). Pulmonary fat embolism: a distinct cause of severe acute chest syndrome in sickle cell anemia. J Am Soc Hematol 83:3107–3112.

33. Christie J, Robinson CM, Pell AC, McBirnie J, Burnett R. (1996). Transcardiac echocardiography during invasive intramedullary procedures. J Bone Joint Surg Br 78:854–855.

34. Takashina M, Ueyama H, Sugano N, Nakata S, Mashimo T. (2007). Incidence of embolic events during acetabular prosthesis insertion in total hip arthroplasty, and effect of intramedullary decompression in preventing embolism: higher risk of embolism with one-piece type of prosthesis. J Anesth 21:459–466.

35. Joist A, Schult M, Ortmann C, Frerichmann U, Frebel T, Spiegel H, Kröpfl A, Redl H. (2004). Rinsing-suction reamer attenuates intramedullary pressure increase and fat intravasation in a sheep model. J Trauma 57:146–151.

36. Kröpfl A, Davies J, Berger U, Hertz H, Schlag G. (1999). Intramedullary pressure and bone marrow fat extravasation in reamed and undreamed femoral nailing. J Orthop Res 17:261–268.

37. Pitto RP, Hamer H, Fabiani R, Radespiel-Troeger M, Koessler M. (2002). Prophylaxis against fat and bone-marrow embolism during total hip arthroplasty reduces the incidence of postoperative deep-vein thrombosis: a controlled, randomized clinical trial. J Bone Joint Surg Am 84:39–48.

38. Hassan BS, Doherty SA, Mockett S, Doherty M. (2002). Effect of pain reduction on postural sway, proprioception, and quadriceps strength in subjects with knee osteoarthritis. Ann Rheum Dis 61:422–428.

11

STRUCTURAL CORRELATES OF OSTEOARTHRITIS PAIN: LESSONS FROM MAGNETIC RESONANCE IMAGING

Philip G. Conaghan

Section of Musculoskeletal Disease, Leeds Institute of Molecular Medicine, University of Leeds, Leeds LS9 7TF, United Kingdom

INTRODUCTION

Magnetic resonance imaging (MRI) has the ability to visualize all the structures of a joint, including soft tissue and cartilage. Initial MRI studies focused on cartilage volume and morphological assessment, with an emphasis on structural progression. Recently, there has been a growing body of work examining the correlation of structural findings with osteoarthritis (OA) symptoms. Painful OA knees have more MRI detected pathology of multiple tissues and these pathologies are often correlated, making individual contributions difficult to assess. However, in large cohort studies, both synovial hypertrophy and large synovial effusions have been demonstrated to be more frequent in patients with OA knee pain. Similarly MRI-determined subchondral bone marrow lesions are associated with OA knee pain. Improved, reliable quantification of the structural features and the availability of large epidemiological OA MRI cohorts will improve structure–pain understanding.

Pain in Osteoarthritis, Edited by David T. Felson and Hans-Georg Schaible

CORRELATION OF STRUCTURAL FINDINGS WITH OSTEOARTHRITIS SYMPTOMS

The individual with OA lives with a syndrome of pain and reduced quality of life. The "structural" OA pathological processes involve the whole joint organ including the cartilage, synovium, subchondral bone, menisci, and ligaments.[1] Trying to understand the relationship between symptoms and structural damage may lead to improved understanding of peripheral origins of OA pain. However, traditional research into such structure–pain associations relied on the conventional radiograph, which predominantly images bone and a surrogate measure of what was presumed to be hyaline cartilage thickness, the joint space. Although the odds for knee pain generally increase with radiographic severity of OA,[2,3] significant discordance between clinical and radiographic changes has been described in community based cohorts.[4–6]

MRI provides the ability to visualize not only all the relevant structures within an OA joint, but its tomographic nature allows for imaging in three dimensions. Hence whole organ evaluation of this complex OA process is possible.[7,8] Until recently, much of the OA MRI literature focused on cartilage with attention to quantitating cartilage volume and morphology.[8] Since the cartilage tissue is relatively aneural, it seems an unlikely primary source of joint pain, although it can produce proinflammatory molecules or mediate increased biomechanical stresses on adjacent tissues. The evaluation of noncartilage structures therefore seems highly important.

The last few years have seen a much needed, rapid growth in OA-related MRI studies, including some large cohort studies that are providing increasing understanding of the OA "phenotype." This chapter focuses on the MRI literature pertaining to OA pathological features and pain; the majority of studies involve the knee and this is therefore reflected in the content. Of course, structure–pain studies will never fully explain the complex and personal pain process in an individual or a given joint.

STRUCTURE–PAIN STUDY LIMITATIONS

Before proceeding, it is worthwhile considering the limitations of studies evaluating structure–pain associations.

1. *How Was Subject Pain Identified and Quantified?* The phasic or episodic nature of pain may interfere in detecting associations, so inclusion criteria specifying duration and frequency of pain may influence study results. Which pain measure is chosen (examples include global, night, or weight-bearing pain) may also influence the outcome. How patient reported outcomes are applied (e.g., to a target joint, or a target limb, or both knees) will influence results.

Few studies take into account likely confounders of how people record pain, including depression.

2. *How Were the Pathological Structures Visualized?* Even using the conventional radiograph of the knee, many studies have imaged only the tibiofemoral joint and not the patellofemoral joint; this may apply to analyses of MRI data as well. Studies employing MRI are also not without complexity and bring a host of novel variables to the analysis, including different magnet strengths, different sequences, and different methods of quantification. This area of MRI is rapidly expanding but care should always be taken in interpreting and comparing studies.

3. *How Were the Pathological Features Quantified?* Semiautomated cartilage volume quantification is now well described and its reliability and sensitivity to change have been reported.[8] There has also been consensus proposals on terminology for describing intra-articular sites in the knee, for cross-study comparisons.[9] At present, there are no well validated quantitative measures for assessing noncartilage features, so a number of semiquantitative knee scores have been developed.[10–12] These share in common a division of the knee into various anatomical subregions, and use varying categorical scales to describe the extent of each of multiple pathological features within these subregions. There remain limited data on the performance metrics of these tools.

4. *How Were the Structure–Pain Associations Made?* One of the complexities of this field is distinguishing if an individual MRI feature is associated with pain, when pathology of multiple features is closely correlated, especially with more advanced disease. This makes statistical analysis complex. It is wise to look at what MRI features were evaluated in a given study and to see what analysis was performed to account for copathologies.

KNEE PAIN VERSUS OSTEOARTHRITIS

The definition of OA can be difficult, especially with the increased phenotypic ability of MRI to add to the complexity. Some recent MRI studies have focused on people with knee pain, rather than requiring a radiographic OA definition for study entry. One group has looked at knee pain in older and younger adults and their associated MRI findings. In a community-based cohort of 500 men and women of mean age 63, the prevalence of knee pain was 48%.[13] After a multivariable analysis, knee pain was significantly associated with medial tibial chondral defects, bone marrow lesions (BMLs), radiographic hip joint space narrowing, greater BMI, and lower knee extension strength. Radiographs were taken in this study (not for inclusion criteria) but radiographic OA was not associated with knee pain. They reported a "dose–response" for a number of severe chondral defects and knee pain. Another report from Tasmania looked at 371 subjects with mean age 45 years, although this study did not include evaluation of BMLs.[14] The prevalence of knee pain was 35% and femoral and patellar chondral defects demonstrated a dose–response significant association with knee pain. Cartilage volume and knee pain did not demonstrate pain associations.

INDIVIDUAL MRI FEATURES AND PAIN

Bone Marrow Lesions

MRI allows the evaluation of the subchondral bone, a richly innervated structure, and for many years considered important in the pain and structural progression of OA.[15,16] The commonest MRI subchondral abnormality is termed a bone marrow lesion or sometimes bone marrow edema. These terms refer to ill-defined high signal areas seen on fat-suppressed T2-weighted or STIR sequences (see Fig. 11.1). It is not known exactly what these lesions represent, and this MRI feature is not specific for OA, with similar MR appearances seen in trauma, osteomyelitis, and rheumatoid arthritis but reflecting different pathological processes.[16–18] Two small studies have matched the histological findings from tibial plateau bone with the site of BMLs in OA patients.[19,20] In the larger of these studies (16 patients) abnormal tissue was only seen in half the sites corresponding to BMLs, with marrow necrosis, fibrosis, and abnormal, remodeled bony trabeculae being the commonest abnormalities.[20]

A link with structural deterioration has been demonstrated for BMLs: in 256 OA knees followed for up to 30 months, there was a strong association between progressive radiographic joint space loss and the presence of BMLs in the same (medial or lateral) compartment of the knee, even when adjusted for a known risk factor, knee alignment.[21] However, these BMLs have also been linked to OA pain. One study described a range of subchondral tibial abnormalities (using T1-weighted images and therefore not directly comparable to other BML studies) in OA patients selected for recent onset of symptoms (mean duration 6 months) and followed for up to 4.5 years.[22] The lesions described by widespread MRI subchondral changes extending into the metaphysis and with MRI appearance similar to BMLs were associated with persistence of pain over the follow-up period.

The most convincing study on the importance of BMLs and pain involved 401 radiographic OA knee participants, 50 of whom had no knee pain.[23] Subjects had coronal T2-weighted fat-suppressed MRI scans and BMLs were graded 0–3 depending on size. As reported in subsequent studies, the frequency

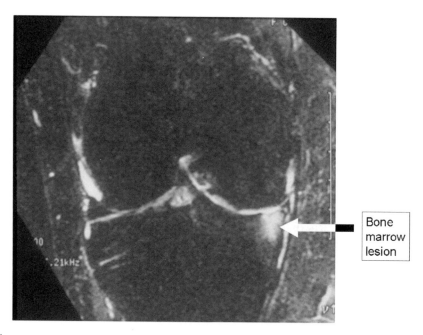

Figure 11.1. Knee MRI of a patient with osteoarthritis showing a bone marrow lesion underneath the medial tibial plateau.

of BMLs increased with radiographic grade (Kellgren and Lawrence grade scored on posteroanterior radiographs only) of OA: 48% of KL grade 0 had BMLs compared with 100% of those with KL grade 4. The BMLs were present in 78% of the painful knees compared with 30% of the nonpainful group ($p < 0.001$), but notably, large lesions (graded 2 or 3) were present in 36% versus 2%, respectively ($p < 0.001$). However, this study did not demonstrate an association of BMLs with pain severity. Another recent study looked at 120 women divided into four groups on the basis of presence or absence of knee pain and presence or absence of radiographic changes.[24] This study used appropriate proton density, fat-suppressed sequences to identify BMLs, which were graded by size on a 0–2 (grade 0 absent, grade $1 < 1\,cm^2$, grade $2 > 1\,cm^2$) scale. Although BMLs were common and their frequency similar in painful and nonpainful OA groups, larger lesions ($> 1\,cm^2$) were more frequent in the painful OA knee group (36% versus 14% in the painless OA group, $p < 0.05$). In common with other studies, women with these large BMLs were more likely to have full thickness cartilage defects; the painful radiographic OA group with full thickness cartilage defects, adjacent subchondral cortical bone abnormalities, and BMLs had significantly greater likelihood of painful OA (OR 3.2).

Recently, Felson and colleagues[25] examined the issue of whether enlarging BMLs are associated with new onset of knee pain by examining subjects from the Multicenter Osteoarthritis Study (MOST), a prospective epidemiologic study of knee OA. They employed a nested case–control study, including participants with no pain at baseline but pain present at 15 months, and defined change in BMLs according to maximal change in WORMS BML score on a compartment-specific basis. Some 49.1% of the 110 cases demonstrated an increase in compartmental BML scores compared with 26.8% of control cases ($n = 220$, $p < 0.001$). Most people with increasing size of BML had BMLs at baseline. Of those with no BMLs at baseline, new BMLs occurred in 32.4% of case compared with 10.8% of controls.

It is important to note that not all studies have demonstrated an association of BMLs with knee pain. One study of 205 people, of whom 35% had symptomatic OA knee and half had radiographic OA, reported that a large knee joint effusion and patellofemoral osteophytes were associated with pain, but chondral defects or BMLs were not.[26] The lack of association of BMLs with pain in this study may well represent the differences in both the cohort inclusion criteria and how the pain was measured compared to the Felson study mentioned previously.[23]

Bone Attrition

Bone attrition is a concept derived initially from radiography and refers to loss of bone contour typically seen in advanced OA; in MRI this refers to a flattening or depression of the articular bone cortex. A MRI study of 1627 knees (1273 subjects) evaluated attrition as part of the WORMS assessment.[27] About a third of this community-based cohort had knee pain, often older females with greater BMI. Definite bone attrition was seen in 28% of painful knees and 10% of painless ($p < 0.0001$; OR adjusted for age, gender, BMI, BMLs, effusions, and KL grade was 1.6 [CI 1.1-2.2]). Not surprisingly, attrition was commonly copresent with BMLs and effusions. Attrition was more closely related to pain in those knees without radiographic OA. Attrition has also been associated with knee pain in a study looking at 143 people with OA knee (KL > 1) and MRI evaluated with the WORMS.[28] Using median quartile regression, they reported pain associations for attrition, BMLs, meniscal tears, and moderate to large effusions.

Synovitis, Effusions, and Synovial Cysts

Synovitis in OA, although secondary, is common (see Fig. 11.2); synovial abnormalities are present from the earliest stages of OA and the severity of synovitis is generally related to the severity of chondropathy in the affected joint.[29–31] Synovitis is best assessed with MRI using the intravenous, para-magnetic-enhancing agent gadolinium,[32] and studies have correlated the MRI synovial hypertrophy seen in OA with microscopic synovial inflammation.[32,33]

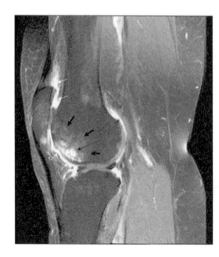

Marked Peripatellar Synovitis (white arrows)

Extensive bone marrow lesion (small black arrows)/bone cysts (long black arrow)

Figure 11.2. Knee MRI of a patient with osteoarthritis showing typical co-occurrence of multiple lesions which could cause pain: bone marrow lesions, cysts and synovitis.

However, for reasons of cost, timing, and potential toxicity, contrast use may be omitted and nongadolinium sequences can be optimized for this purpose.[34]

One large cross-sectional MRI study evaluated synovitis, effusions, and popliteal cysts in a large cohort of OA knee subjects, comparing persons with symptomatic knee OA with persons with radiographic OA but without symptoms.[35] The study employed semiquantitative scoring systems for assessing effusions and cysts, which were graded as absent, small, moderate, or large and correspondingly scored 0–3. Synovial hypertrophy was assessed as present or absent (scored 0 or 1) at three sites: the infrapatella fat pad, intercondylar space, and anterior horn of the lateral meniscus. There was a significant increase in the frequency of both effusions (moderate or large) and synovial hypertrophy in the painful knees compared to those without pain, after adjustment for the radiographic OA severity. In subjects with knee pain and radiographic OA, there was an association between synovitis and pain severity. Popliteal cysts were common ($>20\%$) among those people without knee pain and not surprisingly they were associated with effusions; they were not associated with pain.

Another study from these authors looked at the temporal relationship of pain and synovitis.[36] Using noncontrast detected synovitis scoring at the three sites described previously, they assessed 270 people with painful OA knee at baseline, 15 month, and 30 month time points. Baseline synovitis levels did not correlate with baseline pain levels, but there was a correlation between change in synovitis score and change in pain VAS score ($r = 0.21$, $p < 0.001$). This study did not demonstrate a relationship between synovitis and cartilage loss over the study time course.

Cartilage Pathology

It is worth noting that reduced cartilage volume has been associated with knee pain in a number of studies, although this association is generally not a strong one and often other pathological features are not included in the analysis.[37,38] A recent report of a cohort of men with painful OA knee followed over 30 months has demonstrated that those who are cigarette smokers lose more cartilage and have more severe knee pain.[39]

PERIARTICULAR LESIONS

It is certainly possible that knee pain in OA subjects may arise from extra-articular structures, such as the bursae located around the joint. Hill and colleagues[40] looked at the prevalence and pain relationship of MRI-detected periarticular lesions in their Boston cohort. They categorized abnormalities as being peripatellar (prepatellar, superficial, or deep infrapatella bursitis) or periarticular (including semimembranosus–tibial collateral ligament bursitis, anserine bursitis, iliotibial band syndrome, or tibiofibular cyst). The frequency of peripatellar lesions was not significantly different between participants with radiographic OA with and without knee symptoms (12% vs. 21%, respectively). However, periarticular pathology was seen more frequently in the radiographic OA knee pain group than in the pain-free group (15% vs. 4%, respectively, $p = 0.004$). Neither peripatellar nor periarticular lesions were seen in subjects without pain or radiographic OA.

MENISCI

MRI has long been seen as the best noninvasive test for evaluating meniscal pathology.[41] Meniscal damage and, in particular, meniscectomy have also been associated with subsequent increased risk of symptomatic and radiographic OA.[42,43] Abnormalities of the menisci are very common in OA: one study demonstrated a high prevalence of meniscal tears even in elderly patients without symptoms, and that tears were more common in symptomatic OA knees compared with asymptomatic controls (91% vs. 76%, respectively, $p < 0.005$).[44] This latter study also showed that the frequency of meniscal tears increased with higher KL radiographic grade, but that both pain and function were no different between OA patients with and without meniscal tears. This suggests that meniscal tears are not contributing to pain in OA knees, although they may occasionally contribute to mechanical (locking) symptoms.

A recent study supports these concepts on the role of the menisci. In a cohort from the MOST study of 110 cases with no knee pain at baseline but who developed symptoms by 15 months of follow-up and 220 controls with no symptoms at both time points, meniscal damage was seen in both groups (38% cases, 29% controls).[45] When adjusted for the presence of other OA features, there was no association between meniscal damage and development of new knee pain.

OSTEOPHYTES

Osteophytes are integral to radiographic definitions of OA, and MRI studies have demonstrated correlations between radiographic osteophytes and cartilage defects in all compartments of the knee.[46,47] Radiographic studies have suggested an association between osteophytes and pain.[48] MRI studies have generally not found this association, although the study of Kornaat et al.[26] did demonstrate an association of pain and patellofemoral osteophytes. An interesting hypothesis was investigated by looking at the presence of BMLs in osteophytes and whether such high signal abnormalities were associated with pain.[49] However, after examination of 217 subjects with radiographic OA knee, no associations were found with pain presence, WOMAC severity, or location of pain.

LIGAMENTS

The association of anterior cruciate ligament (ACL) tears with subsequent development and progression of radiographic OA is well described, and combined injuries involving collateral ligaments result in higher incidence of OA.[50,51] Modern MRI cohorts have suggested a surprisingly high frequency of ligamentous abnormalities in OA patients. Data from a large Boston cohort demonstrated a complete ACL tear in 19% of 265 subjects with painful, radiographic OA knee.[52] Analysis of this cohort demonstrated that while the ACL tears were, as expected, associated with increased risk for cartilage loss (possibly mediated by concurrent meniscal injury), they were not associated with worse pain or disability when compared to those subjects without ACL tears, nor was it associated with greater progression of pain over the 30 month follow-up.

EMERGING DATA ON THE HIP

This chapter has reviewed the bulk of publications in this field, which concern knee OA. However, there is some literature on MRI and symptoms in other joint areas. In the hip, there has been a recent description of BMLs in different hip disorders, highlighting the same range of underlying pathologies as are seen at the knee.[54] In 100 people presenting with symptoms (such as pain, clicking, locking, and giving way) who were evaluated using MR arthrography of the hip, cartilage lesions (76%), labral tears (66%), and BMLs (29%) were common. Interestingly, a study that employed the dGEMRIC technique (designed to evaluate glycosaminoglycan content in cartilage) demonstrated a correlation of dGEMRIC index with WOMAC pain in 68 hips with "dysplasia," while conventional radiographic joint space width did not show this association.[53] The authors did not speculate on the nature of this potential relationship.

CONCLUSION

This chapter could not attempt to address the rapid improvements in MRI technology that will improve joint evaluation. As well, it is very difficult for a predominantly static modality (as most current MRI machines are) to allow investigation of the relationship between force, structural pathology, and symptoms. However, the remarkable ability of MRI to visualize all the structures in the OA joint has already dramatically and rapidly increased our understanding of potential sources of OA pain, although such studies have been limited largely to the knee. Important candidate features include synovitis and effusions, BMLs and periarticular lesions such as anserine bursitis. The knowledge emerging from MRI cohorts will help us better understand pain and structural progression and their complex interrelationship, ultimately allowing for a rational basis for therapeutic strategies.

REFERENCES

1. Felson DT, Lawrence RC, Dieppe PA, Hirsch R, Helmick CG, Jordan JM, et al. (2000). Osteoarthritis: new insights. Part 1: the disease and its risk factors. Ann Intern Med 133(8):635–646.
2. Felson DT, Naimark A, Anderson J, Kazis L, Castelli W, Meenan RF. (1987). The prevalence of knee osteoarthritis in the elderly. The Framingham Osteoarthritis Study. Arthritis Rheum 30(8):914–918.
3. Lethbridge-Cejku M, Scott WW Jr, Reichle R, Ettinger WH, Zonderman A, Costa P, et al. (1995). Association of radiographic features of osteoarthritis of the knee with knee pain: data from the Baltimore Longitudinal Study of Aging. Arthritis Care Res 8(3):182–188.
4. Dieppe PA, Cushnaghan J, Shepstone L. (1997). The Bristol "OA500" study: progression of osteoarthritis (OA) over 3 years and the relationship between clinical and radiographic changes at the knee joint. Osteoarthritis Cartilage 5(2):87–97.

5. Creamer P, Hochberg MC. (1997). Why does osteoarthritis of the knee hurt—sometimes? Br J Rheumatol 36(7):726–728.

6. Hannan MT, Felson DT, Pincus T. (2000). Analysis of the discordance between radiographic changes and knee pain in osteoarthritis of the knee. J Rheumatol 27(6):1513–1517.

7. Peterfy C, Kothari M. (2006). Imaging osteoarthritis: magnetic resonance imaging versus X-ray. Curr Rheumatol Rep 8(1):16–21.

8. Eckstein F, Mosher T, Hunter D. (2007). Imaging of knee osteoarthritis: data beyond the beauty. Curr Opin Rheumatol 19(5):435–443.

9. Eckstein F, Ateshian G, Burgkart R, Burstein D, Cicuttini F, Dardzinski B, et al. (2006). Proposal for a nomenclature for magnetic resonance imaging based measures of articular cartilage in osteoarthritis. Osteoarthritis Cartilage 14(10): 974–983.

10. Peterfy CG, Guermazi A, Zaim S, Tirman PF, Miaux Y, White D, et al. (2004). Whole-Organ Magnetic Resonance Imaging Score (WORMS) of the knee in osteoarthritis. Osteoarthritis Cartilage 12(3):177–190.

11. Kornaat PR, Ceulemans RY, Kroon HM, Riyazi N, Kloppenburg M, Carter WO, et al. (2005). MRI assessment of knee osteoarthritis: Knee Osteoarthritis Scoring System (KOSS)—inter-observer and intra-observer reproducibility of a compartment-based scoring system. Skeletal Radiol 34(2):95–102.

12. Hunter DJ, Lo GH, Gale D, Grainger AJ, Guermazi A, Conaghan PG. (2008). The reliability of a new scoring system for knee osteoarthritis MRI and the validity of bone marrow lesion assessment: BLOKS (Boston Leeds Osteoarthritis Knee Score). Ann Rheum Dis 67(2):206–211.

13. Zhai G, Blizzard L, Srikanth V, Ding C, Cooley H, Cicuttini F, et al. (2006). Correlates of knee pain in older adults: Tasmanian Older Adult Cohort Study. Arthritis Rheum 55(2):264–271.

14. Zhai G, Cicuttini F, Ding C, Scott F, Garnero P, Jones G. (2007). Correlates of knee pain in younger subjects. Clin Rheumatol 26(1):75–80.

15. Dieppe P. (1999). Subchondral bone should be the main target for the treatment of pain and disease progression in osteoarthritis. Osteoarthritis Cartilage 7(3):325–326.

16. Bollet AJ. (2001). Edema of the bone marrow can cause pain in osteoarthritis and other diseases of bone and joints. Ann Intern Med 134(7):591–593.

17. Adalberth T, Roos H, Lauren M, Akeson P, Sloth M, Jonsson K, et al. (1997). Magnetic resonance imaging, scintigraphy, and arthroscopic evaluation of traumatic hemarthrosis of the knee. Am J Sports Med 25(2):231–237.

18. Conaghan PG, O'Connor P, McGonagle D, Astin P, Wakefield RJ, Gibbon WW, et al. (2003). Elucidation of the relationship between synovitis and bone damage: a randomized magnetic resonance imaging study of individual joints in patients with early rheumatoid arthritis. Arthritis Rheum 48(1):64–71.

19. Bergman AG, Willen HK, Lindstrand AL, Pettersson HTA. (1994). Osteoarthritis of the knee—correlation of subchondral MR signal abnormalities with histopathologic and radiographic features. Skeletal Radiol 23(6):445–448.

20. Zanetti M, Bruder E, Romero J, Hodler J. (2000). Bone marrow edema pattern in osteoarthritic knees: correlation between MR imaging and histologic findings. Radiology 215(3):835–840.

21. Felson DT, McLaughlin S, Goggins J, Lavalley MP, Gale ME, Totterman S, et al. (2003). Bone marrow edema and its relation to progression of knee osteoarthritis. Ann Intern Med 139(5 Pt 1):330–336.

22. Lotke PA, Ecker ML, Barth P, Lonner JH. (2000). Subchondral magnetic resonance imaging changes in early osteoarthrosis associated with tibial osteonecrosis. Arthroscopy 16(1):76–81.

23. Felson DT, Chaisson CE, Hill CL, Totterman SM, Gale ME, Skinner KM, et al. (2001). The association of bone marrow lesions with pain in knee osteoarthritis. Ann Intern Med 134(7):541–549.

24. Sowers MF, Hayes C, Jamadar D, Capul D, Lachance L, Jannausch M, et al. (2003). Magnetic resonance-detected subchondral bone marrow and cartilage defect characteristics associated with pain and X-ray defined knee osteoarthritis. Osteoarthritis Cartilage 11(6):387–393.

25. Felson DT, Niu J, Guermazi A, Roemer F, Aliabadi P, Clancy M, et al. (2007). Correlation of the development of knee pain with enlarging bone marrow lesions on magnetic resonance imaging. Arthritis Rheum 56(9):2986–2992.

26. Kornaat PR, Bloem JL, Ceulemans RY, Riyazi N, Rosendaal FR, Nelissen RG, et al. (2006). Osteoarthritis of the knee: association between clinical features and MR imaging findings. Radiology 239(3):811–817.

27. Hernandez-Molina G, Neogi T, Hunter DJ, Niu J, Guermazi A, Roemer FW, et al. (2007). The association of bone attrition with knee pain and other MRI features of osteoarthritis. Ann Rheum Dis 67(1):43–47.

28. Torres L, Dunlop DD, Peterfy C, Guermazi A, Prasad P, Hayes KW, et al. (2006). The relationship between specific tissue lesions and pain severity in persons with knee osteoarthritis. Osteoarthritis Cartilage 14(10):1033–1040.

29. Myers SL, Brandt KD, Ehlich JW, Braunstein EM, Shelbourne KD, Heck DA, et al. (1990). Synovial inflammation in patients with early osteoarthritis of the knee. J Rheumatol 17(12):1662–1669.

30. Smith MD, Triantafillou S, Parker A, Youssef PP, Coleman M. (1997). Synovial membrane inflammation and cytokine production in patients with early osteoarthritis. J Rheumatol 24(2):365–371.

31. Loeuille D, Toussaint F, Champigneulles J, Grossin L, Blum A, Chary-Valckenaere I, et al. (2002). MR evaluation of synovial inflammation in knee OA: histological correlation. Arthritis Rheum 46(9):S566–S567.

32. Ostergaard M, Stoltenberg M, Lovgreen-Nielsen P, Volck B, Jensen CH, Lorenzen I. (1997). Magnetic resonance imaging-determined synovial membrane and joint effusion volumes in rheumatoid arthritis and osteoarthritis: comparison with the macroscopic and microscopic appearance of the synovium. Arthritis Rheum 40(10):1856–1867.

33. Fernandez-Madrid F, Karvonen RL, Teitge RA, Miller PR, An T, Negendank WG. (1995). Synovial thickening detected by MR imaging in osteoarthritis of the knee confirmed by biopsy as synovitis. Magn Reson Imaging 13(2):177–183.

34. Peterfy CG, Majumdar S, Lang P, van Dijke CF, Sack K, Genant HK. (1994). MR imaging of the arthritic knee: improved discrimination of cartilage, synovium, and effusion with pulsed saturation transfer and fat-suppressed T1-weighted sequences. Radiology 191(2):413–419.

35. Hill CL, Gale DG, Chaisson CE, Skinner K, Kazis L, Gale ME, et al. (2001). Knee effusions, popliteal cysts, and synovial thickening: association with knee pain in osteoarthritis. J Rheumatol 28(6):1330–1337.

36. Hill CL, Hunter DJ, Niu J, Clancy M, Guermazi A, Genant H, et al. (2007). Synovitis detected on magnetic resonance imaging and its relation to pain and cartilage loss in knee osteoarthritis. Ann Rheum Dis 66(12):1599–1603.

37. Hunter DJ, March L, Sambrook PN. (2003). The association of cartilage volume with knee pain. Osteoarthritis Cartilage 11(10):725–729.

38. Wluka AE, Wolfe R, Stuckey S, Cicuttini FM. (2004). How does tibial cartilage volume relate to symptoms in subjects with knee osteoarthritis? Ann Rheum Dis 63(3):264–268.

39. Amin S, Niu J, Guermazi A, Grigoryan M, Hunter DJ, Clancy M, et al. (2007). Cigarette smoking and the risk for cartilage loss and knee pain in men with knee osteoarthritis. Ann Rheum Dis 66(1):18–22.

40. Hill CL, Gale DR, Chaisson CE, Skinner K, Kazis L, Gale ME, et al. (2003). Periarticular lesions detected on magnetic resonance imaging: prevalence in knees with and without symptoms. Arthritis Rheum 48(10):2836–2844.

41. Cheung LP, Li KC, Hollett MD, Bergman AG, Herfkens RJ. (1997). Meniscal tears of the knee: accuracy of detection with fast spin-echo MR imaging and arthroscopic correlation in 293 patients. Radiology 203(2):508–512.

42. Roos EM, Ostenberg A, Roos H, Ekdahl C, Lohmander LS. (2001). Long-term outcome of meniscectomy: symptoms, function, and performance tests in patients with or without radiographic osteoarthritis compared to matched controls. Osteoarthritis Cartilage 9(4):316–324.

43. Englund M, Roos EM, Lohmander LS. (2003). Impact of type of meniscal tear on radiographic and symptomatic knee osteoarthritis: a sixteen-year followup of meniscectomy with matched controls. Arthritis Rheum 48(8):2178–2187.

44. Bhattacharyya T, Gale D, Dewire P, Totterman S, Gale ME, McLaughlin S, et al. (2003). The clinical importance of meniscal tears demonstrated by magnetic resonance imaging in osteoarthritis of the knee. J Bone Joint Surg Am 85-A(1):4–9.

45. Englund M, Niu J, Guermazi A, Roemer FW, Hunter DJ, Lynch JA, et al. (2007). Effect of meniscal damage on the development of frequent knee pain, aching, or stiffness. Arthritis Rheum 56(12):4048–4054.

46. Boegard T, Rudling O, Petersson IF, Jonsson K. (1998). Correlation between radiographically diagnosed osteophytes and magnetic resonance detected cartilage defects in the tibiofemoral joint. Ann Rheum Dis 57(7):401–407.

47. Boegard T, Rudling O, Petersson IF, Jonsson K. (1998). Correlation between radiographically diagnosed osteophytes and magnetic resonance detected cartilage defects in the patellofemoral joint. Ann Rheum Dis 57(7):395–400.

48. Cicuttini FM, Baker J, Hart DJ, Spector TD. (1996). Association of pain with radiological changes in different compartments and views of the knee joint. Osteoarthritis Cartilage 4(2):143–147.

49. Sengupta M, Zhang YQ, Niu JB, Guermazi A, Grigorian M, Gale D, et al. (2006). High signal in knee osteophytes is not associated with knee pain. Osteoarthritis Cartilage 14(5):413–417.

50. Lundberg M, Messner K. (1997). Ten-year prognosis of isolated and combined medial collateral ligament ruptures. A matched comparison in 40 patients using clinical and radiographic evaluations. Am J Sports Med 25(1):2–6.

51. Gillquist J, Messner K. (1999). Anterior cruciate ligament reconstruction and the long-term incidence of gonarthrosis. Sports Med 27(3):143–156.

52. Amin S, Guermazi A, Lavalley MP, Niu J, Clancy M, Hunter DJ, et al. (2008). Complete anterior cruciate ligament tear and the risk for cartilage loss and progression of symptoms in men and women with knee osteoarthritis. Osteoarthritis Cartilage 16(8):897–902.

53. Kim YJ, Jaramillo D, Millis MB, Gray ML, Burstein D. (2003). Assessment of early osteoarthritis in hip dysplasia with delayed gadolinium-enhanced magnetic resonance imaging of cartilage. J Bone Joint Surg Am 85-A(10):1987–1992.

54. Neumann G, Mendicuti AD, Zou KH, Minas T, Coblyn J, Winalski CS, et al. (2007). Prevalence of labral tears and cartilage loss in patients with mechanical symptoms of the hip: evaluation using MR arthrography. Osteoarthritis Cartilage 15(8):909–917.

12

EVIDENCE OF SENSITIZATION TO PAIN IN HUMAN OSTEOARTHRITIS

Gunnar Ordeberg

Department of Orthopaedics, University Hospital,
SE-751 85 Uppsala, Sweden

INTRODUCTION

Pain is usually characterized as nociceptive, neuropathic, idiopathic, or psychogenic. Different receptors and pain transmitters are involved, and responses to analgesic agents differ in these categories as does the pattern of pain distribution. During the last decade, much attention has been paid to the plasticity in the nervous system regarding pain generation and maintenance, and sensitization of the sensory system.[1,2]

Pain in osteoarthritis (OA) is most frequent in the hip and knee, that is, the big joints under mechanical load. Degenerative changes concomitant with pain are also extremely common in the spine; however, there is often controversy whether the pain is produced from OA in the intervertebral joints, degeneration of disks, or in other structures such as muscles and ligaments.[3] Furthermore, osteophytes, synovitis, and capsular thickening in OA of the intervertebral joints—as well as herniation from the degenerated disk—with mechanical and chemical irritation of the nerve structures may cause pain of peripheral neurogenic origin. This is sometimes not easy to distinguish from degenerative nociceptive pain.[4]

Perceived pain intensity varies greatly even in individuals with similar radiologic severity of OA. This has often been attributed to psychological or social factors.[5] However, it has been shown that individuals with chronic low back pain (LBP) also show lower pain thresholds for mechanical compression of the thumb nail.[6] Our studies presented here support the conclusion that sensitization mechanisms are active in longstanding pain from OA.

PAIN IN OSTEOARTHRITIS

Symptoms of hip OA usually start with localized pain either in the groin or trochanteric region. Pain in the ventral part of the thigh as distal as the knee is also common, and occasionally a patient with hip OA may present with pain predominantly in the knee. The true source of pain is revealed by the clinical examination with restriction and pain with hip rotation along with a normal physical examination of the knee. In the beginning, the patient usually has pain only when the joint is under load. Later, pain at rest may follow. Furthermore, in the beginning, the pain can be eliminated or at least significantly reduced by different kinds of analgesics; later, the response to these pills becomes inadequate or absent. The area with pain will often spread to the thigh and knee, but pain localization in the leg or even widespread pain all over the body is not uncommon. In fact, pain drawings in patients with clinical signs of hip OA have suggested that many patients have a wide pain distribution. Despite this, most patients report almost total pain relief following total hip replacement. Of course, enlargement of the area of pain could be due to concomitant OA in other joints or in the spine. However, we think that sensitization is the most common cause, as the mechanism of increased pain area has also been reported in patients with pain from burns.[7] The wide variation of pain intensity in hip OA, and its poor correlation with the degree of radiological severity as well as of the histological evidence of synovitis, turned our interest to the plasticity of the nervous system and especially to such factors as central sensitization and activation of endogenous pain inhibitory mechanisms for the modulation of pain sensation.

DISTURBANCE OF PAIN INHIBITION

Chronic pain can be associated with reduced central pain modulation. Diffuse noxious inhibitory control (DNIC) is a well recognized CNS pain inhibitory system, by which one acute noxious stimulus inhibits the pain produced by another.[8] Thus DNIC-like heterotopic noxious condition stimulation can induce reduction of pain sensitivity in other parts of the body. Patients with fibromyalgia have exhibited dysfunction with regard to this mechanism,[9] as well as hyperalgesia/allodynia not restricted to painful areas.[10]

We studied the DNIC mechanism in patients with painful hip OA in comparison to healthy controls.[11] Fifteen patients with painful hip OA underwent examination; 13 of them who underwent operation were examined 5 months after surgery when they were almost pain free. Comparison was also made with sex- and age-matched controls. We used a submaximal effort tourniquet test to induce ischemic pain. A blood pressure cuff was applied on the upper arm ipsilateral to the painful hip and inflated to 170 mmHg. The subjects were instructed to perform standard contractions in the same hand which gave rise to ischemic pain in the arm. The pain remained as long as the cuff was inflated. Quantitative sensory testing (QST) was performed

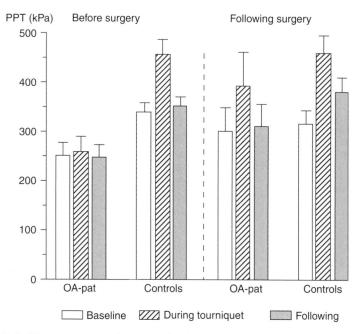

Figure 12.1. Mean pressure pain thresholds (PPTs)($\pm$SEM) in OA patients and healthy controls. Before surgery no statistical significant change in PPTs was seen during tourniquet application in patients. In controls, PPTs increased during tourniquet application ($p < 0.002$), decreased following tourniquet application ($p < 0.001$), and returned to baseline values. Following surgery, PPTs increased during tourniquet application in patients ($p < 0.02$), decreased following tourniquet application in patients ($p < 0.03$), and returned to baseline values. In controls, PPTs increased during tourniquet application ($p < 0.001$) and decreased following tourniquet application ($p < 0.002$), but remained slightly elevated compared to baseline values ($p < 0.01$).

contralateral to the painful area in the leg in the patients and pressure pain thresholds were measured. The minimum pressure at which the patient felt that the stimulus was painful was determined with pressure algometry,[12] while perception thresholds to light touch were assessed using von Frey filaments (Aestesiometer).[13] The thermal sensitivity was analyzed by a Thermotest with cold and warm stimuli.[14] The temperature of the Thermode plate applied to the skin was increased until the patient reported heat pain, and in the same way was lowered until cold pain was felt. Measurements were performed before, during, and 45 minutes following the tourniquet test.

As shown in Figure 12.1, patients had a tendency to lower pressure pain thresholds (PPTs) compared to controls before tourniquet application ($p = 0.05$), while with the tourniquet applied, the PPTs were significantly lower ($p < 0.001$) in patients than in controls, and after tourniquet release, the PPTs were also significantly lower in patients ($p < 0.002$). However, at the second

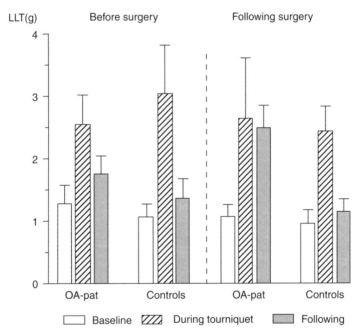

Figure 12.2. Mean light-touch perception thresholds (LTTs) ($\pm$SEM) in OA patients and healthy controls before and following surgery. Before surgery, LTTs increased during tourniquet application in both groups ($p < 0.001$) and decreased following tourniquet application in controls ($p < 0.001$), but not in patients. After tourniquet application LTTs returned to baseline in controls, but there was a strong tendency to elevated LTTs in patients ($p < 0.050$). Following surgery, LTTs increased significantly during tourniquet application in both groups ($p < 0.001$), decreased following tourniquet application in both groups ($p < 0.001$), and returned to baseline values.

registration, after the operation, PPTs increased during tourniquet application in patients and controls alike, and there was no statistically significant differences in PPTs between patients and controls either before, during, or after tourniquet application. Thus the main finding was that the tourniquet produced no modulation of pressure pain sensitivity in patients before surgery, in contrast to controls, suggesting a dysfunction of DNIC mechanisms. However, following surgery, this dysfunction had subsided.

In the same test, perceptions of light-touch thresholds (LTTs) were more similar in patients and controls; before surgery the thresholds increased with tourniquet application in both groups with the only difference being a tendency toward elevated LTTs in patients after tourniquet release (Fig. 12.2). Following surgery, no differences in LTTs were seen between patients and controls.

In the registration of temperature thresholds, there was no effect of tourniquet application on thresholds for the perception of either innocuous warmth or heat pain, before and after surgery. Perception thresholds to innocuous cold increased during tourniquet application in patients as well as controls, and decreased in both groups after tourniquet application before as well as after surgery (Fig. 12.3), with no significant differences found between the groups.

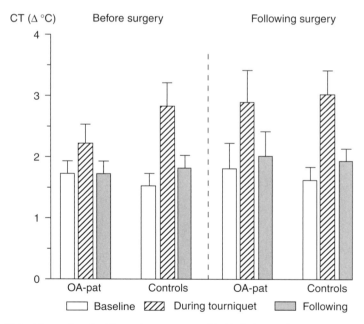

Figure 12.3. Mean thresholds to innocuous cold (CTs) ($\pm$SEM) in OA patients and healthy controls before and following surgery. Before, as well as following surgery, CTs increased during tourniquet application in both groups ($p < 0.001$), decreased following surgery in both groups ($p < 0.001$), and returned to baseline.

In another study of hyperalgesia,[15] in 14 of the patients with painful hip OA, quantitative sensory testing was performed in the most painful area (for most patients this was the trochanteric region), and in their respective controls (see Table 12.1) before and (in the 12 patients who had subsequent operation) after surgery. Pressure pain sensitivity was assessed with a pressure algometer and thermal sensitivity with a Thermotest. Compared to controls, patients had increased sensitivity to pressure with a lower threshold for pain ($p < 0.002$), and increased sensitivity to innocous warmth ($p < 0.03$) and cold pain ($p < 0.05$), and a tendency to increased sensitivity to heat pain ($p = 0.054$) before surgery. However, at the second examination after surgery, no significant differences in sensitivity of any kind were seen between patients and controls. Furthermore, patients also had reduced PPTs on the contralateral side before surgery. These was also normalized following surgery. Interestingly, the same type of sensory aberrations seen before surgery in these patients with hip OA have previously

TABLE 12.1   Quantitative Sensory Testing in Patients with Osteoarthritis of the Hip and in Healthy Controls[a]

	Before Surgery (n = 14)		Following Surgery (n = 12)	
Measurements[b]	Pain Side	Contralateral Side	Pain Side	Contralateral Side
PPT (kPa)				
Patients	198.8 ± 22.7**[†]	252.8 ± 30.1	290.8 ± 44.7[†]	298.7 ± 52.7
Controls	338.7 ± 26.3	333.2 ± 22.0	333.8 ± 32.3	315.4 ± 29.8
LTT log 10 (mg)				
Patients	3.25 ± 0.4	3.11 ± 0.2	3.01 ± 0.3[††]	3.03 ± 0.2
Controls	3.06 ± 0.2	3.00 ± 0.2	3.03 ± 0.3	2.97 ± 0.2
CT ($\Delta°C$)				
Patients	1.4 ± 0.2	1.6 ± 0.2	1.6 ± 0.3	1.8 ± 0.4
Controls	1.6 ± 0.3	1.6 ± 0.2	1.5 ± 0.2	1.6 ± 0.1
WT ($\Delta°C$)				
Patients	2.5 ± 0.4*	3.0 ± 0.5*	3.8 ± 0.5†	3.8 ± 0.8[‡]
Controls	4.2 ± 0.7	3.8 ± 0.5	3.2 ± 0.3	3.2 ± 0.3
CT + WT ($\Delta°C$)				
Patients	3.8 ± 0.5	4.6 ± 0.6	5.5 ± 0.7	5.6 ± 1.1
Controls	5.8 ± 0.9	5.4 ± 0.6	4.6 ± 0.4	4.8 ± 0.3
HPT ($\Delta°c$)				
Patients	41.2 ± 0.8	41.2 ± 0.7	43.1 ± 1.0	43.3 ± 0.9
Controls	42.9 ± 0.6	42.8 ± 0.8	42.8 ± 0.7	43.0 ± 0.6

[a]Mean $\pm$ Standard error of mean.
[b]PPT = pressure–pain threshold; LTT = light-touch perception threshold; CT = perception threshold to innocuous cold; WT = perception threshold to innocuous warmth; (CT + WT) = sum of innocuous thermal thresholds; HPT = heat pain threshold. Statistically significant difference are indicated: (a) between groups, *$p < 0.05$; **$p < 0.01$; (b) between treatments, †$p < 0.05$, ††$p < 0.01$; (c) between sides, ‡$p < 0.05$.

been reported in patients with fibromyalgia.[10] However, these abnormalities have not been found in similar studies of patients with rheumatoid arthritis and with trapezius myalgia.[16,17]

CEREBROSPINAL FLUID ANALYSES OF SUBSTANCE P

It is known from several studies that patients with fibromyalgia have increased substance P-like activity (SPLI) in cerebrospinal fluid (CSF).[18] In earlier investigations we also analyzed CSF samples from 11 patients with painful hip or knee OA for SPLI and compared them to a group of 9 pain-free controls and 9 patients with radiating pain from a herniated lumbar disk.[19]

The SPLI in CSF from the OA patients was increased in comparison to the controls (Fig. 12.4) but also in comparison to the patients with radiating pain.

As shown in Figure 12.5, there was a correlation between SPLI and pain score as recorded preoperatively, but the increased SPLI was less than that seen in patients with fibromyalgia.[20] The OA patients in the study were all candidates for joint replacement and had another CSF sample 5 months after the operation. SPLI had decreased but was still higher than in the controls.

These findings thus suggest a gradual transition in OA from uncomplicated nociceptive pain to secondary sensory disturbances having similarities with findings in patients with fibromyalgia.

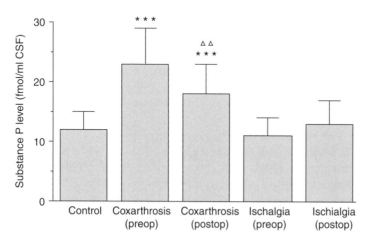

Figure 12.4. Substance P levels in cerebrospinal fluid from patients with hip OA(coxarthrosis) and ischialgia (radiating pain from herniated lumbar disk) ($M \pm$SEM). ***Patient groups compared to control group ($p < 0.001$). $^{\triangle\triangle}$ Postoperative activity compared to preoperative values ($p < 0.01$).

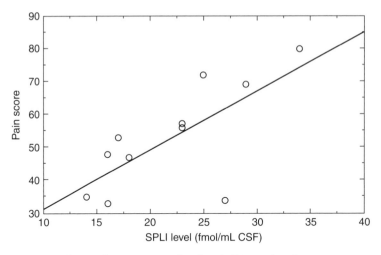

Figure 12.5. Correlation between CSF levels of SPLI and pain scores as recorded preoperatively. $y = 1.78 + 13.9$; $r^2 = 0.51$ ($p < 0.01$).

DISCUSSION

Long standing pain impulses may induce changes in neuronal structures, and this can be a mechanism in sensitization. We have shown that long-lasting pain in OA is accompanied by disturbances in the central inhibition of pain. The study indicates the presence of allodynia (exaggerated response to normally nonnoxious stimuli) in patients suffering from long-lasting OA pain as reduced thresholds for pain in the affected area and its contralateral counterpart. Moreover, the acute induced pain in the DNIC procedure did not affect pain thresholds in another body region in the patients, as it was supposed to do from previous studies of the DNIC system and also did in the controls. Allodynia and disturbed central inhibition are both known to be important factors in the generation of pain.[21]

There is also evidence that the process of pain sensitization is influenced by external factors such as fear and psychosocial stress.[5] However, little is known about when and to what extent this sensitization is reversible and the role of constitutional factors. There is conflicting evidence on whether a wide distribution of pain (suggestive of disturbed pain inhibitory mechanisms) will affect the outcome of surgery in pain conditions. In the orthopedic literature, especially regarding patients with back pain, wide pain distribution is often regarded as a sign of behavioral symptoms.[22] However, in a study of patients, operated on by fusion for presumed lumbar pain of segmental origin, no difference in clinical result was observed 2 years after surgery between patients with localized pain on their preoperative pain drawings and those with pain spread also to other regions.[23]

It is possible that long-lasting pain could be produced either by profound degenerative changes or by disturbances affecting pain sensitization. In a Danish study of patients with low back pain, patients with a high frequency of tender points had less radiological degeneration than the rest, but among patients with no or only few tender points, there was a correlation between degree of radiological degeneration and pain intensity on the VAS scale.[24] This is in contrast to almost all previous studies on patients with back pain, where no or only a very weak correlation has been found between back pain intensity and the degree of radiological degeneration.[25]

While the pain inhibition mechanism we studied was reversible in our patients, we do not know whether this always holds true even after prolonged pain impulses and additional sensitization mechanisms.

It is well known that widespread pain, for example, in patients with a diagnosis of fibromyalgia, is very difficult to counteract. Accordingly, there is a reluctance to perform surgical treatment on patients with widespread pain, even in the presence of a morphologic and potentially pain-inducing lesion.[26]

In conclusion, pain in OA is multifaceted and pain intensity has a limited correlation to the degree of OA. One reason for this is a disturbance of central inhibitory impulses and sensitization. Further studies are needed in order to improve our knowledge of these and other pain-related mechanisms.

ACKNOWLEDGMENTS

The author thanks Prof. Erik Torebjörk for generously providing laboratory facilities at the Department of Clinical Neurophysiology, Uppsala University Hospital. The author has received grant support from the Swedish Medical Society, Olle Höök's Foundation, and Tore Nilsson's Foundation.

REFERENCES

1. McCormack K. (1999). Fail-safe mechanisms that perperuate neuropathic pain. Pain Clin Updates VII(3):1–4.
2. Lidbeck J. (2002). Central hyperexcitability in chronic musculoskeletal pain: a conceptual breakthrough with multiple clinical implications. Pain Res Manage 7:881–892.
3. Schwarzer AC, Aprill CN, Derby R, Fortin J, Kine G, Bogduk N. (1994). The relative contributions of the disc and zygapophyseal joint in chronic low back pain. Spine 19(7):801–806.
4. Brisby H, Olmarker K, Larsson K, Nutu M, Rydevik B. (2002). Proinflammatory cytokines in cerebrospinal fluid and serum in patients with disc herniation and sciatica. Eur Spine J 11(1):62–66.

5. Turk DC. (2003). Cognitive-behavioral approach to the treatment of chronic pain patients. Reg Anesth Pain Med 28(6):573–579.

6. Giesecke T, Gracely RH, Grant MA, Nachemson A, Petzke F, Williams DA, Clauw DJ. (2004). Evidence of augmented central pain processing in idiopathic chronic low back pain. Arthritis Rheum 50(2):613–623.

7. Pedersen JL. (2000). Inflammatory pain in experimental burns in man. Dan Med Bull 47(3):168–195.

8. Edwards RR, Ness TJ, Weigent DA, Fillingim RB. (2003). Individual differences in diffuse noxious inhibitory controls (DNIC): association with clinical variables. Pain 106(3):427–437.

9. Kosek E, Hansson P. (1997). Modulatory influence on somatosensory perception from vibration and heterotopic noxious conditioning stimulation (HNCS) in fibromyalgia patients and healthy subjects. Pain 70:41–51.

10. Kosek E, Ekholm J, Hansson P. (1996). Sensory dysfunction in fibromyalgia patients with implications for pathogenic mechanisms. Pain 68:375–383.

11. Kosek E, Ordeberg G. (2000). Lack of pressure pain modulation by heterotopic noxious conditioning stimulation in patients with painful osteoarthritis before, but not following, surgical pain relief. Pain 88(1):69–78.

12. Jensen K, Andersen HO, Olesen J, Lindblom U. (1986). Pressure–pain threshold in human temporal region. Evaluation of a new pressure algometer. Pain 25(3): 313–323.

13. Weinstein S. (1992). Tactile sensitivity of the phalanges. Percept Motor Skills 1962(14):351–354.

14. Hansson P, Ekblom A, Lindblom U, Marchettini P. (1988). Does acute intraoral pain alter cutaneous sensibility? J Neurol Neurosurg Psychiatry 51(8):1032–1036.

15. Kosek E, Ordeberg G. (2000). Abnormalities of somatosensory perception in patients with painful osteoarthritis normalizes following sucessful treatment. Eur J Pain 4(3):229–238.

16. Leffler AS, Kosek E, Lerndal T, Nordmark B, Hansson P. (2002). Somatosensory perception and function of diffuse noxious inhibitory controls (DNIC) in patients suffering from rheumatoid arthritis. Eur J Pain 6:161–176.

17. Leffler AS, Hansson P, Kosek E. (2002). Somatosensory perception in a remote pain-free area and function of diffuse noxious inhibitory controls (DNIC) in patients suffering from long-term trapezius myalgia. Eur J Pain 6:149–159.

18. Vaeroy H, Helle R, Forre O, Kass E, Terenius L. (1988). Elevated CSF levels of substance P and high incidence of Raynaud phenomenon in patients with fibromyalgia: new features for diagnosis. Pain 32(1):21–26.

19. Lindh C, Zhurong L, Lyrenäs S, Ordeberg G, Nyberg F. (1997). Elevated cerebrospinal substance P-like immunoreactivity in patients with painful osteoarthritis, but not in patients with rhizopathic pain from a herniated lumbar disc. Scand J Rheumatol 26:468–472.

20. Russell IJ, Orr MD, Littman B, Vipraio GA, Alboukrek D, Michalek JE, Lopez Y, MacKillip F. (1994). Elevated cerebrospinal fluid levels of substance P in patients with the fibromyalgia syndrome. Arthritis Rheum 37(11):1593–1601.

21. Staud R. (2005). Predictors of clinical pain intensity in patients with fibromyalgia syndrome. Curr Pain Headache Rep 9(5):316–321.

22. Waddell G, Richardson J. (1992). Observation of overt pain behaviour by physicians during routine clinical examination of patients with low back pain. J Psychosom Res 36(1):77–87.

23. Hagg O, Fritzell P, Hedlund R, Moller H, Ekselius L, Nordwall A. (2003). Swedish Lumbar Spine Study. Pain-drawing does not predict the outcome of fusion surgery for chronic low-back pain: a report from the Swedish Lumbar Spine Study. Eur Spine J 12(1):2–11.

24. Jensen OK, Nielsen CV, Stengaard-Pedersen K. (2007). Sensitization of the nociceptive system in patients with low back pain and sickness abscence. Eur Spine J 16 Suppl(1):34–35.

25. Witt I, Vestergaard A, Rosenklint A. (1984). A comparative analysis of X-ray findings of the lumbar spine in patients with and without lumbar pain. Spine 9(3):298–300.

26. Voorhies RM, Jiang X, Thomas N. (2007). Predicting outcome in the surgical treatment of lumbar radiculopathy using the Pain Drawing Score, McGill Short Form Pain Questionnaire, and risk factors including psychosocial issues and axial joint pain. Spine J 7(5):516–524.

13

CURRENT PERSPECTIVES ON THE CLINICAL PRESENTATION OF JOINT PAIN IN HUMAN OSTEOARTHRITIS

Paul Creamer

Consultant Rheumatologist, Southmead Hospital, Bristol BS10 5NB, United Kingdom

INTRODUCTION

Pain is the commonest symptom of osteoarthritis (OA), the principal reason why individuals seek medical care and a major determinant of other outcomes such as disability and joint replacement. Most studies have examined knee OA: little is known about the cause of pain in other sites affected by knee OA. Community studies indicate only a modest relationship between structural change on X-ray and reporting of pain. Many community subjects, for example, fail to complain of pain despite extensive X-ray change, while others report pain with normal X-rays. Pain severity of patients attending hospital is even less related to X-ray change, being more dependent on body mass index (BMI), coping strategies, and psychosocial variables. Magnetic resonance imaging (MRI) is proving to be a valuable tool with which to investigate the relationship between pain and structure. Many patients can identify more than one type of pain. It is increasingly clear that OA pain is heterogeneous, being

---

Pain in Osteoarthritis, Edited by David T. Felson and Hans-Georg Schaible
Copyright © 2009 Wiley-Blackwell.

classifiable on the basis of location, precipitating factors, response to anti-inflammatory and steroid medication, and effect of local anesthetic and other local therapies. This potential to classify OA pain represents a useful tool with which to test hypotheses regarding structural origin of pain.

OSTEOARTHRITIS

Osteoarthritis (OA) is a disorder of synovial joints characterized by destruction of articular cartilage and overgrowth of marginal and subchondral bone.[1] Research into OA has been limited by difficulties in defining the disease. An epidemiological approach evaluates the incidence, prevalence, and associations of OA, using radiographs to define disease. Clinicians concentrate on the smaller number of individuals with symptoms, who elect to present to medical care. Finally, basic scientists have traditionally studied cartilage biomechanics and biochemistry (although cartilage is only one of several tissues to be affected in OA).

Individuals with OA who become symptomatic almost always present with pain, although stiffness (usually after inactivity, also know as "gelling"), limitation of movement, crepitus, joint line tenderness, and joint swelling are also seen. Pain, however, is the principal symptom of OA and the major reason why subjects seek medical attention, which may include costly interventions such as joint replacement.[2] Pain is also the most significant determinant of disability. Given the current lack of disease-modifying drugs for OA, the treatment of OA is essentially the treatment of OA pain.

OA can affect any synovial joint but most of our knowledge of pain in OA derives from the knee. It is important to note that mechanisms may vary from joint to joint, and data from the knee may not necessarily be transferable to other joints. Most frequently, affected joints include the apophyseal joints of the spine, interphalangeal joints and first carpometacarpal joint in the hand, knee (particularly medial tibiofemoral and lateral patellofemoral joints), hip, and first tarsometatarsal joint. Ankle and shoulder are rarely affected. The distribution is therefore highly defined—even within individual joints. The pathophysiology underlying such specificity may reflect a discordance between the demands made on a joint and the ability in terms of structure, function, evolutionary adaptation, and genetic predisposition to withstand such load.

KNEE PAIN IN THE COMMUNITY

Knee pain is usually assessed as a dichotomous variable (present or absent) using, for example, the NHANES-I screening question: "Have you ever had pain in or around the knee on most days for at least one month?" Subtle changes in the phrasing of the question can result in large differences in apparent prevalence of pain, but in general about 24–28% of community dwellers aged 40–70 respond positively to such a question.[3] Prevalence of knee pain increases with radiographic severity of OA.[4–8] In the NHANES-I study, for example, among subjects aged 65–74, knee pain was reported by 8.8% of subjects with normal X-rays, 20.4% with Kellgren and Lawrence (K + L) grade 1 OA, 36.9% with grade 2, and 60.4% with grades 3–4.[9] Similar findings of a progressive increase in the risk of pain reporting with worsening radiographic change have been reported at other joint sites (Table 13.1). The relationship between knee pain and radiographic change differs between ethnic groups: joint pain in African American women is more likely to be associated with radiographic OA knee as compared with Caucasian women.[12]

It is clear that there are many subjects in whom X-ray changes and reported pain are discordant.[13] Pain may be reported in the absence of X-ray changes— the prevalence of self-reported knee pain with normal X-rays is about 10.0%. There are several potential reasons for this. First, most studies utilize only supine or weight-bearing views of the tibiofemoral joint; failure to assess the patellofemoral joint could result in a subject being classified as "X-ray negative" when in fact changes were present but not seen. Indeed, up to 24% of females reporting knee pain have isolated patellofemoral disease and if lateral views are included the predictive value of pain for radiographic change increases.[14] Second, a positive response to the NHANES-I knee question does not differentiate between isolated knee pain and widespread pain of which the knee is but a part. The prevalence of "widespread chronic pain" is about 11%.[15] Such patients may answer affirmatively about knee pain but this would not necessarily imply local pathology. Third, X-rays are relatively insensitive: they may be normal when other diagnostic studies such as arthroscopy show clear evidence of OA.[16] X-rays do not allow visualization of nonbony sources of pain, such as capsule, synovium, or ligaments. Finally, not all knee pain is due to OA: causes such as anserine bursitis, internal derangements, and referred pain from hip or spine would not be identified on X-rays of the knees.

The second group consists of subjects who are X-ray positive but do not report pain. Pain reporting in grade 3–4 OA ranges from 40% to 79%: thus up

TABLE 13.1 Prevalence (%) of Reported Pain by Radiographic Severity at First Carpometacarpal (ICMC), Distal (DIP), and Proximal (PIP) Interphalangeal and Hip Joints

Radiographic Severity (KL Grade)	Joint Site		
	ICMC[a]	DIP/PIP[a]	Hip[b]
0/1	10.6	15.2	8.0 (M), 12.0 (F)
2	34.2	48.7	10.0 (M), 14.0 (F)
3/4	65.1	80.9	44.0 (M), 86.0 (F)

[a]From Hart.[10]

[b]From Lawrence.[11]

TABLE 13.2   Clinical and Imaging Correlates of Knee Pain Reporting

Variable Associated with KP Reporting	Reference
Correlates of Knee Pain (KP) as a Dichotomous Variable (present/absent).[a]	
Global radiographic severity	Felson 1987, Hochberg 1989, Carman 1989, Davis 1992, Spector 1993, Lethbridge-Cejku 1995 and others
Osteophyte severity	Spector 1993, Lethbridge 1995, Cicuttini 1996
Synovitis on MRI	Hill 2001
Bone marrow oedema on MRI	Felson 2001
Psychological well being (GWB)	Davis 1992
Health status	Davis 1992
Anxiety (women only)	Creamer 1999a
Feeling "low" or "very low" in spirits	Hochberg 1989
Hypochondriasis	Lichtenberg 1986
Negative affect	Dekker 1993
Lower educational level	Hannon 1992

Pain Measure	Independent Variable	Reference
Correlates of Knee Pain Severity as a Continuous Variable[b]		
WOMAC	BMI	Creamer 1999b
	Helplessness (AAI)	Creamer 1999b
	Circadian rhythm	Bellamy 1990
MPQ	Age	Creamer 1999b
	BMI	Creamer 1999b
	Education	Creamer 1999b
	Depression (CES-D)	Creamer 1999b
	Depression (BDI)	Summers 1998
	Anxiety (SSTAI)	Summers 1998
	Anxiety (Zung)	Salaffi 1991
	Depression (Zung)	Salaffi 1991
	Pain coping (CSQ)	Keefe 1987
VAS	Duration	Creamer 1999b
	Helplessness (AAI)	Creamer 1999b
	Muscle weakness (dynamometer)	van Baar 1998*
	Pain coping (PCI)	van Baar 1998*
	Psychosocial disability (SIP)	Hopman Rock 1996*
	Sclerosis on X ray	Szebenyi 2006*

[a]Data generally derived from community studies.

[b]Data derived from hospital patients (asterisked studies included community subjects).

WOMAC = Western Ontario and McMaster Universities Osteoarthritis Index; MPQ = McGill Pain Questionnaire; VAS = Visual Analogue Scale

AAI = Arthritis Attitudes Index; BDI = Beck Depression Inventory; CES-D = Center for Epidemiologic Studies-Depression; CSQ = Coping Strategies Questionnaire; GWB = General Well Being Instrument; PCI = Pain Coping Inventory; SIP = Sickness Impact Profile; SSTAI = Spielberger Stait Trait Anxiety Index; Zung = Zung Anxiety (Depression) Inventory

to half the patients in the community with, by any standard, established radiographic OA deny pain. The relationship improves if osteophytes rather than global change are used.[7,8,17] The precise question that is asked may affect the response in terms of pain reporting. The NHANES-I question may underestimate prevalence: patients may have had pain but not on "most days of a month" or they may simply fail to recall previous episodes of pain. Further more, OA may be a phasic condition with episodes of pain separated by remissions: the question may fail to capture the painful episode.

Another approach to examining the relationship between structural change and pain is to consider the prevalence of X-ray change in those presenting with joint pain. A community survey of 4057 subjects aged 40–70 years found a point prevalence of knee pain of 28.3%. Of these, 74% had at least grade 1 osteophyte and 40.9% had at least grade 2.[3] In 195 subjects aged over 40 presenting to their physician with a first episode of hip pain, Birrel et al.[18] found 44% had a KL grade ≥ 2 and 34% had KL≥ 3. A minimum joint space of ≤ 2.5 mm was seen in 30%. By the time subjects present to primary care with hip pain, a significant number will already have established OA change on X-ray.

Radiographic change is thus only a small risk factor for pain reporting in OA in the community (see Table 13.2). Psychological well-being and health status,[9] anxiety (in women only),[19] feeling "low" or "very low" in spirits,[5] hypochondriasis,[20] and "negative affect"[21] have all been associated with higher levels of knee pain reporting. Lower educational level is an independent risk factor for pain reporting.[22]

OSTEOARTHRITIS PAIN IN THE CLINIC

Some individuals with knee or hip pain elect to present to medical care. The reasons for this choice are unclear but comorbidity (especially psychosocial), coping beliefs, social support, availability of services, and degree of empower-ment are all likely to be more important than pain severity, radiographic change, age, or functional limitation. A community study of subjects with hip or knee pain found that depression scores were significantly higher in those who had elected to seek medical care.[23] A similar role for psychological factors in the promotion of healthcare seeking behavior has been suggested in other conditions such as fibromyalgia.

It is safe to assume that almost all individuals with OA presenting to healthcare will have pain. Although pain is clearly important to patients and is discussed at 98% of consultations, potential causes are discussed minimally or not at all in up to 46% cases.[24] Furthermore, physicians and patients may disagree about the severity of their pain and effect on life.[25] Suarez-Almazor et al.[26] in a study of 105 patients with musculoskeletal disease found that intraclass correlation coefficient (ICC) for agreement on pain severity between doctors and their patients was only 0.42. Physicians tended to rate their patients' health status higher than the patients themselves and were less willing to gamble on the risk of death versus perfect health. The *importance* of pain to patients with OA and the relationship between *pain severity and its importance* has been little studied but clearly has great relevance.

For patients presenting to healthcare, pain becomes a continuous variable—pain severity. A major advance in OA pain research has been the adoption of standardized, validated questionnaires such as the WOMAC, Lequesne Index, McGill Pain Questionnaire (MPQ), or a simple Visual Analog Scale (VAS). The WOMAC has recently been shown to be more responsive than SF-36[27] and the Lequesne Index[28] and appears not to be influenced by anxiety and depression as much as the McGill Pain Questionnaire (MPQ).[29] It also allows pain occurring in different situations to be separately assessed. The risk factors for pain severity are different from those for pain as a dichotomous variable (see Table 13.2). It is important to note that risk factors may differ according to the definition of the factor being studied (e.g., different measures may be used to assess depression) and the pain severity measure being used as an outcome (e.g., WOMAC, McGill Pain Questionnaire, or simple VAS). In a group of hospital outpatients with knee OA,[29] risk factors for pain severity after adjustment for confounding variables included obesity, helplessness, and low educational attainment. Age, disease duration, and quality of life are not usually related to severity of pain. Others have reported links between pain severity and psychological factors: Summers et al.[30] reporting on 65 patients with OA of hip or knee found that depression (as measured by the Beck Depression Inventory) and anxiety correlated with some measures of the MPQ. Another study of 61 patients with knee OA found significant correlations between MPQ and Zung Anxiety and Depression Inventory scores.[31] In the community, chronicity and severity of knee pain were associated with higher psychosocial disability (as measured by subscales of the Sickness Impact Profile) compared to age and sex matched controls from the same community.[32] Coping mechanisms may not only influence reported pain severity but may predict future pain (and disability).[33]

Just as X-ray change is only weakly related to pain reporting as a dichotomous variable (present or absent), it has almost no relation to pain severity in subjects presenting to medical care.[19,29,34,35] Szebenyi et al.[36] in a cross-sectional study of 167 community-based subjects with knee OA, found no difference in VAS pain severity score between those subjects with normal X-rays and those with radiographic OA (KL 1–4) in either tibiofemoral or patellofemoral joints (although there was a weak increase in severity if changes were present in both compartments). In this study, the presence of subchondral bone sclerosis was associated with increased pain severity, although other studies have found osteophytes to be more closely linked to pain severity. It may be that a certain threshold of structural disease needs to be reached for joints to become painful, but beyond that, other factors (coping strategies, depression, co morbidity, BMI) determine the perceived severity for an individual.

MRI has the ability to image structures not seen on plain X-ray but which may be responsible for pain. In general, the presence of radiographic OA is associated with more MR change in a variety of structures[35,37] but, as with plain X-ray, there is little correlation with pain severity. The main exception to this is the presence of subchondral bone marrow lesions, which are associated with knee pain in cross sectional[38] and longitudinal[39] studies. (See Chapters 11, 14, and 17 in this volume.)

THE NATURE AND NATURAL HISTORY OF OSTEOARTHRITIS PAIN

Generally quoted descriptions of OA pain are largely anecdotal, supported by surprisingly little patient-based evidence. "Typical" OA pain is said to be insidious, variable, and intermittent ("good days and bad days"); mainly occurring on use, movement, or weight bearing and later in the day. Nearly all symptomatic patients have use-related pain, but many also have rest or night pain. The natural history is one of slow progression, although this may occur in "bursts" or "flares" rather than as a continuous process.

Knee pain is generally felt anteriorly or medially, especially after prolonged standing or walking. It may radiate down the shin. Getting from sitting to standing is especially painful, although this may last only for a few minutes. Many patients define more than one type of knee pain — usually a chronic background ache with shorter, sharper bursts of pain on certain movements. Limitation of range of movement and weakness of quadriceps contribute, with pain, to disability.

Pain due to hip OA classically is felt in the groin, on walking, but may radiate to the knee. Sometimes the knee is the only site of pain (a source of diagnostic confusion), while pain may also be felt in buttock or lateral thigh. Stiffness and difficulty with function are also common.

Hand OA is extremely common and often asymptomatic. Thumb base OA is more likely to cause pain than interphalangeal OA and may be felt diffusely "around the wrist," often with major functional consequences. Interphalangeal OA may present simply with gradually enlarging nodes at DIP or PIP, although a more acute, inflammatory pattern with severe pain is recognized. This pattern, often occurring around the time of menopause, results in individual joints being painful and swollen for a few months, then settling to be replaced by another inflamed joint.

A diurnal variation has been described at both the knee[40] and the hand[41] (See Fig. 13.1) with pain being worse in the evenings and easier in mornings. Gender affects within and across day pain reporting in OA, with women being more likely than men to show an increase in pain during the day and men being more likely to show an increase in coping efficacy over the day.[42] This study also confirmed differences in the way men and women react to pain in terms of coping strategies. Day-to-day variation in pain severity also occurs. The

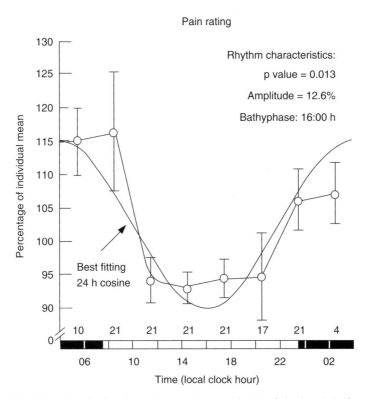

Figure 13.1. Circadian rhythm for pain in patients with OA of the hand. Self–measurements/ratings were made by 20 or 21 patients every 24 hours during waking for 10 days. Individual values had trends removed and were converted to a percentage of the mean before combining for group analysis by population mean cosinor. For rhythm characteristics, p value is from the zero amplitude test; amplitude = half peak–trough difference of cosine; bathyphase = lowest point of cosine (referenced from 0000). p Values < 0.001 for each variable from ANOVA for time effect. (From Ref. 41 with permission.)

influence of weather or barometric pressure is often cited by patients. Strusberg et al.[43] found that OA pain correlated with low temperature ($r = -0.23$, $p < 0.001$) and high humidity ($r = 0.24$, $p < 0.001$); other reports have linked pain with rising barometric pressure in women with hand OA.[44] Seasonal variation (worse in winter) is often reported but this may be more due to perception than reality since reported symptoms do not necessarily agree with measured clinical scores.[45] Pain may also be reported more strongly at weekends.[40]

Most patients with OA describe their pain as "aching," with "stabbing," "cramping," and "shooting" also chosen in one study.[46] Some authors have suggested that terminology may allow differentiation between OA and other joint pains (e.g., patients with RA may choose "throbbing" and "burning" more often): however, there is much overlap between conditions and pain descriptors are rarely useful clinically.

Longitudinal studies show that most (but not all) patients feel that their pain gets worse with time. In the Bristol OA 500 study,[47] for example, the proportion of subjects with knee OA reporting their pain to be "severe" was 25% at baseline, 17% at 3 years, and 27% at 8 years. However, 80% of patients felt they had worsened overall. Other studies[48] have indicated that about 25% patients report significant improvements in pain over a 7 year period, although this was not reflected in changes in structure on X-ray.

PAIN PATTERNS IN OSTEOARTHRITIS

Although the cause remains uncertain, it is increasingly clear that pain in OA is heterogeneous, varying between individuals and with different phases of the disease. In simple terms, some patients may have local sources of pain while in others the pain is centrally driven. Recently, efforts have been made to identify different *patterns of pain*, in the hope that they may indicate different pathological or anatomical processes. The location of pain at the knee, for example, is not random, but falls into two well-defined groups: generalized anterior pain and localized inferomedial pain. These differences are not explicable by radiographic change and may represent local bony or soft tissue sources.[49,50] Another example is the response to local anesthetic:[51,52] in many patients this will abolish pain temporarily while in others no effect is seen. Further evidence for a local source of pain in some patients with knee OA comes from studies showing that a locally applied anesthetic[53] or NSAID[54] patch applied locally to the skin over the knee can reduce pain, as can intra-articular injections of morphine.[55] Some patients may have a more inflammatory cause for their pain, perhaps explaining the variation in response to intra-articular steroids[56] or systemic NSAIDs (although it seems that clinical features of "inflammation" in OA do not seem to reliably predict response to these treatments).

Night pain represents another pattern of OA pain. Often used by orthopedic surgeons as an indicator of the need for joint surgery, night pain is said to be an unusual feature, limited to advanced disease. We found[49,50] that 43% subjects with knee OA reported pain of ≥ 30 mm on a VAS for night pain and 14.7% actually felt the night to be the most painful time. Also, 27.9% felt that resting in bed made their pain worse. We were unable to confirm a relationship between night pain and overall disease severity of the patient's OA; the latter being measured by global pain, disability, findings on examination, or changes on X-ray. A modest relationship with disease duration was seen, but most significantly, night pain was associated with high levels of helplessness and worse perceived quality of life, perhaps due to underlying fatigue.

The complexity of pain mechanisms is further emphasized by the fact that intra-articular anesthetic can also abolish pain in contralateral, untreated joints, implying central or spinal mechanisms.[51]

EFFECT OF PAIN ON DISEASE

We have considered the risk factors for pain reporting, but what about the effect pain may have on the underlying disease? Reduction in pain, for example, by intra-articular anesthetic, results in increased maximum voluntary contraction (MVC) of quadriceps.[52] The influence of pain on other potential risk factors such as proprioception and balance is unclear: Hassan et al.[52] reported that pain reduction did not result in improvements in proprioception or static postural stability. Jadelis et al.[57] examined dynamic balance in a cross-sectional study of older patients with knee OA. Balance was most strongly related to quadriceps strength, but in those subjects with weak quadriceps pain severity became an independent predictor of poor balance. The influence of chronic OA pain on the neuroendocrine system is controversial, with recent studies failing to find an increase in ACTH, cortisol, or testosterone in men with painful OA compared to controls.[58]

We do not know if long-term pain reduction can reduce progression of disease but there is some evidence that pain predicts incident knee OA and that subjects with pain progress faster than those with similar radiographic change without pain. Hart et al.[59] found odds ratios of 1.91 (95% CI 1.18–3.09) for knee pain predicting development of osteophyte at follow-up. Cooper et al.[60] in a follow-up study of 354 community subjects found that baseline knee pain predicted incident knee OA at 5 years (OR 2.9 (1.2–6.7) for KL≥1; OR 1.3 (0.6–2.7) for KL≥2). Knee pain also predicted progression over 5 years.

CAUSES OF PAIN IN OSTEOARTHRITIS

The anatomic cause of pain in OA remains unknown.[61] Any theory has to consider that the principal structure involved (cartilage) possesses few pain-sensitive fibers. Bone pain may be a factor in many subjects: perhaps via osteophyte growth with stretching of periosteum, raised intraosseous pressure, or microfractures. The relation of bone pathology to knee pain is reviewed in Chapter 11 in this volume.

Other sources of pain include muscle hypersensitivity,[62] ligament damage, capsular tension, meniscal injury, and synovitis. Inflammation may be present in OA and may cause pain either by direct stimulation of primary afferent peripheral afferent nociceptive fibers (PANs) or by sensitizing PANs to mechanical or other stimuli. Systemic markers of inflammation such as CRP are raised in many patients with OA and may predict future progression of disease.[63] In addition, there is a central component to pain and influences such as anxiety, depression and co-morbidity are likely to operate in some patients as described previously.

CONCLUSION

Many questions remain about OA pain. What makes a person with OA pain seek medical attention? Is it worsening of the disease (little evidence for this)? Loss of coping skills? Socioeconomic or financial factors? What would be the effect of early aggressive pain control in reducing intensity or duration of chronic pain—in other words, does control of pain affect the natural history of the disease? To what extent is pain protective and to what extent does it reduce function and result in physical deconditioning? How can we improve our understanding of our patients' health perceptions and risk–benefit preferences so that we may suggest more appropriate interventions? Many individuals with radiographic OA do not report pain and perhaps we should ask not "why is OA painful?" but "why is it so often pain free?"

Much effort is being expended on finding drugs capable of modifying the disease process, notably on cartilage loss. We would expect an effective disease-modifying drug to also have an effect on pain but, given the poor correlation currently seen between structural change (at least on X-ray) and symptoms, a word of caution might reasonably be sounded. There are grounds to at least consider the wisdom of investing large resources in expensive technologies designed to reduce structural change when this may not, in fact, affect the problems that are important for the patient.

REFERENCES

1. Felson DT. (2004). An update on the pathogenesis and epidemiology of osteoarthritis. Radiol Clin North Am 42:1–9.
2. Dieppe PA, Lohmander S. (2005). Pathogenesis and management of pain in osteoarthritis. Lancet 365:965–974.
3. O'Reilly SC, Muir KR, Doherty M. (1996). Screening for pain in knee osteoarthritis: which question? Ann Rheum Dis 55:931–933.
4. Felson DT, Naimark A, Anderson J, Kazis L, Castelli W, Meenan RF. (1987). The prevalence of knee osteoarthritis in the elderly: the Framingham Osteoarthritis Study. Arthritis Rheum 30:914–918.
5. Hochberg MC, Lawrence RC, Everett DF, Cornoni-Huntley J. (1989). Epidemiological associations of pain in osteoarthritis of the knee. Semin Arthritis Rheum 18 (suppl 2):4–9.

6. Carman WJ. (1989). Factors associated with pain and osteoarthritis in the Tecumseh Community Health Study. Semin Arthritis Rheum 18:10–13.

7. Spector TD, Hart DJ, Byrne J, Harris PA, Dacre JE, Doyle DV. (1993). Definition of osteoarthritis for epidemiological studies. Ann Rheum Dis 52:70–74.

8. Lethbridge-Cejku M, Scott WW Jr, Reichle R, et al. (1995). Association of radiographic features of osteoarthritis of the knee with knee pain: data from the Baltimore Longitudinal Study of Aging. Arthritis Care Res 8:182–188.

9. Davis M, Ettinger W, Neuhaus J, Barclay J, Degal M. (1992). Correlates of knee pain among US adults with and without radiographic knee osteoarthritis. J Rheumatol 19:1943–1949.

10. Hart DJ, Spector TD, Ewggar P, Coggan D, Cooper C. (1994). Defining osteoarthritis of the hand for epidemiological studies: the Chingford Study. Ann Rheum Dis 53:220–223.

11. Lawrence JS. (1977). *Rheumatism in Populations*. London: William Heinemann.

12. Lachance L, Sowers M, Jamadar D, Jannausch M, Hochberg M, Crutchfield M. (2001). The experience of pain and emergent osteoarthritis of the knee. Osteoarthritis Cartilage 9:527–532.

13. Hannan MT, Felson DT, Pincus T. (2000). Analysis of the discordance between radiographic changes and knee pain in osteoarthritis of the knee. J Rheumatol 27:1513–1517.

14. McAlindon T, Cooper C, Kirwan J, Dieppe PA. (1993). Determinants of disability in osteoarthritis of the knee. Ann Rheum Dis 52:258–262.

15. Croft P, Rigby AS, Boswell R, Schollum J, Silman A. (1993). The prevalence of chronic widespread pain in the general population. J Rheumatol 20:710–713.

16. Fife RS, Brandt K, Braunstein E, et al. (1991). Relationship between arthroscopic evidence of cartilage damage and radiographic evidence of joint space narrowing in early osteoarthritis of the knee. Arthritis Rheum 34:377–382.

17. Cicuttini FM, Baker J, Hart D, Spector TD. (1996). Association of pain with radiological changes in different compartments and views of the knee joint. Osteoarthritis Cartilage 4:143–147.

18. Birrell F, Croft P, Cooper C, Hosie G, Macfarlane GJ, Silman A. (2000). Radiographic change is common in new presenters in primary care with hip pain. Rheumatology 39:772–775.

19. Creamer P, Lethbridge-Cejku M, Costa P, Herbst J, Tobin J, Hochberg M. (1999). The relationship of anxiety and depression with self reported knee pain in the community: data from the Baltimore Longitudinal Study of Aging. Arthritis Care Res 12:3–7.

20. Lichtenberg PA, Swensen CH, Skehan MW. (1986). Further investigation of the role of personality, lifestyle and arthritic severity in predicting pain. J Psychosom Res 30:327–337.

21. Dekker J, Tola P, Aufdemkampe G, Winckers M. (1993). Negative affect, pain and disability in osteoarthritis patients: the mediating role of muscle weakness. Behav Res Ther 31:203–206.

22. Hannon MT, Anderson JJ, Pincus T, Felson DT. (1992). Educational attainment and osteoarthritis: differential associations with radiographic changes and symptom reporting. J Clin Epidemiol 45:139–147.

23. Dexter P, Brandt K. (1994). Distribution and predictors of depressive symptoms in osteoarthritis. J Rheumatol 21:279–286.

24. Bellamy N, Bradley L. (1996). Workshop on chronic pain, pain control and patient outcomes in rheumatoid arthritis and osteoarthritis. Arthritis Rheum 39:357–362.

25. Hodgkins M, Albert D, Daltroy L. (1985). Comparing patients and their physicians assessments of pain. Pain 23:273–277.

26. Suarez-Almazor ME, Conner-Spady B, Kendall CJ, Russell AS, Skeith K. (2001). Lack of congruence in the ratings of patients' health status by patients and their physicians. Med Decision Making 21:113–121.

27. Davies GM, Watson DJ, Bellamy N. (1999). Comparison of the responsiveness and relative effect size of the WOMAC Osteoarthritis Index and the short-form Medical Outcomes Study Survey in a randomised, clinical trial of osteoarthritis patients. Arthritis Care Res 12:172–179.

28. Theiler R, Sangha O, Schaeren S, Michel BA, Tyndall A, Dick W, Stucki G. (1999). Superior responsiveness of the pain and function sections of the WOMAC as compared to the Lequesne-algofunctional Index in patients with osteoarthritis of the lower extremities. Osteoarthritis Cartilage 7:515–519.

29. Creamer P, Lethbridge-Cejku M, Hochberg MC. (1999). Determinants of pain severity in knee osteoarthritis: effect of demographic and psychosocial variables using 3 pain measures. J Rheumatol 26:1785–1792.

30. Summers MN, Haley WE, Reveille JO, Alarcon GS. (1988). Radiographic assessment and psychological variables as predictors of pain and functional impairment in osteoarthritis of the knee or hip. Arthritis Rheum 31:204–209.

31. Salaffi F, Cavalieri F, Nolli M, Ferraccioli G. (1991). Analysis of disability in knee osteoarthritis. Relationship with age and psychological variables but not with radiographic score. J Rheumatol 18:1581–1586.

32. Hopman-Rock M, Odding E, Hofman A, et al. (1996). Physical and psychosocial disability in elderly subjects in relation to pain in the hip and/or knee. J Rheumatol 23:1037–1044.

33. Steultjens MP, Dekker J, Bijlsma JW. (2001). Coping, pain, and disability in osteoarthritis: a longitudinal study. J Rheumatol 28:1068–1072.

34. Bruyere O, Honore A, Rovati LC, et al. (2002). Radiologic features poorly predict clinical outcomes in knee osteoarthritis. Scand J Rheumatol 31:13–16.

35. Link T, Steinbach L, Ghosh S, et al. (2003). Osteoarthritis: MR imaging findings in different stages of disease and correlation with clinical findings. Radiology 226:373.

36. Szebenyi B, Hollander A, Dieppe P, et al. (2006). Associations between pain, function, and radiographic features in osteoarthritis of the knee. Arthritis Rheum 54:230–235.

37. Kornaat P, Bloem J, Ceulemans R, et al. (2006). Osteoarthritis of the knee: association between clinical features and MR imaging findings. Radiology 239:811–817.

38. Felson DT, Chaisson CE, Hill CL, Totterman SM, Gale ME, Skinner KM, Kazis L, Gale DR. (2001). The association of bone marrow lesions with pain in knee osteoarthritis. Ann Intern Med 134:541–549.

39. Felson DT, Niu J, Guermazi A, et al. (2007). Osteoarthritis: correlation of the development of knee pain with enlarging bone marrow lesions on magnetic resonance imaging. Arthritis Rheum 56:2986–2992.

40. Bellamy N, Sothern R, Campbell J. (1990). Rhythmic variations in pain perception in osteoarthritis of the knee. J Rheumatol 17:364–372.

41. Bellamy N, Sothern R, Campbell J, Buchanan W. (2002). Rhythmic variations in pain, stiffness and manual dexterity in hand osteoarthritis. Ann Rheum Dis 61: 1075–1080.

42. Keefe FJ, Affleck G, France CR, et al. (2004). Gender differences in pain, coping, and mood in individuals having osteoarthritic knee pain: a within-day analysis. Pain 110:571–577.

43. Strusberg I, Mendelberg RC, Serra HA, Strusberg AM. (2002). Influence of weather conditions on rheumatic pain. J Rheumatol 29:335–338.

44. Wilder F, Hall B, Barrett J. (2003). Osteoarthritis pain and weather. Rheumatology 42:955–958.

45. Hawley DJ, Wolfe F, Lue FA, Moldofsky H. (2001). Seasonal symptom severity in patients with rheumatic diseases: a study of 1,424 patients. J Rheumatol 28: 1900–1909.

46. Wagstaff S, Smith O, Wood P. (1985). Verbal pain descriptors used by patients with arthritis. Ann Rheum Dis 44:262–265.

47. Dieppe P, Cushnaghan J, Tucker M, Browning S, Shepstone L. (2000). The Bristol OA 500 study: progression and impact of the disease after 8 years. Osteoarthritis Cartilage 8:63–68.

48. Johnson SR, Archibald A, Davis AM, Badley E, Wright JG, Hawker GA. (2007). Is self-reported improvement in osteoarthritis pain and disability reflected in objective measures? J Rheumatol 34:159–164.

49. Creamer P, Lethbridge-Cejku M, Hochberg M. (1998). What is the significance of night pain in knee osteoarthritis? Br J Rheumatol 37(Suppl 1):153.

50. Creamer P, Lethbridge-Cejku M, Hochberg MC. (1998). Where does it hurt? Pain localisation in osteoarthritis of the knee. Osteoarthritis Cartilage 6:318–323.

51. Creamer P, Hunt M, Dieppe P. (1996). Pain mechanisms in osteoarthritis of the knee: effect of intraarticular anaesthetic. J Rheumatol 23:1031–1036.

52. Hassan BS, Doherty SA, Mockett S, Doherty M. (2002). Effect of pain reduction on postural sway, proprioception, and quadriceps strength in subjects with knee osteoarthritis. Ann Rheum Dis 61:422–428.

53. Burch F, Codding C, Patel N, Sheldon E. (2004). Lidocaine patch 5% improves pain, stiffness, and physical function in osteoarthritis pain patients: a prospective, multicenter, open-label effectiveness trial. Osteoarthritis Cartilage 12:253–255.

54. Brühlmann P, Michel BA. (2003). Topical diclofenac patch in patients with knee osteoarthritis: a randomized, double-blind, controlled clinical trial. Clin Exp Rheumatol 21:193–198.

55. Likar R, Schafer M, Paulak F, et al. (1997). Intraarticular morphine analgesia in chronic pain patients with osteoarthritis. Anesth Analg 84:1313–1317.

56. Bellamy N, Campbell J, Robinson V, Gee T, Bourne R, Wells G. (2006). Intraarticular corticosteroid for treatment of osteoarthritis of the knee (Cochrane Review) Cochrane. Database Syst Rev 19(2):CD005328.

57. Jadelis K, Miller ME, Ettinger WH Jr, Messier SP. (2001). Strength, balance, and the modifying effects of obesity and knee pain: results from the Observational Arthritis Study in Seniors (OASIS). J Am Geriatr Soc 49:884–891.

58. Khoromi S, Muniyappa R, Nackers L, et al. (2006). Effects of chronic osteoarthritis pain on neuroendocrine function in men. J Clin Endocrinol Metab 91:4313–4318.

59. Hart DJ, Doyle DV, Spector TD. (1999). Incidence and risk factors for radiographic knee osteoarthritis in middle-aged women: the Chingford Study. Arthritis Rheum 42:17–24.

60. Cooper C, Snow S, McAlindon TE, Kellingray S, Stuart B, Coggon D, Dieppe PA. (2000). Risk factors for the incidence and progression of radiographic knee osteoarthritis. Arthritis Rheum 43:995–1000.

61. Felson D. (2005). The sources of pain in knee osteoarthritis. Curr Opin in Rheumatol 17:624–628.

62. Bajaj P, Graven-Nielsen T, Arendt-Nielsen L. (2001). Osteoarthritis and its association with muscle hyperalgesia: an experimental controlled study. Pain 93:107–114.

63. Spector TD, Hart DJ, Nandra D. (1997). Low level increases in serum C-reactive protein are present in early osteoarthritis of the knee and predict progressive disease. Arthritis Rheum 40:723–727.

PART III

TREATMENT OF OSTEOARTHRITIC PAIN

14

GENERAL APPROACH TO TREATING OSTEOARTHRITIC PAIN: TARGETING BIOMECHANICS INFLAMMATION AND NOCICEPTION

David T. Felson

Boston University School of Medicine, 650 Albany Street, Boston, Massachusetts 02118, USA

INTRODUCTION

Joint pain or discomfort from osteoarthritis affects a large percentage of middle age and elderly persons in all countries. It stands out as a major reason for limitations in physical functioning and accounts for many visits to physicians for treatment. While pain is the most common moniker for joint symptoms, it is not the only one. Patients also frequently label their joint symptoms as discomfort or stiffness, and the pathophysiology of these symptoms is similar to the pathophysiology of "pain."

Pain in Osteoarthritis, Edited by David T. Felson and Hans-Georg Schaible
Copyright © 2009 Wiley-Blackwell.

FOCUS

In considering treatment for osteoarthritic pain, we focus on knees, hips, and hands, where pain and the occurrence of disease are correlated. While back pain and neck pain are extraordinarily common, it is not yet clear that pain in these two regions is related to the occurrence or development of osteoarthritis,[1] and these sites of pain will therefore not be a focus here. While much of our discussion of treatment will include approaches to hip and hand osteoarthritis, the treatment of pain in these joints is not nearly as well studied as the treatment of pain in osteoarthritis of the knee. The pathophysiology of pain is likely to be the same in all of these joints, and therefore general conceptual approaches to the knee will likely apply to hips and hands.

While we recognize that pain and discomfort of the joint are the most common presenting symptoms, they are not the only symptoms of osteoarthritis. Recent evidence[2] suggests that in knees, at least, symptoms reflecting joint instability are highly prevalent and may, like pain, produce their own functional limitations. Severe malalignment across the joint may, independent of pain, produce difficulty in carrying out activities and functional limitations.[3]

EVALUATING JOINT PAIN

Furthermore, patients presenting with pain that they insist originates in the joint may, on close observation, not have joint pain at all, but rather pain emanating from a periarticular structure. In the knee the most common periarticular pains emanate from the anserine bursa and the iliotibial band. An experienced clinician should examine and evaluate these sites in patients presenting with knee pain. For hip pain, trochanteric bursitis, which causes pain in the lateral hip, is far more prevalent than hip osteoarthritis itself. In hands, tendinitis and compression neuropathy can cause discomfort or pain. Thus all pain in hands, hips, and knees does not emanate from the joint.

Similarly, when the joint is the source of pain, it may not be from osteoarthritis. Obviously, acute injuries need to be ruled out, but other forms of arthritis frequently cause pain in hip, knee, and hand joints. These include crystal-induced arthritis and chronic inflammatory arthritis such as rheumatoid arthritis. Generally, synovial fluid examination is the best way to diagnose other forms of arthritis in the joint, especially crystal-induced arthritis such as gout and pseudogout (although the latter is associated with the occurrence of osteoarthritis). Also, rheumatoid arthritis and other forms of inflammatory arthritis should be considered if the patient has chronic pain with prolonged morning stiffness.

Regardless of the source of pain, patients may present to the physician complaining of pain for reasons that have little to do with articular pathology.

Depressed persons are often overwhelmed by pain. The failure to identify and manage the underlying depression may lead to failure of treatment. Similarly, fibromyalgia, which causes generalized pain, can accentuate the pain affecting a person who might have otherwise minimally painful osteoarthritis. Secondary gain from disability payments may lead to an exaggeration by patients of their symptoms. Understanding the patient's motivation in complaining of pain may be needed.

To determine if the pain is from osteoarthritis, all of these other sources of pain need to be ruled out. Even more, however, the clinician should confirm that the pain is typical in its nature of osteoarthrtitic pain. Described by Creamer in Chapter 13 in this volume, osteoarthritic pain is typically pain with activity. For example, the knee does not hurt until one gets up from a chair; it may not hurt with standing, but rather hurts with walking or going up and down stairs. Also, hip osteoarthritis symptoms may not arise except with bending over to tie one's shoe or when one gets out of a deep chair. The hand joints are not painful until one tries to pinch something strongly or perform demanding manual tasks. Symptoms gradually result after the activity has been completed. When the day is full of pain-causing activities, pain often persists at the end of the day, resolving only with a good night's sleep. While nocturnal pain can occur in osteoarthritis, it tends to be present only when disease is far advanced.

The most common mistake made by clinicians is to assume that an older patient presenting with knee or hip pain will almost certainly have knee or hip osteoarthritis as a cause. While osteoarthritis accounts for the majority of chronic joint pain in older people, there are many exceptions and appropriate treatment of pain involves a careful dissection of the possible reasons for that pain and that targeted treatment for the appropriate clinical syndrome. When the clinician has become confident that the patient's pain is in fact osteoarthritic in its etiology, a conceptual approach focusing on the potential sources of pain within the joint is needed.

OSTEOARTHRITIC PAIN

Osteoarthritic pain is triggered by excess joint loading, which causes the characteristic activity-related pain. A particular mechanopathology that developed as a consequence of the osteoarthritic process makes a joint vulnerable to specific activities, activities that did not cause pain before the onset of osteoarthritis. For example, in a normal knee, weight-bearing joint loading is distributed broadly across the medial and, to a lesser extent, the lateral tibiofemoral compartments. When, as a consequence of osteoarthritis, the knee develops varus malalignment, weight-bearing load is transmitted over only a tiny sliver of the inner medial joint. Walking and other weight-bearing activities confer high loads over that small area and these loads are likely to be painful. Since cartilage does not contain pain fibers, the specific means by which this high load causes pain is unknown but may include stimulating nociceptors in bone or synovium, or inceasing tension within the joint capsule. Thus the causes of pain in osteoarthritic joints are a function of both the activity that causes the pain and the joint's vulnerability to that specific activity. Added to that is the particular nociceptive environment within the joint.

Contributing to the likelihood of pain is the presence of inflammation, which lowers the threshold for nociception and makes it more likely that a given stimulus will cause a painful response. The consequence of this mechanism of pain development is that, in a nonvulnerable knee with an absence of inflammation, where nociceptive tissues are not cranked up to fire more often or at lower threshold than normal, a high level of activity will be necessary to cause pain. Examples might include a long run or climbing multiple flights of stairs. On the other hand, when inflammation exists within the joint and perhaps in other structures around the joint, this inflammation lowers the threshold for nociception, and much less vigorous activity triggers pain. A clinical example might be an older woman with severely varus malaligned knees and an effusion, whose knees become painful when she walks around her house.

To abrogate the pain in all of these circumstances, we need to address potential intervention points in this pain framework. These intervention points include biomechanical manipulations, so as to lower the amount of load in focal areas within an affected joint (e.g., bracing to decrease the malalignment of the knee). Another intervention point would be to diminish inflammation. Doing so might secondarily raise the threshold for nociception within a joint. Lastly, because nociceptive thresholds are likely to be critical in contributing to osteoarthritic pain, we could focus on nociception itself, attempting to modulate the firing of receptors that are overstimulated in osteoarthritis.

The chapters that follow expand on each of these possible approaches, offering a conceptual framework for understanding how each mechanism contributes to pain and suggesting opportunities for treatment.

REFERENCES

1. Lawrence RC, et al. (2008). Estimates of the prevalence of arthritis and other rheumatic conditions in the United States. Part II. Arthritis Rheum 58(1):26–35.
2. Felson DT, et al. (2007). Knee buckling: prevalence, risk factors, and associated limitations in function. Ann Intern Med 147(8):534–540.
3. Sharma LSJ, Felson DT, Cahue S, Shamiyeh E, Dunlop DD. (2001). The role of knee alignment in disease progression and functional decline in knee osteoarthritis. JAMA 286:188–195.

15

NEUROBIOLOGICAL MECHANISMS OF OSTEOARTHRITIC PAIN AND ANALGESIC TREATMENT

Tuhina Neogi

Boston University School of Medicine, 650 Albany Street, Boston, Massachusetts 02118, USA

Joachim Scholz

Department of Anesthesia and Critical Care, Massachusetts General Hospital, Neural Plasticity Research Group, 149 13th Street, Charlestown, Massachusetts 02129, USA

INTRODUCTION

Pain is the major clinical symptom in osteoarthritis (OA). It contributes to functional limitations and reduces quality of life. Knee OA is the leading cause of disability in the elderly population in the United States.[1] Approximately 25% of people older than 55 years report persistent knee pain[2] and, based on radiographic criteria, OA is prevalent in 30% of the population aged 65–74 years.[3] However, traditional approaches to evaluating the association between radiographic changes and presence or severity of knee pain have not shown strong associations; persons with clearly abnormal joint radiographs may have

Pain in Osteoarthritis, Edited by David T. Felson and Hans-Georg Schaible

no or only mild pain,[4,5] while others with pain may not have radiographic OA.[6] Interindividual differences in pain sensitivity may add to the discrepancy between radiographic findings and pain ratings. Genetic predisposition,[7,8] prior experience,[9,10] expectations about analgesic treatment,[11,12] current mood,[13] and social and cultural environment[14–16] all contribute to a person's response to pain. One way to eliminate the influence of such factors is to examine the association of radiographic features of OA with knee pain within individuals who have one knee that has pain while the other does not. In these individuals with knees that are discordant for the presence or severity of pain, a strong association between pain and radiographic features of OA was found.[17] Although much treatment focus has been on targeting structural abnormalities that occur in OA, such agents have been largely unsuccessful in limiting progression of disease. Nonetheless, it is still unclear which structural lesions actually *cause* joint pain in OA, and whether the nature of the pain is nociceptive or inflammatory. Satisfactory pain reduction is rarely achieved. A better understanding of the mechanisms that underlie the manifestation and persistence of joint pain will be necessary to make progress and develop strategies for targeted pain management in OA. In this chapter we review nociceptive pathways involved in the processing of joint pain and neurobiological mechanisms that are responsible for increased pain after joint lesions and inflammation. We summarize the mechanisms of action of current analgesic therapies and highlight potential future treatments for osteoarthritic pain.

JOINT INNERVATION AND NOCICEPTIVE PATHWAYS

Ligaments and the fibrous joint capsule are richly innervated by thinly myelinated Aδ fibers and unmyelinated C fibers that respond to noxious mechanical, thermal, and chemical stimuli (nociceptors).[18] For example, articular branches of the tibial nerve that innervate the posterior knee contain between 70% and 78% unmyelinated axons, approximately half of them belonging to C fiber nociceptors, the other half to postganglionic sympathetic nerve fibers.[19] Nociceptors are also found in menisci, adipose tissue of the joint, the synovium, and the periosteum, but are absent from cartilage. Many nociceptors of the joint respond to innocuous movements but are increasingly activated when movements exceed the physiological working range, whereas other nociceptors are active exclusively during noxious movements.[20] A third group of so-called silent nociceptors are normally inactive and respond only under pathological circumstances such as inflammation.[21]

The central axons of nociceptors terminate in the dorsal horn, the first relay station for somatosensory information in the central nervous system. Projections of Aδ fiber nociceptors synapse predominantly in the superficial dorsal horn (Rexed lamina I), but some Aδ nociceptors also have projections to deeper layers (laminae V and X).[22] Other afferents from articular nerves including C fiber nociceptors terminate in laminae II and III. Dorsal horn neurons that respond exclusively to noxious stimulation of deep tissue and neurons with converging input from skin, joint, and muscle participate in the processing of nociceptive information.[23–25] However, these neurons have receptive fields that are not specific for a particular tissue or anatomical structure, but include joint and adjacent muscles. Transmission neurons of the dorsal horn convey sensory input from deep tissue through the spinothalamic tract to predominantly the ventroposterolateral nucleus and the region between the ventroposterolateral and the ventrolateral nuclei of the thalamus. Animal studies have shown that convergence of nociceptive signals from joints and other anatomical structures on thalamic neurons is common, although the actual size of the receptive field varies between species.[26] Thalamic neurons forward nociceptive information from joints to the primary and secondary somatosensory cortex on the contralateral side and the primary somatosensory cortex on the ipsilateral side.[27]

INCREASED PAIN SENSITIVITY AFTER TISSUE DAMAGE AND INFLAMMATION

Tissue injury and inflammation lead to a decrease in the excitation threshold and an increase in the responsiveness to suprathreshold stimuli of Aδ and C fiber nociceptors (peripheral sensitization).[28–30] As a consequence, noxious mechanical and thermal stimuli begin to evoke an exaggerated response at the injury site (primary hyperalgesia).[31] The inflammation-induced drop in the activation threshold of joint nociceptors may be substantial so that even weak mechanical stimuli such as normally innocuous palpation or movement within the normal working range of the joint provoke pain.[21,32–34] Moreover, initially insensitive nociceptors begin to respond to joint movements and pressure after joint injury or inflammation.[32,34] In addition, nociceptors become spontaneously active and develop ongoing discharges, potentially facilitated by the exposure to chemical mediators of inflammation such as bradykinin, prostaglandins, and serotonin.[35–37]

Several mechanisms contribute to peripheral sensitization. Membrane excitability increases as transient receptor potential (TRP) channels, which respond to chemical and thermal stimuli, are recruited from intracellular stores and inserted in the axonal membrane at peripheral terminals. Redistribution of voltage-gated sodium channels along the axon leads to amplified membrane depolarization. Cells disrupted by mechanical injury, mast cells, and invading immune cells such as macrophages and lymphocytes release multiple proinflammatory substances, including protons, adenosine triphosphate (ATP), kinins, amines, prostaglandins, growth factors, and cytokines. These mediators act directly on nociceptors and trigger intracellular signaling cascades, many of them resulting in phosphorylation and thus activation of TRP and sodium channels. As a consequence, the responsiveness of nociceptors to external stimuli rises.[29,30]

Changes in the central nervous system are mainly responsible for the enhanced sensitivity to mechanical (but not thermal) stimuli that develops outside the area of the injury (secondary hyperalgesia).[31,38,39] Intense nociceptor activity after tissue injury or inflammation promotes insertion of α-amino-3-hydroxy-5-methyl-4-isoxazolepropionic acid (AMPA)-type glutamate receptors in the plasma membrane of pain transmission neurons in the dorsal horn of the spinal cord. Glutamate and neuropeptide co-release from nociceptors produces a cumulative depolarization of these transmission neurons, which leads to the opening of voltage-gated calcium channels and release of a magnesium blockade of N-methyl-D-aspartic acid (NMDA)-type glutamate receptors. As a result, transmission neurons become increasingly responsive to peripheral input (central sensitization).[40] Once established, central sensitization is maintained by low-level noxious and even nonnociceptive input from the periphery.[41]

Central sensitization increases afferent signal transmission through changes that are either restricted to activated synapses (homosynaptic potentiation) or spread to adjacent synapses (heterosynaptic potentiation). One form of homosynaptic potentiation is wind-up, a progressive increase in discharges of dorsal horn neurons in response to repetitive afferent stimulation (temporal summation). Heterosynaptic potentiation manifests as an increase in the number of dorsal horn neurons responding to afferent input, in part attributable to the recruitment of previously subthreshold Aβ fiber input. This causes a reduction in the threshold for mechanically induced pain and an expansion of the receptive field of dorsal horn neurons (spatial summation).[40,42] Lasting modifications of central pain processing pathways are generated by signaling cascades similar to those involved in long-term potentiation in the hippocampus[43,44] and transcriptional changes such as the induction of cyclooxygenase 2 (COX-2) in the central nervous system.[45] To prevent the disruption of the normal relationship between stimulus and response and avoid the development of persistent pain, early interventions that avert the establishment of these long-term modifications of nociceptive pathways would be required.

NOCICEPTIVE VERSUS INFLAMMATORY JOINT PAIN

OA is considered a degenerative joint disease. Absence of systemic markers of inflammation differentiates it from inflammatory arthritides.[46,47] What causes pain in OA is unclear.[46–48] Damage to the articular cartilage itself cannot be painful because cartilage lacks sensory afferents. Structural changes involving the subchondral bone, increased intraosseus pressure, and stretching of the periosteum caused by the growth of osteophytes are believed to be potentially major sources of the pain.[49–52] (For more detail, see Chapter 11 in this volume.) Pain in OA may therefore be primarily nociceptive and have a protective function by alerting the individual to mechanical limitations of joint movements and a reduced ability of the joint to cope with the additional pressure applied during movement or increases in static weight bearing. That the pain is usually localized to the affected joint, correlates with exercise and weight bearing, and is relieved during rest supports the notion that pain plays an important role in preventing further structural damage. However, the discrepancy of radiographic findings with the severity of pain in some individuals and the absence of pain in some persons with clear structural damage of the joint strongly indicate the involvement of other, nonnociceptive mechanisms. The occurrence of spontaneous pain, pain at rest, and night pain in advanced OA also suggest that pain no longer reflects the presence of a noxious stimulus.

OA is defined as a primarily noninflammatory disease. Yet swelling, indicative of underlying joint effusion, and stiffness of the joint are clinical signs suggesting an inflammatory component contributing to the pathogenesis of OA in some patients.[53] The presence of synovitis in biopsy samples indicates that inflammation is involved in the persistence of OA, if not in its etiology. Monocytes and other immune cells infiltrating the synovium, synovial effusion, and elevation of cytokines and complement factors have all been described in osteoarthritic joints, although these inflammatory changes are clearly less prominent than in, for example, rheumatoid arthritis (see Chapter 4 in this volume). Mechanisms of inflammatory pain may therefore explain some of the symptoms in OA. Peripheral sensitization of nociceptors is likely to contribute to the pain provoked by normally innocuous pressure and movements within the working range of the joint (allodynia). Radiating pain—for example, pain in the groin, the buttocks, or the knee associated with hip OA—suggests spatial summation, a feature of central sensitization. Central sensitization may also account for reduced pain thresholds in unaffected joints and muscles; such generalized somatosensory abnormalities are, in some patients, relieved by local therapy of the affected joint.[54–56] The analgesic efficacy of nonsteroidal anti-inflammatory drugs (NSAIDs) strongly suggests involvement of inflammatory pain mechanisms. NSAIDs provide better pain relief than acetaminophen, which is primarily analgesic but lacks anti-inflammatory activity.[57–59] Pain reduction by selective inhibitors of cyclooxygenase 2 (COX-2), the inducible isoform of cyclooxygenase,[60] further supports the notion that pain in OA is caused in part by inflammation. A more detailed discussion of the evidence for the efficacy of these agents can be found in Chapter 4 in this volume.

ANIMAL MODELS OF OA PAIN

Several distinct animal models have been developed to elucidate the cause of joint damage in OA, determine the contribution of inflammatory changes, evaluate diagnostic techniques, and test disease-modifying therapies.[61,62] Cartilage lesions similar to those observed in humans are generated by transection of articular ligaments, most commonly the anterior cruciate ligament of the knee, and partial resection of menisci to produce joint instability in large animals (sheep, dog) and rodents (rabbit, rat, mouse). Nonsurgical models include spontaneous joint degeneration in aged animals, ovariectomy-induced estrogen deficiency, and gene mutations such as deletion of procollagen, type II, and alpha 1 (*Col2a1*) or overexpression of matrix metalloproteinase 13.[61,62] Most experimental studies have focused on the exploration of mechanisms responsible for structural damage in OA; only a few have examined the induction of pain. Recently, however, injections of the chondrocyte toxin monosodium iodoacetate (MIA) into the rat knee joint have been employed to provoke mechanical allodynia and hyperalgesia and changes in weight bearing of the hind paw similar to the clinical signs of OA in humans.[63–65] Cartilage damage after the injection of MIA,[64] increased expression of genes such as *COX2* and *interleukin-1β*,[66] and response to analgesic treatment with, for example, celecoxib and morphine[63,65] indicate that this model may provide a valid tool for future studies on pain mechanisms and the development of targeted analgesic treatment in OA.

Joint pain in animals used to be evaluated indirectly by measuring changes in static and dynamic weight bearing, foot posture, spontaneous mobility, and gait.[67] Hypersensitivity of the hind paw to mechanical stimulation with calibrated von Frey filaments, pressure, or heat was recorded as a parameter of secondary hyperalgesia developing in response to joint inflammation.[67] Recently, more specific measures have been developed to improve the assessment of joint pain in animal models. A calibrated forceps for quantifiable mechanical stimulation of the joint allows direct determination of the threshold for pressure-induced pain. Withdrawal of the hind limb[68] and vocalizations in the audible and ultrasonic range[69] are recorded as outcome measures of this test. In animal models of OA, pain-like behavior is also evoked by passive movement of the knee. Here, the knee is extended until the animal starts to withdraw the leg. The maximum angle of tolerated extension is then recorded as "struggle threshold."[69] Such increased specificity of phenotyping pain responses should improve the characterization of pain related to OA in these animal models.

CLINICAL ASSESSMENT OF JOINT PAIN

The spectrum of clinical symptoms and signs and radiographic findings indicates differences in the manifestation of OA across patients. This heterogeneity is inadequately reflected in current methods of OA pain assessment, which hinders distinguishing between pain mechanisms related to nociception versus inflammation.

Pain, physical function, and the patient's global assessment are recommended clinical outcome measures for research trials on OA.[70,71] Pain is typically measured on a visual analogue, verbal, or numerical rating scale either with a global pain intensity score or by specifically inquiring about pain intensity during rest and physical activities such as walking or stair climbing. The most commonly used questionnaires are the Western Ontario and McMaster Universities Osteoarthritis Index (WOMAC),[72] the Lequesne index,[73] the Knee Injury and Osteoarthritis Outcome Score (KOOS),[74] and the Hip Disability and Osteoarthritis Outcome Score (HOOS).[75] Interference of pain with physical functioning, emotional well-being, and social functioning is measured in the Medical Outcomes Study 36-Item Short Form Health Survey (SF-36)[76] and the Brief Pain Inventory (BPI).[77,78]

Global pain intensity scores and the currently used indices of movement-induced pain and pain interfering with physical activities fail to reveal the diversity of pain manifestations in OA. Furthermore, these instruments do not capture short-term fluctuations in OA-related pain.[79] To elucidate the nature of OA pain in the individual patient, a more detailed assessment of pain-related symptoms and signs would be required. Given the complexity of OA pain, analysis of its sensory property (quality) alone, for example, in the McGill Pain Questionnaire[80,81] cannot be expected to identify pain subtypes. The assessment of OA pain should include a physical examination that differentiates between pain at the joint, adjacent muscles, and skin; pain at rest and during standardized passive and active movements; pain caused by the application of calibrated pressure at defined anatomical sites of the joint; and cutaneous allodynia and hyperalgesia evoked by mechanical and thermal stimuli. A standardized evaluation of signs such as swelling and stiffness would help assess inflammation. Evaluation of these symptoms and signs is necessary to distinguish clinically between pain that is predominantly nociceptive and pain that is caused by mechanisms associated with inflammation, which could have important implications for therapeutic management of the pain.

GENETICS AND PAIN SENSITIVITY

Although there are a number of association studies linking genetic variations and mutations to an increased risk for OA, particularly hand OA,[46,82] these associations may not account for discrepancies in the experience of pain. However, there are genetic determinants of pain sensitivity that may, at least partially, explain these differences. A polymorphism of the estrogen receptor α gene is associated with an increased risk for moderate or severe pain in female patients with temporomandibular OA.[83] The risk of developing painful temporomandibular OA depends furthermore on haplotype variants of the gene encoding *catechol-O-methyltransferase (COMT)*, an enzyme that regulates catecholamine and enkephalin levels.[84]

COMT haplotypes are also associated with differences in mechanical and thermal pain thresholds of healthy individuals,[85] indicating that genetic variants may determine both overall pain sensitivity and the susceptibility to develop chronic pain in a disease. A similar genetic association exists between pain sensitivity and back pain. A haplotype of the gene encoding guanosine triphosphate (GTP) cyclohydrolase that correlates inversely with the experience of pain during noxious stimulation in healthy volunteers also protects against persistent back pain. GTP cyclohydrolase is the rate-limiting enzyme for the synthesis of 6(R)-L-erythro-5,6,7,8-tetrahydrobiopterin (BH4), an enzyme cofactor involved in catecholamine, serotonin, and nitric oxide synthesis, which increases in inflammatory and neuropathic pain.[86] Twin studies also suggest genetic factors contributing to the risk for low back pain and neck pain.[87,88]

Differences in pain sensitivity and the response to analgesic treatment have been linked to gender,[89] race, and ethnicity,[90–92] further indicating that overall pain sensitivity may be in part genetically determined. It is, however, necessary to take into account that these differences may be influenced by and reflect shared psychosocial and cultural factors, and disparities in the access to health care.[93,94]

PSYCHOLOGICAL FACTORS

Pain is a complex experience, involving emotional distress, fear, and anxiety. The response to chronic pain further depends on its impact on the quality of life and social and work interactions. Patients treated for chronic OA pain show higher depression scores and depression may be one reason for electing to seek medical care for hip or knee pain.[95] Many individuals with OA develop coping strategies that are characterized by anxiety and a feeling of helplessness,[96] and heightened pain experience in some individuals has been associated with catastrophizing, which is a tendency to focus on and exaggerate the threat posed by a painful stimulus and to negatively evaluate one's own ability to cope with pain.[97,98] These emotional and cognitive aspects of the experience of pain may partly explain differences in the reporting of joint pain between patients with comparable pathological changes. In a recent study of 12 persons with knee OA, the arthritic pain state was compared to an experimental pain state and the pain-free state using positron emission tomography (PET) with ^{18}F-fluorodeoxyglucose to measure metabolic activity in the brain as a correlate of neuronal activity, with a focus on the lateral and medial pain systems. During arthritic pain, although both the medial and lateral systems were activated, the medial system was more active than during the experimental application of a painful heat stimulus, indicating an increased affective, aversive conditioning, and motivational response aspect of the pain experience.[99] In another small study also examining functional imaging in individuals with and without knee OA, ^{133}Xe single photon emission computed tomography (SPECT) of the brain was performed after application of pressures that were calibrated to each individual's pain threshold. Persons with OA showed activation in brain regions involved in the emotional dimension of pain and processing of pain affect.[97] These studies suggest affective and motivational responses to OA-related pain, which should adequately be addressed to effectively manage chronic pain in OA.

ANALGESIC TREATMENT

A better understanding of the neurobiological mechanisms that are responsible for OA pain will be essential to facilitate the development of novel therapies and improve the management of pain. Here, we briefly review pharmacological and nonpharmacological treatments that specifically target nociceptive pathways.

Pharmacologic Treatment

Nonsteroidal Anti-inflammatory Drugs and Acetaminophen

Nonsteroidal anti-inflammatory drugs (NSAIDs) are the most commonly used class of analgesic drugs in OA. They inhibit the synthesis of prostaglandins by blocking either nonselectively the constitutively expressed isoform of COX (COX-1) and the inducible isoform COX-2, or selectively COX-2, which is upregulated after tissue injury and inflammation. The analgesic effect of NSAIDs is mediated largely through blockade of COX-2.[100] One major proinflammatory prostanoid is prostaglandin E_2 (PGE_2). In the periphery, PGE_2 increases the responsiveness of nociceptors to mechanical and chemical stimuli.[101,102] But tissue injury and inflammation also induce PGE_2 synthesis in the spinal cord, where this prostanoid modulates the excitability of dorsal horn neurons and synaptic processing.[45,103] Consequently, NSAIDs produce analgesia by inhibiting both peripheral and central sensitization.

Acetaminophen has analgesic and antipyretic efficacy similar to those of NSAIDs, but substantially less anti-inflammatory activity.[100] Compared to NSAIDs, acetaminophen is a weak COX inhibitor in the presence of peroxides, which are found in high concentrations at sites of inflammation.[104] In the absence of inflammatory mediators, however, acetaminophen blocks COX-2 activity similar to selective inhibitors of this isoform.[105] Acetaminophen may also produce analgesia through a central mechanism of action, as it reaches higher concentrations in the central nervous system than acetic NSAIDs and inhibits the spinal release of PGE_2 after noxious stimulation.[106] The main advantage of acetaminophen over NSAIDs is its safety, especially the lack of gastrointestinal side effects. It is therefore recommended as first-line analgesic treatment in OA, although NSAIDs may provide better pain relief and improve functional outcome.[107]

Recently developed drugs in this class include new COX-2-selective inhibitors, dual inhibitors of COX and lipoxygenase (so-called "COX/LOX"), and NSAIDs coupled to nitric oxide-donating moieties. These are primarily anti-inflammatory agents with improved gastrointestinal safety profiles,[108] but COX-2 inhibitors are associated with an increased risk of myocardial ischema.

A detailed discussion of the analgesic efficacy and side effects of NSAIDs and acetaminophen in OA can be found in Chapter 4 in this volume.

Opioids

Primary sensory afferents, including nociceptors, and neurons of the brain and the spinal cord that are involved in the processing of nociceptive input express G protein-coupled receptors (μ, δ, and κ) for opioid analgesics. In humans, the analgesic effect of opioids such as morphine, fentanyl, and codeine is mainly achieved through activation of the μ receptor. Opioids reduce the release of excitatory transmitters from primary afferents and inhibit the transmission of nociceptive information by dorsal horn neurons. Opioids also enhance pain control through inhibitory pathways descending from brainstem nuclei.[109] Tramadol, a synthetic codeine analogue prescribed for mild to moderate pain, has dual action as a weak μ receptor agonist and inhibitor of serotonin and norepinephrine uptake.

Opioids have been included in treatment guidelines for OA by both the American College of Rheumatology and Osteoarthritis Society Research International (OARSI). A recent meta-analysis of the analgesic efficacy of opioids in OA demonstrated a pooled effect size of all opioids of −0.79 (95% CI −0.98 to −0.59), indicating a large effect, but there was substantial heterogeneity between the studies.[110] In contrast, the pooled effect size for physical function was −0.31 (95% CI −0.39 to −0.24), indicating a small effect. The number of patients needed to be treated to cause one harmful event (number needed to harm; NNH) was 5, with the most frequent adverse events being nausea, constipation, dizziness, somnolence, and vomiting. Other important side effects of opioids include tolerance, dependence, and respiratory suppression in cases of overdosing or intoxication. Opioids can be injected directly into the affected joint, where they attenuate pain by acting on peripheral receptors with a substantially reduced risk of systemic side effects.[111] Opioids with fewer systemic side effects are currently under development but not yet studied in OA.

Cannabinoids

Cannabinoids are alkaloids derived from the hemp plant *Cannabis sativa*, which bind to the G protein-coupled cannabinoid receptors CB1 and CB2, and other receptors including the transmitter-gated TRP vanilloid type 1 (TRPV1) and TRPA1 receptor channels.[112,113] CB1 receptors are abundantly expressed by neurons of the central nervous system and at a lower level, primary sensory afferents, whereas CB2 receptors are found mainly on immune cells.[114] TRPV1 and TRPA1 are predominantly found on nociceptors.[115] The CB1 and TRPV1 agents, arachidonyl-2-chloroethylamide (ACEA) reduces the increased responsiveness of knee joint afferents to mechanical stimuli that develops in rats after intra-articular MIA injections.[116] These results indicate that cannabinoids may produce analgesia by limiting peripheral sensitization in the osteoarthritic joint. Clinical studies have not been performed to date.

Capsaicin

A natural alkaloid derivative from capsicum, capsaicin (trans-8-methyl-N-vanillyl-6-nonenamide) is the active ingredient responsible for the burning sensation often experienced when eating hot chilli peppers.[117] Capsaicin binds to TRPV1 and activates nociceptors, inducing the release of glutamate and peptides such as substance P and calcitonin gene related peptide from central terminals. Repeated topical application of capsaicin produces analgesia by depleting nociceptors of transmitter peptides.[118]

The analgesic efficacy of topical capsaicin has been evaluated in some clinical trials of hand and knee osteoarthritis,[119–122] and a positive analgesic effect over placebo has been reported in a pooled meta-analysis.[123] However, the results of these trials need to be interpreted with caution, because the application of capsaicin is inevitably associated with a burning sensation that prevents proper blinding and produces high placebo effects. Burning dysesthesia is also the reason for poor compliance with this treatment.[124] Combining capsaicin with QX-314, a lidocaine derivative that passes through the TRPV1 channel after it has been opened by capsaicin, provides a nociceptor-specific local anesthetic block and eliminates the burning sensation.[125] This novel pharmacological strategy is still at an experimental stage, but it demonstrates that targeted inhibition of nociceptive pathways is possible.

Nerve-Growth Factor Antagonists

Nerve growth factor (NGF) plays an important role for neuronal survival during embryonic and early postnatal development. In the adult nervous system, NGF is no longer required to prevent neuronal cell death; instead, it modulates nociceptor function through activation of the tyrosine kinase A (TRKA).[126] NGF is elevated after tissue injury and inflammation. Signaling pathways downstream of TRKA lead to phosphorylation of TRPV1, activation of mitogen-activated protein kinases, and increased synthesis of neurotransmitters, including substance P. Furthermore, NGF acts on mast cells, provoking the release of prostaglandins, bradykinin, and proinflammatory cytokines such as interleukin-1 and tumor necrosis factor.[127] NGF contributes to the development of hyperalgesia in animal models of acute and persistent inflammatory pain.[128]

RN624 (Rinat Neuroscience and Pfizer, San Francisco, CA), a humanized neutralizing monoclonal antibody directed against NGF, reduces pain in a rodent model of arthritis.[128] In patients with knee OA, RN624 provides pain relief and improves joint function for up to 3 months, with treatment response according to OARSI (Outcome Measures for Arthritis Clinical Trials OMER-ACT) criteria being 1.7 to 4.2 times more likely than in patients treated with placebo. In a phase 2 trial of tanezumab (Pfizer) among individuals with knee OA who had failed NSAIDs or were candidates for total joint replacement, a dose-response relation was noted, with the OARSI-OMERACT response criteria being met at 4 months in up to 87.5% compared with 49.3% in placebo.[129–131] The most frequent side effects reported in the two trials completed so far were transient dysesthesia and allodynia.

Outlook

Antidepressants and anticonvulsants are commonly used to treat pain caused by a lesion or disease affecting the somatosensory system (neuropathic pain). Antidepressants are also recommended for pain management in musculoskeletal disorders such as fibromyalgia. Pain relief is achieved independent of the antidepressive activity of these drugs. By increasing the synaptic concentrations of monoamine neurotransmitters, particularly norepinephrine and serotonin, antidepressants increase the activity of inhibitory pathways that descend from brainstem nuclei and modulate pain transmission in the spinal cord.[132] The analgesic effect of antidepressants in OA was initially noted in an early case report of persons taking imipramine,[133] and amitripyline was shown to reduce joint pain in an animal model of OA.[134] Clinical studies of efficacy in humans are being conducted with venlafaxine and duloxetine, with the latter recently reported as being efficacious.[135]

The anticonvulsant pregabalin may improve treatment of knee and hip pain but there is as yet no evidence evaluating this possibility. Pregabalin binds to the $\alpha_2\delta$ subunit of voltage-gated calcium channels, which is upregulated in primary sensory neurons after peripheral nerve injury. Pregabalin attenuates pain presumably by reducing the release of glutamate, norepinephrine, and substance P from the central terminals of these neurons.[136]

Nonpharmacologic Treatment

Transcutaneous Electrical Nerve Stimulation and Acupuncture

Transcutaneous electrical nerve stimulation (TENS) is recommended as treatment for pain relief in 8 out of 10 existing guidelines for the management of knee OA,[137] as well as the recent OARSI guidelines.[138] TENS is thought to produce presynaptic inhibition in the dorsal horn of the spinal cord by modulating the release of endorphins, enkephalins, and dynorphins,[139,140] yet the precise mechanism of its action is unknown. A Cochrane review[141] and a recent meta-analysis[142] found short-term efficacy of TENS in knee OA without major side effects. However, most studies on the analgesic efficacy of TENS in OA were small, were inadequately blinded, and involved different stimulation protocols so that it is difficult to adequately evaluate and compare the results of these trials.

Similarly, acupuncture is believed to modulate nociceptive pathways through peripheral stimulation, although the exact mechanism of action is unknown. Acupuncture has been endorsed in 5 out of 8 guidelines in which it was considered.[137] The recent OARSI guidelines report an effect size of 0.51 (95% CI 0.23–0.79).[138] However, this assessment is based on studies that are difficult to interpret because of their small sample sizes and concerns regarding adequate blinding. Acupuncture has a high placebo effect related to the provider's communication style and the patient's expectation for benefit.[143] Furthermore, a recent meta-analysis demonstrated that acupuncture does not produce a clinically relevant improvement in pain when compared with sham acupuncture in persons with knee OA for either relief of short-term (8–12 weeks) or long-term (3–6 months) pain (standardized mean differences of −0.35 and −0.13, respectively).[144]

CONCLUSION

Although pain is recognized as the most important clinical symptom of OA, pain management remains unsatisfactory for many patients. The discordance between structural lesions, functional deficits, and pain suggests that treatment strategies focusing on structural modification and prevention of joint damage will not necessarily also provide pain relief. In order to make progress, we need to understand better what causes pain in OA so that we can specifically target the nociceptive and inflammatory pain mechanisms involved.

REFERENCES

1. Guccione AA, Felson DT, Anderson JJ, Anthony JM, Zhang Y, Wilson PW, et al. (1994). The effects of specific medical conditions on the functional limitations of elders in the Framingham Study. Am J Public Health 84(3):351–358.

2. Peat G, McCarney R, Croft P. (2001). Knee pain and osteoarthritis in older adults: a review of community burden and current use of primary health care. Ann Rheum Dis 60(2):91–97.

3. Felson DT, Naimark A, Anderson J, Kazis L, Castelli W, Meenan RF. (1987). The prevalence of knee osteoarthritis in the elderly. The Framingham Osteoarthritis Study. Arthritis Rheum 30(8):914–918.

4. Davis MA, Ettinger WH, Neuhaus JM, Barclay JD, Segal MR. (1992). Correlates of knee pain among US adults with and without radiographic knee osteoarthritis. J Rheumatol 19(12):1943–1949.

5. Lawrence JS, Bremner JM, Bier F. (1966). Osteo-arthrosis. Prevalence in the population and relationship between symptoms and X-ray changes. Ann Rheum Dis 25(1):1–24.

6. Hannan MT, Felson DT, Pincus T. (2000). Analysis of the discordance between radiographic changes and knee pain in osteoarthritis of the knee. J Rheumatol 27(6):1513–1517.

7. Zubieta JK, Smith YR, Bueller JA, Xu Y, Kilbourn MR, Jewett DM, et al. (2001). Regional mu opioid receptor regulation of sensory and affective dimensions of pain. Science 293(5528):311–315.

8. Mogil JS. (1999). The genetic mediation of individual differences in sensitivity to pain and its inhibition. Proc Natl Acad Sci USA 96(14):7744–7751.

9. Vase L, Riley JL 3rd, Price DD. (2002). A comparison of placebo effects in clinical analgesic trials versus studies of placebo analgesia. Pain 99(3):443–452.

10. Colloca L, Benedetti F. (2006). How prior experience shapes placebo analgesia. Pain 124(1-2):126–133.

11. Fields HL. (2000). Pain modulation: expectation, opioid analgesia and virtual pain. Prog Brain Res 122:245–253.

12. Wager TD. (2005). Expectations and anxiety as mediators of placebo effects in pain. Pain 115(3):225–226.

13. Villemure C, Slotnick BM, Bushnell MC. (2003). Effects of odors on pain perception: deciphering the roles of emotion and attention. Pain 106(1-2):101–108.

14. Giardino ND, Jensen MP, Turner JA, Ehde DM, Cardenas DD. (2003). Social environment moderates the association between catastrophizing and pain among persons with a spinal cord injury. Pain 106(1-2):19–25.

15. Gamsa A. (1990). Is emotional disturbance a precipitator or a consequence of chronic pain? Pain 42(2):183–195.

16. Deshields TL, Tait RC, Gfeller JD, Chibnall JT. (1995). Relationship between social desirability and self-report in chronic pain patients. Clin J Pain 11(3): 189–193.

17. Negoi T, Felson D, Niu J, et al. (2008). Radiographic features of osteoarthritis are strongly associated with knee pain in two cohorts: MOST and Framingham. *Arthritis Rheum* 58:S436.

18. Julius D, Basbaum AI. (2001). Molecular mechanisms of nociception. Nature 413(6852):203–210.

19. Hines AE, Birn H, Teglbjaerg PS, Sinkjaer T. (1996). Fiber type composition of articular branches of the tibial nerve at the knee joint in man. Anat Rec 246(4):573–578.

20. Schaible HG, Schmidt RF. (1983). Responses of fine medial articular nerve afferents to passive movements of knee joints. J Neurophysiol 49(5):1118–1126.

21. Coggeshall RE, Hong KA, Langford LA, Schaible HG, Schmidt RF. (1983). Discharge characteristics of fine medial articular afferents at rest and during passive movements of inflamed knee joints. Brain Res 272(1):185–188.

22. Craig AD, Heppelmann B, Schaible HG. (1988). The projection of the medial and posterior articular nerves of the cat's knee to the spinal cord. J Comp Neurol 276(2):279–288.

23. Janig W. (1987). Neuronal mechanisms of pain with special emphasis on visceral and deep somatic pain. Acta Neurochir Suppl (Wien) 38:16–32.

24. Schaible HG, Schmidt RF, Willis WD. (1986). Responses of spinal cord neurones to stimulation of articular afferent fibres in the cat. J Physiol 372:575–593.

25. Yu XM, Mense S. (1990). Response properties and descending control of rat dorsal horn neurons with deep receptive fields. Neuroscience 39(3):823–831.

26. Hutchison WD, Luhn MA, Schmidt RF. (1992). Knee joint input into the peripheral region of the ventral posterior lateral nucleus of cat thalamus. J Neurophysiol 67(5):1092–1104.

27. Heppelmann B, Pawlak M, Just S, Schmidt RF. (2001). Cortical projection of the rat knee joint innervation and its processing in the somatosensory areas SI and SII. Exp Brain Res 141(4):501–506.

28. Gold MS, Flake NM. (2005). Inflammation-mediated hyperexcitability of sensory neurons. Neurosignals 14(4):147–157.

29. Hucho T, Levine JD. (2007). Signaling pathways in sensitization: toward a nociceptor cell biology. Neuron 55(3):365–376.

30. Woolf CJ, Ma Q. (2007). Nociceptors—noxious stimulus detectors. Neuron 55(3):353–364.

31. Kilo S, Schmelz M, Koltzenburg M, Handwerker HO. (1994). Different patterns of hyperalgesia induced by experimental inflammation in human skin. Brain 117 (Pt 2):385–396.

32. Grigg P, Schaible HG, Schmidt RF. (1986). Mechanical sensitivity of group III and IV afferents from posterior articular nerve in normal and inflamed cat knee. J Neurophysiol 55(4):635–643.

33. Schaible HG, Schmidt RF. (1985). Effects of an experimental arthritis on the sensory properties of fine articular afferent units. J Neurophysiol 54(5):1109–1122.

34. Schaible HG, Schmidt RF. (1988). Time course of mechanosensitivity changes in articular afferents during a developing experimental arthritis. J Neurophysiol 60(6):2180–2195.

35. Neugebauer V, Schaible HG, Schmidt RF. (1989). Sensitization of articular afferents to mechanical stimuli by bradykinin. Pflugers Arch 415(3):330–335.

36. Schaible HG, Schmidt RF. (1988). Excitation and sensitization of fine articular afferents from cat's knee joint by prostaglandin E2. J Physiol 403:91–104.

37. Schepelmann K, Messlinger K, Schaible HG, Schmidt RF. (1992). Inflammatory mediators and nociception in the joint: excitation and sensitization of slowly conducting afferent fibers of cat's knee by prostaglandin I2. Neuroscience 50(1):237–247.

38. Koltzenburg M. (2000). Neural mechanisms of cutaneous nociceptive pain. Clin J Pain 16(3 Suppl):S131–S138.

39. Schaible HG, Ebersberger A, Von Banchet GS. (2002). Mechanisms of pain in arthritis. Ann NY Acad Sci 966:343–354.

40. Woolf CJ, Salter MW. (2000). Neuronal plasticity: increasing the gain in pain. Science 288(5472):1765–1769.

41. Woolf CJ. (1983). Evidence for a central component of post-injury pain hypersensitivity. Nature 306(5944):686–688.

42. Grubb BD, Stiller RU, Schaible HG. (1993). Dynamic changes in the receptive field properties of spinal cord neurons with ankle input in rats with chronic unilateral inflammation in the ankle region. Exp Brain Res 92(3):441–452.

43. Ikeda H, Stark J, Fischer H, Wagner M, Drdla R, Jager T, et al. (2006). Synaptic amplifier of inflammatory pain in the spinal dorsal horn. Science 312(5780): 1659–1662.

44. Ji RR, Kohno T, Moore KA, Woolf CJ. (2003). Central sensitization and LTP: do pain and memory share similar mechanisms? Trends Neurosci 26(12):696–705.

45. Samad TA, Moore KA, Sapirstein A, Billet S, Allchorne A, Poole S, et al. (2001). Interleukin-1beta-mediated induction of Cox-2 in the CNS contributes to inflammatory pain hypersensitivity. Nature 410(6827):471–475.

46. Dieppe PA, Lohmander LS. (2005). Pathogenesis and management of pain in osteoarthritis. Lancet 365(9463):965–973.

47. Kidd BL. (2006). Osteoarthritis and joint pain. Pain 123(1-2):6–9.

48. Felson DT. (2005). The sources of pain in knee osteoarthritis. Curr Opin Rheumatol 17(5):624–628.

49. O'Neill TW, McCloskey EV, Kanis JA, Bhalla AK, Reeve J, Reid DM, et al. (1999). The distribution, determinants, and clinical correlates of vertebral osteophytosis: a population based survey. J Rheumatol 26(4):842–848.

50. Simkin PA. (2004). Bone pain and pressure in osteoarthritic joints. Novartis Found Symp 260:179–186; discussion 86–90, 277–279.

51. Szebenyi B, Hollander AP, Dieppe P, Quilty B, Duddy J, Clarke S, et al. (2006). Associations between pain, function, and radiographic features in osteoarthritis of the knee. Arthritis Rheum 54(1):230–235.

52. van der Kraan PM, van den Berg WB. (2007). Osteophytes: relevance and biology. Osteoarthritis Cartilage 15(3):237–244.

53. Yuan GH, Masuko-Hongo K, Kato T, Nishioka K. (2003). Immunologic intervention in the pathogenesis of osteoarthritis. Arthritis Rheum 48(3):602–611.

54. Kosek E, Ordeberg G. (2000). Lack of pressure pain modulation by heterotopic noxious conditioning stimulation in patients with painful osteoarthritis before, but not following, surgical pain relief. Pain 88(1):69–78.

55. Creamer P, Hunt M, Dieppe P. (1996). Pain mechanisms in osteoarthritis of the knee: effect of intraarticular anesthetic. J Rheumatol 23(6):1031–1036.

56. Kosek E, Ordeberg G. (2000). Abnormalities of somatosensory perception in patients with painful osteoarthritis normalize following successful treatment. Eur J Pain 4(3):229–238.

57. Pincus T, Koch G, Lei H, Mangal B, Sokka T, Moskowitz R, et al. (2004). Patient Preference for Placebo, Acetaminophen (paracetamol) or Celecoxib Efficacy Studies (PACES): two randomised, double blind, placebo controlled, crossover

clinical trials in patients with knee or hip osteoarthritis. Ann Rheum Dis 63(8):931–939.

58. Pincus T, Koch GG, Sokka T, Lefkowith J, Wolfe F, Jordan JM, et al. (2001). A randomized, double-blind, crossover clinical trial of diclofenac plus misoprostol versus acetaminophen in patients with osteoarthritis of the hip or knee. Arthritis Rheum 44(7):1587–1598.

59. Wegman A, van der Windt D, van Tulder M, Stalman W, de Vries T. (2004). Nonsteroidal antiinflammatory drugs or acetaminophen for osteoarthritis of the hip or knee? A systematic review of evidence and guidelines. J Rheumatol 31(2):344–354.

60. Bjordal JM, Ljunggren AE, Klovning A, Slordal L. (2004). Non-steroidal antiinflammatory drugs, including cyclo-oxygenase-2 inhibitors, in osteoarthritic knee pain: meta-analysis of randomised placebo controlled trials. BMJ 329(7478):1317.

61. Ameye LG, Young MF. (2006). Animal models of osteoarthritis: lessons learned while seeking the "Holy Grail." Curr Opin Rheumatol 18(5):537–547.

62. van den Berg WB. (2001). Lessons from animal models of osteoarthritis. Curr Opin Rheumatol 13(5):452–456.

63. Fernihough J, Gentry C, Malcangio M, Fox A, Rediske J, Pellas T, et al. (2004). Pain related behaviour in two models of osteoarthritis in the rat knee. Pain 112(1-2):83–93.

64. Kobayashi K, Imaizumi R, Sumichika H, Tanaka H, Goda M, Fukunari A, et al. (2003). Sodium iodoacetate-induced experimental osteoarthritis and associated pain model in rats. J Vet Med Sci 65(11):1195–1199.

65. Pomonis JD, Boulet JM, Gottshall SL, Phillips S, Sellers R, Bunton T, et al. (2005). Development and pharmacological characterization of a rat model of osteoarthritis pain. Pain 114(3):339–346.

66. Dumond H, Presle N, Pottie P, Pacquelet S, Terlain B, Netter P, et al. (2004). Site specific changes in gene expression and cartilage metabolism during early experimental osteoarthritis. Osteoarthritis Cartilage 12(4):284–295.

67. Neugebauer V, Han JS, Adwanikar H, Fu Y, Ji G. (2007). Techniques for assessing knee joint pain in arthritis. Mol Pain 3:8.

68. Skyba DA, Radhakrishnan R, Sluka KA. (2005). Characterization of a method for measuring primary hyperalgesia of deep somatic tissue. J Pain 6(1):41–47.

69. Yu YC, Koo ST, Kim CH, Lyu Y, Grady JJ, Chung JM. (2002). Two variables that can be used as pain indices in experimental animal models of arthritis. J Neurosci Methods 115(1):107–113.

70. Brooks P, Hochberg M. (2001). Outcome measures and classification criteria for the rheumatic diseases. A compilation of data from OMERACT (Outcome Measures for Arthritis Clinical Trials), ILAR (International League of Associations for Rheumatology), regional leagues and other groups. Rheumatology (Oxford) 40(8):896–906.

71. Pham T, van der Heijde D, Altman RD, Anderson JJ, Bellamy N, Hochberg M, et al. (2004). OMERACT-OARSI initiative: Osteoarthritis Research Society International set of responder criteria for osteoarthritis clinical trials revisited. Osteoarthritis Cartilage 12(5):389–399.

72. Bellamy N, Buchanan WW, Goldsmith CH, Campbell J, Stitt LW. (1988). Validation study of WOMAC: a health status instrument for measuring clinically important patient relevant outcomes to antirheumatic drug therapy in patients with osteoarthritis of the hip or knee. J Rheumatol 15(12):1833–1840.

73. Lequesne MG. (1997). The algofunctional indices for hip and knee osteoarthritis. J Rheumatol 24(4):779–781.

74. Roos EM, Roos HP, Lohmander LS, Ekdahl C, Beynnon BD. (1998). Knee Injury and Osteoarthritis Outcome Score (KOOS)—development of a self-administered outcome measure. J Orthop Sports Phys Ther 28(2):88–96.

75. Nilsdotter AK, Lohmander LS, Klassbo M, Roos EM. (2003). Hip disability and osteoarthritis outcome score (HOOS)—validity and responsiveness in total hip replacement. BMC Musculoskelet Disord 4:10.

76. Ware JE Jr, Sherbourne CD. (1992). The MOS 36-item short-form health survey (SF-36). I. Conceptual framework and item selection. Med Care 30(6):473–483.

77. Mendoza T, Mayne T, Rublee D, Cleeland C. (2006). Reliability and validity of a modified Brief Pain Inventory short form in patients with osteoarthritis. Eur J Pain 10(4):353–361.

78. Williams VS, Smith MY, Fehnel SE. (2006). The validity and utility of the BPI interference measures for evaluating the impact of osteoarthritic pain. J Pain Symptom Manage 31(1):48–57.

79. Hutchings A, Calloway M, Choy E, Hooper M, Hunter DJ, Jordan JM, et al. (2007). The Longitudinal Examination of Arthritis Pain (LEAP) study: relationships between weekly fluctuations in patient-rated joint pain and other health outcomes. J Rheumatol 34(11):2291–2300.

80. Grafton KV, Foster NE, Wright CC. (2005). Test–retest reliability of the Short-Form McGill Pain Questionnaire: assessment of intraclass correlation coefficients and limits of agreement in patients with osteoarthritis. Clin J Pain 21(1):73–82.

81. Wagstaff S, Smith OV, Wood PH. (1985). Verbal pain descriptors used by patients with arthritis. Ann Rheum Dis 44(4):262–265.

82. Ikegawa S. (2007). New gene associations in osteoarthritis: what do they provide, and where are we going? Curr Opin Rheumatol 19(5):429–434.

83. Kang SC, Lee DG, Choi JH, Kim ST, Kim YK, Ahn HJ. (2007). Association between estrogen receptor polymorphism and pain susceptibility in female temporomandibular joint osteoarthritis patients. Int J Oral Maxillofac Surg 36(5): 391–394.

84. Diatchenko L, Slade GD, Nackley AG, Bhalang K, Sigurdsson A, Belfer I, et al. (2005). Genetic basis for individual variations in pain perception and the development of a chronic pain condition. Hum Mol Genet 14(1):135–143.

85. Slade GD, Diatchenko L, Bhalang K, Sigurdsson A, Fillingim RB, Belfer I, et al. (2007). Influence of psychological factors on risk of temporomandibular disorders. J Dent Res 86(11):1120–1125.

86. Tegeder I, Costigan M, Griffin RS, Abele A, Belfer I, Schmidt H, et al. (2006). GTP cyclohydrolase and tetrahydrobiopterin regulate pain sensitivity and persistence. Nat Med 12(11):1269–1277.

87. MacGregor AJ, Andrew T, Sambrook PN, Spector TD. (2004). Structural, psychological, and genetic influences on low back and neck pain: a study of adult female twins. Arthritis Rheum 51(2):160–167.

88. Battie MC, Videman T, Levalahti E, Gill K, Kaprio J. (2007). Heritability of low back pain and the role of disc degeneration. Pain 131(3):272–280.

89. Mogil JS, Wilson SG, Chesler EJ, Rankin AL, Nemmani KV, Lariviere WR, et al. (2003). The melanocortin-1 receptor gene mediates female-specific mechanisms of analgesia in mice and humans. Proc Natl Acad Sci USA 100(8):4867–4872.

90. Edwards CL, Fillingim RB, Keefe F. (2001). Race, ethnicity and pain. Pain 94(2):133–137.

91. Edwards RR, Doleys DM, Fillingim RB, Lowery D. (2001). Ethnic differences in pain tolerance: clinical implications in a chronic pain population. Psychosom Med 63(2):316–323.

92. Edwards RR, Fillingim RB. (1999). Ethnic differences in thermal pain responses. Psychosom Med 61(3):346–354.

93. Green CR, Anderson KO, Baker TA, Campbell LC, Decker S, Fillingim RB, et al. (2003). The unequal burden of pain: confronting racial and ethnic disparities in pain. Pain Med 4(3):277–294.

94. Greenspan JD, Craft RM, LeResche L, Arendt-Nielsen L, Berkley KJ, Fillingim RB, et al. (2007). Studying sex and gender differences in pain and analgesia: a consensus report. Pain 132(Suppl 1):S26–S45.

95. Dexter P, Brandt K. (1994). Distribution and predictors of depressive symptoms in osteoarthritis. J Rheumatol 21(2):279–286.

96. Creamer P, Lethbridge-Cejku M, Hochberg MC. (2000). Factors associated with functional impairment in symptomatic knee osteoarthritis. Rheumatology (Oxford) 39(5):490–496.

97. Bradley LA. (2004). Recent approaches to understanding osteoarthritis pain. J Rheumatol Suppl 70:54–60.

98. Sullivan MJ, Thorn B, Haythornthwaite JA, Keefe F, Martin M, Bradley LA, et al. (2001). Theoretical perspectives on the relation between catastrophizing and pain. Clin J Pain 17(1):52–64.

99. Kulkarni B, Bentley DE, Elliott R, Julyan PJ, Boger E, Watson A, et al. (2007). Arthritic pain is processed in brain areas concerned with emotions and fear. Arthritis Rheum 56(4):1345–1354.

100. Hinz B, Brune K. (2004). Pain and osteoarthritis: new drugs and mechanisms. Curr Opin Rheumatol 16(5):628–633.

101. Lin CR, Amaya F, Barrett L, Wang H, Takada J, Samad TA, et al. (2006). Prostaglandin E2 receptor EP4 contributes to inflammatory pain hypersensitivity. J Pharmacol Exp Ther 319(3):1096–1103.

102. Southall MD, Vasko MR. (2001). Prostaglandin receptor subtypes, EP3C and EP4, mediate the prostaglandin E2-induced cAMP production and sensitization of sensory neurons. J Biol Chem 276(19):16083–16091.

103. Bar KJ, Natura G, Telleria-Diaz A, Teschner P, Vogel R, Vasquez E, et al. (2004). Changes in the effect of spinal prostaglandin E2 during inflammation: prostaglandin E (EP1-EP4) receptors in spinal nociceptive processing of input from the normal or inflamed knee joint. J Neurosci 24(3):642–651.

104. Boutaud O, Aronoff DM, Richardson JH, Marnett LJ, Oates JA. (2002). Determinants of the cellular specificity of acetaminophen as an inhibitor of prostaglandin H(2) synthases. Proc Natl Acad Sci USA 99(10):7130–7135.

105. Hinz B, Cheremina O, Brune K. (2008). Acetaminophen (paracetamol) is a selective cyclooxygenase-2 inhibitor in man. FASEB J 22(2):383–390.

106. Muth-Selbach US, Tegeder I, Brune K, Geisslinger G. (1999). Acetaminophen inhibits spinal prostaglandin E2 release after peripheral noxious stimulation. Anesthesiology 91(1):231–239.

107. Zhang W, Jones A, Doherty M. (2004). Does paracetamol (acetaminophen) reduce the pain of osteoarthritis? A meta-analysis of randomised controlled trials. Ann Rheum Dis 63(8):901–907.

108. Wieland HA, Michaelis M, Kirschbaum BJ, Rudolphi KA. (2005). Osteoarthritis—an untreatable disease? Nat Rev Drug Discov 4(4):331–344.

109. Schumacher MA, Basbaum AI, Way WL. (2007). Opioid analgesics & antagonists. In Katzung BG (ed.). *Basic & Clinical Pharmacology*, 10th ed. New York: McGraw-Hill.

110. Avouac J, Gossec L, Dougados M. (2007). Efficacy and safety of opioids for osteoarthritis: a meta-analysis of randomized controlled trials. Osteoarthritis Cartilage 15(8):957–965.

111. Stein A, Yassouridis A, Szopko C, Helmke K, Stein C. (1999). Intraarticular morphine versus dexamethasone in chronic arthritis. Pain 83(3):525–532.

112. Rice AS. (2001). Cannabinoids and pain. Curr Opin Investig Drugs 2(3): 399–414.

113. Akopian AN, Ruparel NB, Patwardhan A, Hargreaves KM. (2008). Cannabinoids desensitize capsaicin and mustard oil responses in sensory neurons via TRPA1 activation. J Neurosci 28(5):1064–1075.

114. Pertwee RG. (2001). Cannabinoid receptors and pain. Prog Neurobiol 63(5): 569–611.

115. Kobayashi K, Fukuoka T, Obata K, Yamanaka H, Dai Y, Tokunaga A, et al. (2005). Distinct expression of TRPM8, TRPA1, and TRPV1 mRNAs in rat primary afferent neurons with adelta/c-fibers and colocalization with trk receptors. J Comp Neurol 493(4):596–606.

116. Schuelert N, McDougall JJ. (2008). Cannabinoid-mediated antinociception is enhanced in rat osteoarthritic knees. Arthritis Rheum 58(1):145–153.

117. Caterina MJ, Julius D. (2001). The vanilloid receptor: a molecular gateway to the pain pathway. Annu Rev Neurosci 24:487–517.

118. Mason L, Moore RA, Derry S, Edwards JE, McQuay HJ. (2004). Systematic review of topical capsaicin for the treatment of chronic pain. BMJ 328(7446):991.

119. Deal CL, Schnitzer TJ, Lipstein E, Seibold JR, Stevens RM, Levy MD, et al. (1991). Treatment of arthritis with topical capsaicin: a double-blind trial. Clin Ther 13(3):383–395.

120. Altman RD, Aven A, Holmburg CE, Pfeiffer LM, Sack M, Young GT. (1994). Capsaicin cream 0.025% as monotherapy for osteoarthritis: a double-blind study. Semin Arthritis Rheum 23(Suppl 3):25–33.

121. Schnitzer T, Morton C, Coker S. (1994). Topical capsaicin therapy for osteoarthritis pain: achieving a maintenance regimen. Semin Arthritis Rheum 23(Suppl 3):34–40.

122. McCarthy GM, McCarty DJ. (1992). Effect of topical capsaicin in the therapy of painful osteoarthritis of the hands. J Rheumatol 19(4):604–607.

123. Zhang WY, Li Wan Po A. (1994). The effectiveness of topically applied capsaicin. A meta-analysis. Eur J Clin Pharmacol 46(6):517–522.

124. Stitik TP, Altschuler E, Foye PM. (2006). Pharmacotherapy of osteoarthritis. Am J Phys Med Rehabil 85(11 Suppl):S15–S28; quiz S9–S31.

125. Binshtok AM, Bean BP, Woolf CJ. (2007). Inhibition of nociceptors by TRPV1-mediated entry of impermeant sodium channel blockers. Nature 449(7162): 607–610.

126. Davies AM. (2003). Regulation of neuronal survival and death by extracellular signals during development. EMBO J 22(11):2537–2545.

127. Hefti FF, Rosenthal A, Walicke PA, Wyatt S, Vergara G, Shelton DL, et al. (2006). Novel class of pain drugs based on antagonism of NGF. Trends Pharmacol Sci 27(2):85–91.

128. Shelton DL, Zeller J, Ho WH, Pons J, Rosenthal A. (2005). Nerve growth factor mediates hyperalgesia and cachexia in auto-immune arthritis. Pain 116(1-2): 8–16.

129. Lane N, Webster L, Lu S, Gray M, Hefti FF, Walicke PA. (2005). RN624 (Anti-NGF) improves pain and function in subjects with moderate knee osteoarthritis: a phase I study. Arthritis Rheum 52(9 Suppl):S461.

130. Mokhtarani M, Zhao C, Gray M, Chan C, Hefti FF. (2006). RN264 (anti-nerve growth factor antibody) effectively reduces pain and improves function in subjects with knee osteoarthritis. Osteoarthritis Cartilage 14(Suppl B):S41.

131. Lane NE, Schnitzer TJ, Smith MD, Brown MT. (2008). Tanezumab relieves moderate to severe pain due to osteoarthritis (OA) of the knee: A phase 2 trial. *Arthritis Rheum* 58:S896.

132. Mico JA, Ardid D, Berrocoso E, Eschalier A. (2006). Antidepressants and pain. Trends Pharmacol Sci 27(7):348–354.

133. Kuipers RK. (1962). Imipramine in the treatment of rheumatic patients. Acta Rheumatol Scand 8:45–51.

134. Butler SH, Weil-Fugazza J, Godefroy F, Besson JM. (1985). Reduction of arthritis and pain behaviour following chronic administration of amitriptyline or imipramine in rats with adjuvant-induced arthritis. Pain 23(2):159–175.

135. Chappell AS, Ossanna MJ, Liu-Seifert H, Collins H. (2008). Duloxetine 60 to 120 mg versus placebo in the treatment of patients with osteoarthritis knee pain. Arthritis Rheum 58:S486.

136. Rogawski MA, Loscher W. (2004). The neurobiology of antiepileptic drugs for the treatment of nonepileptic conditions. Nat Med 10(7):685–692.

137. Zhang W, Moskowitz RW, Nuki G, Abramson S, Altman RD, Arden N, et al. (2007). OARSI recommendations for the management of hip and knee osteoarthritis, Part I: critical appraisal of existing treatment guidelines and systematic review of current research evidence. Osteoarthritis Cartilage 15(9):981–1000.

138. Zhang W, Moskowitz RW, Nuki G, Abramson S, Altman RD, Arden N, et al. (2008). OARSI recommendations for the management of hip and knee osteoar-thritis, Part II: OARSI evidence-based, expert consensus guidelines. Osteoarthritis Cartilage 16(2):137–162.

139. Bushnell MC, Marchand S, Tremblay N, Duncan GH. (1991). Electrical stimula-tion of peripheral and central pathways for the relief of musculoskeletal pain. Can J Physiol Pharmacol 69(5):697–703.

140. Sluka KA, Walsh D. (2003). Transcutaneous electrical nerve stimulation: basic science mechanisms and clinical effectiveness. J Pain 4(3):109–121.

141. Osiri M, Welch V, Brosseau L, Shea B, McGowan J, Tugwell P, et al. (2000). Transcutaneous electrical nerve stimulation for knee osteoarthritis. Cochrane Database of Systematic Reviews Issue 4, Art. No. CD002823. DOI: 10.1002/14651858.CD002823.

142. Bjordal JM, Johnson MI, Lopes-Martins RA, Bogen B, Chow R, Ljunggren AE. (2007). Short-term efficacy of physical interventions in osteoarthritic knee pain. A systematic review and meta-analysis of randomised placebo-controlled trials. BMC Musculoskelet Disord 8:51.

143. Suarez-Almazor M, Looney C, Street R, Liu Y, Cox V, Pietz K, et al. (2007). A randomized controlled trial of acupuncture for osteoarthritis of the knee: effects of provider communication style. Arthritis Rheum 56(9 Suppl):S315.

144. Manheimer E, Linde K, Lao L, Bouter LM, Berman BM. (2007). Meta-analysis: acupuncture for osteoarthritis of the knee. Ann Intern Med 146(12):868–877.

16

EXERCISE, TAPING, AND BRACING AS TREATMENTS FOR KNEE OSTEOARTHRITIS PAIN

Kim Louise Bennell, Michael Anthony Hunt, and
Rana Shane Hinman

*Centre for Health, Exercise & Sports Medicine, School of Physiotherapy,
The University of Melbourne, 202 Berkeley Street,
Melbourne, Victoria 3010, Australia*

INTRODUCTION

Pain associated with osteoarthritis (OA) of the knee is the most common complaint of those affected by the condition. The chronicity of the disorder often leads to muscle weakness, joint stiffness and/or instability, and reduced physical function, with subsequent losses in functional independence and health-related quality of life. As a result, many groups advocate the implementation of early treatment strategies to minimize symptoms and slow disease progression. In particular, the consensus is for the initial use of nonpharmacological interventions to achieve these goals. The potential role of physiotherapy interventions in this regard is receiving growing interest in the biomedical literature and in established clinical guidelines.

Pain in Osteoarthritis, Edited by David T. Felson and Hans-Georg Schaible
Copyright © 2009 Wiley-Blackwell.

This chapter outlines evidence of the effectiveness of several common physiotherapy treatment options available for individuals with knee OA: exercise, taping, and bracing. The influence of these interventions on mechanical factors associated with knee joint loading—a commonly cited risk factor for disease progression—is also discussed. Additionally, practical considerations for each modality are highlighted as they pertain to optimal reduction of symptoms and disease progression.

OVERVIEW OF PHYSIOTHERAPY FOR THE TREATMENT OF OSTEOARTHRITIS

Physiotherapy incorporates a wide range of potential treatment options that are tailored to a patient's unique clinical presentation. Indeed, given the heterogeneity in patient symptoms, even for those with similar radiographic evidence of disease severity, it is unrealistic to develop generic treatment programs to be used by all. Instead, many factors relating to a patient's anatomical and mechanical environment, psychosocial variables including patient attitudes, and environmental factors all must be considered when deciding on the best treatment approach. There is much evidence to support the use of various types of physiotherapy treatments, but little to suggest the superiority of one particular type used in isolation, nor a particular mode of delivery. As a result, many authors and leading health advocates suggest a combination of physiotherapy treatments to be used in conjunction with other treatment approaches including patient education,[1,2] especially given the absence of a known cure for OA.

KNEE LOADING IN THE PATHOPHYSIOLOGY OF KNEE OSTEOARTHRITIS

It is well accepted that localized knee loading is an important contributor to the breakdown of articular cartilage and subsequent reports of knee pain. Indirect correlates of joint load such as body mass[3] and occupational tasks[4] have been shown to be risk factors for knee OA development or progression and suggest a likely role for joint load in the disease pathogenesis. Additionally, animal studies investigating the in vitro response of cartilage to repeated load have found a direct relationship between prolonged loading and rate of cartilage degeneration.[5] Given the difficulties in the measurement of load in vivo, particularly during functional movements, researchers have had to employ more indirect methods of quantifying knee joint load. Quantitative motion analysis provides an accurate and noninvasive means to achieve this goal and, importantly, can be used to measure dynamic loading characteristics experienced during everyday activities such as walking.

Studies employing gait analysis in investigation of knee OA typically report the magnitude of the external adduction moment about the knee, an indirect measure of medial compartment tibiofemoral joint load.[6] The knee adduction moment (KAM) during stance has been shown to be higher in knees affected with OA than those without,[7] is positively related to the known changes in bone mineral density in response to load,[8] and is associated with measures of disease severity such as Kellgren and Lawrence grade of disease severity and joint space width.[9,10] Reports of changes in the magnitude of the KAM based on intensity of knee pain provide further evidence for the clinical utility of this measure.[11–13] Additionally, two longitudinal studies examining onset of knee pain or disease progression have been published that report the KAM. Amin et al.[14] examined 80 community-dwelling elders without knee pain over a span of 3–4 years and found that the 7 individuals who developed chronic knee pain between testing sessions had significantly higher peak KAM magnitudes at baseline. Miyazaki et al.[15] found a strong relationship between baseline KAM magnitude in 74 patients with radiographically confirmed knee OA and reduction in joint space width in subsequent follow-up visits, and reported a 6.46 times increase in the risk of OA progression with every unit increase in the KAM (normalized to percentage of body weight times height) at baseline.

Given the links between knee joint load, severity of pain, and articular cartilage degeneration, many clinical interventions aim to attenuate or redistribute the loads experienced within the knee joint. Accordingly, many recent studies examining the efficacy of available treatments for knee OA measure changes in the KAM to determine the utility of each treatment.[12,16–19] However, little is known about the effects of physiotherapy interventions on knee joint loading. Instead, most studies use clinical characteristics such as self-reported patient symptoms and function as the main outcome measures when examining these interventions. Therefore our knowledge of the long-term effects of physiotherapy on OA progression is limited in this regard. The following sections outline the known effects of exercise, taping, and bracing on symptoms such as pain and describe the rationale behind their use for the modification of knee joint load.

EXERCISE FOR KNEE OSTEOARTHRITIS

Exercise can take many forms, including muscle strengthening, stretching/range of motion, and aerobic conditioning. Additionally, the exercise can be land based or water based, can involve expensive, specialized equipment, or no equipment at all, and can be delivered in a group setting or individually. Certainly the mode of exercise delivery is dependent on patient-specific factors such as disease characteristics, goals of treatment, and availability of equipment.

Exercise for patients with knee OA has a large potential to reduce symptoms and improve physical functioning (Table 16.1). Importantly, exercise represents

TABLE 16.1   Summary of Evidence Supporting the Use of Exercise in the
Treatment of Knee Osteoarthritis

Results	Muscle Strengthening	Aerobic Exercise	Combination Exercise
Decreased knee pain	Refs. 29–35	Refs. 31, 44, 45, and 48	Refs. 32, 56, 57, and 63
Improved physical function	Refs. 29 and 31	Refs. 31 and 46–48	Refs. 32, 56, and 63
Improved muscle strength	Refs. 29–35 and 40	Ref. 31	Refs. 32, 56, and 63
Increased aerobic capacity	Ref. 31	Refs. 31 and 47–49	
Reduced knee joint load	Ref. 25		Ref. 19
Prevents OA development	Refs. 26 and 36 (no strength intervention)	Via reduced body mass	
Reduces OA progression	Refs. 40 and 42 (indirect evidence for Ref. 42)	Via reduced body mass	

a method of treatment that is accompanied by few contraindications or adverse effects in individuals with knee OA.[20] Typical physiological changes following exercise may include improvements in muscle strength, neuromuscular control, range of motion, and joint stability. In addition to the potential for symptom reduction and functional gains, the effects on overall health and well-being of the patient after commencing an exercise regimen cannot be understated.

Muscle Strengthening

Patients with knee OA typically exhibit reductions in muscle strength possibly as a consequence of reductions in physical activity and disuse or pain inhibition.[21–24] Conversely, inadequate strength, particularly of the quadriceps muscle group, may reduce the ability to sufficiently absorb load during dynamic activities[25] and therefore plays a role in the development of knee OA.[21,26] Consequently, many studies have investigated the effects of lower limb strengthening on clinical symptoms such as pain and function in patients with knee OA.

Biomechanically, the loads passing through a joint from external forces must be counteracted by the generation of internal forces to achieve equilibrium. During walking, the ground reaction force (GRF) and inertial properties of the lower limb result in loads experienced within the knee joint of up to three times that of body weight.[27] These loads are then distributed to various structures within the joint including subchondral bone, cartilage, menisci, ligaments, and muscles. The distribution of the load is dependent on the orientation of the external forces as well as the capacity of each structure to absorb the loads. Clearly, active force generation (i.e., from the muscles) is of particular interest given that it can be consciously controlled by the individual and can be improved with training. Indeed, for a given external load, increasing the force generated by contraction of muscles has the potential to unload passive structures, such as the cartilage and subchondral bone, and is paramount to the protection of such structures against degradation.

Quadriceps Strengthening

The quadriceps are the largest group of muscles crossing the knee joint and have the greatest potential to generate forces at the knee. A recent biomechanical modeling study[28] found that much of the internal force generated to counteract the external KAM in early stance originates from the quadriceps. Minimal force generation comes from the ligaments or the joint capsule, and only the gastrocnemius muscles exert large amounts of force during late stance. Interestingly, the findings indicate that although the frontal plane moment arm from the quadriceps to the knee joint center is very small, the substantial magnitude of the overall quadriceps force is sufficient to balance the tendency of the shank to adduct due to the GRF. Furthermore, the findings provide evidence to support the inclusion of quadriceps strengthening as part of the treatment program for knee OA.

Many clinical studies have examined the effects of strength training on measures of pain and physical function in the osteoarthritic population. Although some studies focus solely on improvement of quadriceps strength,[29,30] others include the quadriceps among a group of muscles to be targeted.[31-34] These studies have shown consistent improvements in isokinetic and isometric knee extension strength after training as well as reductions in pain and physical disability. A recent meta-analysis[35] confirmed these findings; however it indicated that no particular method of strength training was superior. Additionally, the authors suggested that although strengthening exercises alone provide relief of pain and improvement in physical function, effectiveness was increased when strengthening was combined with other exercises such as stretching, functional balance training, and aerobic conditioning.

Hip Muscle Strengthening

Very little is known about the role that the hip musculature plays in the pathophysiology of knee OA. Indeed, there is no research examining the associations between hip strength and measures of pain or function. Although research in this area is limited, there is a theoretical rationale to improve the strength of the hip abductors and adductors of those affected with knee OA. These muscles are known to control pelvic motion in the frontal plane during gait. During stance, those with insufficient stance limb hip abductor strength to control the pelvis will exhibit a contralateral pelvic drop, known as a Trendelenburg sign.[36] This drop will theoretically shift the body's center of mass away from the stance limb toward the swing limb, thereby increasing the distance between the GRF vector and the knee joint center of rotation and subsequent KAM. This has been supported by recent studies using gait analysis in patients with knee OA. However, we are unaware of any studies that have measured hip abduction strength in individuals with knee OA or the potential benefit of hip abductor muscle strengthening in this patient population.

To our knowledge, only one study has been published examining hip adductor strength in patients with knee OA. Yamada et al.[37] measured isometric hip adductor strength in a group of 32 women with medial compartment knee OA and 13 healthy age-matched women. The OA group exhibited significantly greater hip adductor strength than controls as well as significantly higher hip adductor to hamstrings strength ratios. Given the additional findings of increasing hip adductor strength and varus malalignment in more severely diseased knees, the authors attributed the increase in hip adductor strength to their potential role in resisting lateral thrust and the KAM during gait in malaligned lower limbs. Although this is a biomechanical possibility, it is speculative and further exploration into the role of hip adductor strengthening in the reduction of knee joint load and knee pain is warranted.

Aerobic Exercise

Aerobic exercise involves exercising for prolonged periods of time at an elevated intensity (approximately 60–80% of maximum heart rate). Common activities include swimming, walking, and cycling and all have been found to be effective in reducing symptoms of knee OA. Structured walking programs have received particular interest in the treatment of knee OA given the familiarity and minimal need for equipment. When compared to control groups, walking programs have been shown to reduce knee joint pain,[31,38,39] improve physical functioning during activities such as stair climbing,[40] increase aerobic capacity[41] and physical endurance,[42,43] and improve gait characteristics.[43] Additionally, Sharma et al.[44] found that the amount of aerobic exercise per week was predictive of long-term physical function (WOMAC physical function and time required for 5 chair stands) in a 3 year longitudinal cohort study of 236 individuals with knee OA.

Aerobic exercise also has the potential to reduce body mass — a well-known risk factor for knee OA development and progression.[3,45–47] Given the strong associations among body mass, knee joint loading, and articular cartilage degeneration, exercise programs that promote weight loss through aerobic activity appear warranted. Indeed, many clinicians advocate the use of some form of aerobic activity for individuals with knee OA, particularly those who are obese, and weight loss consistently appears in clinical guidelines for the treatment of knee OA.[2]

Combination Exercise Therapy

Although studies examining single exercise interventions (e.g., walking programs, quadriceps strengthening) provide valuable information on the effectiveness of these particular treatment methods, they may be impractical in isolation given the use of multiple interventions within clinical practice. In fact, physiotherapists rarely advocate the use of a single intervention for the rehabilitation of most pathologies. This is especially relevant given that previous research has failed to find clear evidence to support one type of exercise over another.[31,41,48,49] In contrast, the presumption that clinical outcome is maximized by the combination of different types of exercise or with other intervention strategies has been supported by much research.

Rogind et al.[32] and Suomi and Collier[50] conducted studies investigating changes in pain and function after the implementation of exercise programs that included strengthening, endurance, balance, range of motion, coordination, and general fitness. Both studies found favorable effects of the combination exercise programs with significant reductions in pain and improvements in strength, walking speed, and self-reported physical function. Suomi and Collier[50] also reported significantly decreased perceptions of pain and difficulty during activities of daily living (ADL) after the completion of only 8 weeks of training. This latter finding is especially important given the decreased functional independence typically reported by elderly patients with knee OA resulting from a reduced ability to perform ADL.

Bennell et al.[51] conducted a randomized, controlled trial of 119 individuals with knee OA which employed a novel, multifaceted physiotherapy program with an emphasis on functional exercise, balance training, knee taping, and manual therapy. Significant improvements were found after 12 weeks in pain (42% reduction measured on a visual analogue scale) and self-reported function (WOMAC and SF-36). Although 70% of patients in the physiotherapy group reported global improvement immediately following the intervention, 72% of those in the placebo group (who received inactive ultrasound and the application of an inert gel) reported similar changes and there were no significant differences between groups in any outcome measure. Placebo effects and the novelty of the physiotherapy program (i.e., emphasis on motor control rather than strengthening or aerobic fitness) may have accounted for the nonsignificant findings. Although the program was standardized, and highlights the potential importance of individualized treatment, there are assumed benefits of exercise interventions targeting functional control and coordination in addition to strength and endurance.

Many authors advocate the use of exercises emphasizing motor control strategies for individuals with knee OA. Fitzgerald and Oatis[52] highlight the combination of sensory and motor dysfunction in this patient population that contribute to the physical impairments commonly observed. They suggest that programs focusing on techniques to improve balance and coordination may be beneficial for these patients to improve skills required for ADL. Indeed, Hurley[53] argues that maximizing strength gains are of little value if the individual lacks the neuromuscular control to perform functional activities. Instead, he suggests that the effects of exercise can be optimized by combining strength and endurance exercises with coordination and functional performance training and/or patient education. With evidence to suggest that individuals with knee OA exhibit altered neuromuscular control strategies during tasks such as force targeting,[54] walking,[55,56] and stair ascent/descent[55] compared to those without joint disease, more research into the efficacy of exercise programs aiming to enhance motor control is needed.

The effects of combination exercise therapies are not limited to strengthening programs. Messier et al.[57] showed in a trial of 316 overweight individuals with radiographic evidence of knee OA that those receiving dietary advice combined with aerobic and resistance exercise experienced significantly more improvement in pain, function, and mobility after 18 months than groups of participants receiving either diet advice or exercise given in isolation. Additionally, those who received the exercise plus dietary advice lost more weight (5.7%) than those who received only dietary advice (4.9%) or exercise (3.7%), and significantly more than those who received healthy lifestyle education (1.2%). These results suggest that anatomical factors associated with knee OA (i.e., body mass) and clinical measures of symptoms and function can both be optimized with the combination of effective therapies.

Modes of Delivery

There is little consensus on the preferred method of exercise in individuals with knee OA. As indicated previously, it appears as though treatment regimens employing a variety of exercise types are more beneficial than focusing on a single aspect of exercise. Much of this research has reported on the effects of land-based exercise with little attention to other forms of exercise. Aquatic exercise, for example, is commonly used for individuals with knee OA and has been shown to provide improvements in strength, physical function, and symptoms.[58,59] Importantly, the impact loading experienced at the knee is greatly reduced during aquatic therapy and may be a preferred method of exercising for those with painful knees. However, Foley et al.[58] caution that some patients may benefit from the functional loading only achieved in land-based exercise and suggest that aquatic-based exercise may be more suitable for improving aerobic function, while land-based exercise may be desirable for strength gains.

Given the concerns over the rising cost of providing effective treatment for patients, much research has been conducted on the effectiveness of home-based exercise programs. Evcik and Sonel[39] compared groups assigned to either a home-based strengthening program, home-based walking program, or control group for 3 months. They found significant improvements in pain and self-reported function in both exercise groups compared to the control group, but no differences between the strengthening and walking groups. Baker et al.[60] also investigated the benefits of a partially supervised home strengthening program. Forty-six patients were randomized to either a home-based strength training program or to a nutrition education program for 4 months. Significant improvements in pain, strength, and physical function were observed in the strengthening program compared to the education program.

What is less clear, however, is whether a home-based exercise program gives similar outcomes as group-based exercise. Advantages of group-based exercise programs include the social aspects of group therapy, which may increase compliance, and the ability to minimize resources required to treat a large group of patients. Little research to date has been conducted to ascertain the differences between the two modes of delivery. Although not home based, Fransen et al.[29] did not observe differences in subjective or objective measures of physical function between groups receiving group (maximum 6 patients) or individual physical therapy after 8 weeks of training. It must be noted that both groups exhibited significant improvements over a third group that received no treatment.

McCarthy et al.[61] studied the effects of supplementing a home-based exercise program with physiotherapist-supervised exercise for 8 weeks. At the 12 month follow-up assessment, patients who received the home-based program supplemented with the 8 week group exercise class exhibited significant improvements in locomotor function and walking pain. Therefore optimal improvements in symptoms and function may be achieved through the use of both individualized and group treatment sessions and this approach may alleviate some of the financial burdens associated with patient care in this population.

Dosage

Another consideration is the frequency and duration of the exercise program. Although many studies have reported a definitive dose-based response to exercise, there may be issues with maintaining high compliance in programs with long durations. Most exercise guidelines would suggest a physiological response can be attained with as little as 3 exercise sessions per week, and research into the effectiveness of exercise programs in individuals with knee OA have shown improvements after 8 or 12 week programs.[32,33,41,42,50,51]

Factors Influencing Outcome

Several factors have the potential to alter outcomes of an exercise intervention in individuals with knee OA. One of the most commonly cited factors is patient compliance. Many studies have reported significant differences in outcome response after an exercise intervention based on the number of completed sessions,[31,62–66] with those individuals exhibiting higher adherence to the program achieving more beneficial results. As a result, examination of the factors that contribute to compliance rates for exercise programs in individuals with knee OA has received interest in the literature.

Intensity and frequency of exercise appears to influence compliance in elderly patients. Perri et al.[67] performed a randomized controlled trial of 379 healthy sedentary individuals and found that compliance was greater in those who exercised 5–7 times per week than those allocated to moderate frequency (3–4 times per week). Conversely, they found that walking intensity was inversely correlated to compliance as those who walked at a moderate intensity (44–55% of maximum heart rate) were more compliant than those who walked at a high intensity (65–75% of maximum heart rate). The type of exercise, however, does not appear to be related to compliance as Minor et al.[41] reported no differences in compliance between those randomized to either walking, aerobic aquatics, or range of motion treatment arms.

Patient monitoring has also been shown to affect compliance rates in exercise programs. It is often observed that compliance is higher when patients receive attention from health professionals rather than a primarily home-based exercise program. Accordingly, directed exercise programs have been shown to have superior outcomes in self-reported locomotor function, pain, and patient satisfaction compared to nonsupervised programs.[68] Additionally, participation in physical activity tends to decrease after completion of a study protocol or prescribed program when patients are no longer monitored or when advice is no longer given regarding exercise progression. More research is needed to identify effective methods to maintain participation in exercise for long durations.

Without doubt, much of the research into factors influencing compliance has focused on psychosocial attributes of the individual. Patient attitudes toward exercise, and OA in general, have been cited as factors associated with the uptake of exercise. Campbell et al.[69] performed a qualitative analysis of individuals with knee OA who had undergone a trial consisting of initial visits to a physiotherapist and then primarily of home-based strengthening exercises. They found that compliance was positively related to perception of more severe knee symptoms, belief in the effectiveness of the intervention, and understanding of the pathogenesis of knee OA (those who were less compliant tended to believe that OA was part of the natural ageing process or that it was simply a "wear and tear" disease). Higher self-efficacy, a belief in one's own ability to perform tasks, has been shown to be associated with higher compliance and better exercise outcome[70] and with better performance on measures of mobility such as 6 minute walk distance and the timed-up-and-go test.[71]

One strategy suggested to improve patient compliance with exercise includes catering the exercise program to the unique requirements of the patient as well as ensuring availability of resources. While some patients may prefer the social outlet provided through group exercise sessions, there is little evidence that compliance differs between group and individual exercise. Other methods to improve compliance include monitoring via telephone contact[72] or self-reported diary,[73–75] graphic feedback,[76] or lifestyle retraining.[73] While monitoring from a health care professional is the preferred method of contact, patients can rely on their own social support network when an appropriate health care professional is unavailable.[73,77,78] Additionally, self-monitoring via positive feedback loops based on level of physical function and attainment of goals may be useful for some patients.

These strategies are necessary to ensure a successful treatment effect both during and following cessation of an exercise program. Studies have shown that while patients can generally achieve favorable outcomes after an exercise intervention, follow-up assessments tend to show regression of gains without continued physical training.[31,32] The requirement for continued participation in physical activity to achieve gains or maintenance is not unique to individuals with knee OA. However, given the known consequences of discontinued activity on symptoms and overall physical functioning in this patient population, more steps must be taken to ensure continued compliance with prescribed treatment regimens.

KNEE TAPING

Taping the knee, in particular, the patella, is a physical therapy treatment strategy recommended in the management of knee OA by clinical guidelines[79] and by expert clinical consensus.[80] Knee taping involves the application of adhesive rigid strapping tape to the patella and/or associated soft tissue structures. Taping aims to realign the patella so as to reduce patellofemoral joint stress and to unload painful soft tissues around the knee joint, with the ultimate intention of reducing knee pain.

Patellofemoral Joint: An Important Source of Symptoms in Knee Osteoarthritis

The patellofemoral joint (PFJ) is commonly affected by OA. Authors of a community-based study of knee OA comparing compartmental changes observed a higher frequency of radiographic osteophytes in the PFJ compared to the tibiofemoral joint (TFJ).[81] Another investigation of individuals with knee pain revealed the most common radiographic pattern of OA to be combined TFJ and PFJ degenerative change.[82] It also appears that the PFJ is an important source of symptoms associated with knee OA, and possibly more important than the TFJ. Kornaat et al.[83] recently evaluated the association between structural abnormalities on magnetic resonance imaging and knee pain and stiffness in a large group of individuals with and without knee OA.

Osteophytes in the PFJ were significantly associated with knee pain, whereas tibiofemoral osteophytes were not. Similar findings have been reported by others.[84–88]

Patellar Tracking

In order to understand the rationale behind knee taping, an understanding of PFJ biomechanics is necessary. The manner in which the patella articulates and moves within the femoral trochlear groove may be referred to as patellar tracking. Patellar tracking results from the interaction between passive and active structures. The passive osseous anatomical anomalies most likely to alter the alignment and motion of the patella are a shallow femoral trochlea groove[89] and patella alta.[90] Soft tissue tensions in medial and lateral retinaculae, joint capsule, and ligaments also contribute to maintaining patellar alignment.[91] Active structures, namely, the vastus medialis obliquus (VMO) and the vastus lateralis (VL), are also important contributors to the maintenance of proper patellar tracking. As these two vasti quadriceps muscles have antagonistic effects on mediolateral patellar stability, their timely and coordinated contraction is essential to ensure mediolateral stability.[92] Weakness of one of these muscles, or disruption to their neuromotor control, may result in abnormalities in patellar tracking, which may ultimately alter the distribution of PFJ contact areas and cause localized increases in PFJ stress (load per unit area). Abnormalities in patellar tracking are often observed as patellar malalignment.

Patellar Malalignment

Patellar malalignment is commonly manifested as lateral patellar tilt, lateral patellar displacement/subluxation, or a combination of the two. Research has shown that indices of patellar alignment are associated with radiographic features of PFJ OA, such as osteophytosis and joint space narrowing,[93] as well as MRI features of disease, such as cartilage thickness loss and bone marrow lesions.[94] This suggests that patellar malalignment is a possible contributor to increased stress on the PFJ, potentially leading to the development of osteoarthritic change within the joint. Additionally, patellar malalignment has been implicated in PFJ disease progression.[95] Medial displacement and tilt of the patella predisposes to progression of medial joint space narrowing, while lateral displacement is predictive of progression of lateral joint space narrowing. The congruence angle—a measure of patellar subluxation— correlates with radiographic severity of PFJ OA[96] in that medial subluxation tends to be associated with medial PFJ OA, while lateral subluxation primarily results in arthritic changes laterally. Patellar subluxation is commonly observed clinically,[96] and given that lateral subluxation shifts the PFJ contact area laterally and reduces contact area magnitude by 50%,[97] strategies aimed at

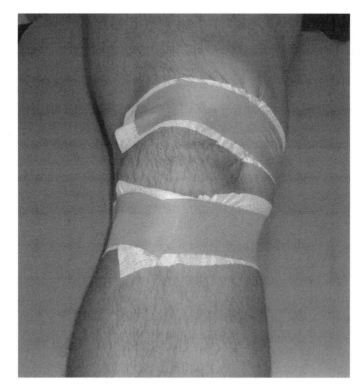

Figure 16.1. Taping resulting in medial displacement of the patella. The tape is applied to prevent lateral displacement of the patella during movement and to reduce lateral patellar joint stress.

normalizing patellar alignment may be of particular importance in treatment of PFJ OA. Indeed, although a wide variety of taping techniques can be used, the most common technique for PFJ OA is applied to correct excessive lateral patellar displacement/subluxation and tilt (Fig. 16.1).

Effects on Pain

While taping was first published as a treatment for knee OA in 1994,[98] it has been used clinically by physiotherapists for many years.[99] Several studies have demonstrated the effectiveness of knee taping for patients with knee OA. Using a within-subjects crossover trial design, Cushnaghan et al.[98] evaluated the effects of three types of patellar tape on pain in 14 subjects with symptomatic and radiographic PFJ OA. Neutral, medial, and laterally directed patellar tape patterns were applied each for 4 days, with 3 days of no tape between taping conditions. Average pain was measured 1 hour following tape application, and daily thereafter. While no difference in pain severity was evident 1 hour following tape application, a significant difference was observed from day 2 onwards, with medially directed patellar taping resulting in approximately 25% less pain than either neutral or laterally directed taping. A subsequent study of 18 participants with TFJ OA and varying degrees of PFJ OA confirmed these findings.[100] Using a combination therapeutic taping technique designed to correct lateral displacement and tilt as well as unload the infrapatellar fat pad, Hinman et al.[100] demonstrated immediate reductions in knee pain by up to 50% during various functional tasks.

Results of these small studies were subsequently confirmed in a larger randomized controlled trial.[101] Eighty-seven participants with tibiofemoral OA and varying degrees of patellofemoral OA were randomly allocated to receive 3 weeks of either therapeutic tape (correction of lateral patellar displacement and tilt as well as unloading of the infrapatellar fat pad), control tape (sham condition with no correction of patellar position or unloading of soft tissues), or no tape. Tape was applied by trained physiotherapists and participants wore the tape continuously before it was reapplied at weekly intervals. After 3 weeks of treatment, the therapeutic tape group showed a significantly greater reduction in pain than the control and no tape groups. Following intervention, the therapeutic tape group demonstrated 40% less pain on movement compared to baseline. This was significantly greater than the 16% reduction in pain reported by the control tape group and the no tape group, whose pain remained unchanged. Furthermore, reductions in pain continued for at least 3 weeks after taping treatment had ceased, suggesting extended short-term benefits of knee taping.

Mechanisms of Pain Reduction

It is not known definitively how taping relieves knee pain. The largely nonsignificant effects of control tape demonstrated by Hinman and colleagues[100,101] show that therapeutic tape has a direct effect on knee pain that cannot be attributed to placebo (e.g., attention by physiotherapist, use of tape) or cutaneous stimulation alone. Although tape has been proposed to alter proprioceptive acuity at the knee,[102] studies in knee OA have not demonstrated an effect of knee taping on joint position sense.[103]

It is most likely that taping results in subtle changes in patellar alignment as some research has shown improvements in healthy individuals and those with patellofemoral pain syndrome.[104–107] Unfortunately, this has yet to be confirmed in those with PFJ OA. Improved patellar alignment is likely to unload the lateral patellar facet, leading to redistribution of PFJ contact pressures. Improvement in patellar alignment has also been postulated to enhance the function and activation of VMO, in particular, its onset timing relative to that of VL, which would further serve to improve patellar tracking. Such effects of tape, however, have only been demonstrated in those with patellofemoral pain syndrome[108] and have not been observed in patients with knee OA.[103]

Additionally, taping that unloads the infrapatellar fat pad — known to be pain sensitive and proposed to be a source of pain in knee OA[109] — by shortening the soft tissue may relieve pain based on the principle that inflamed soft tissue does not respond well to stretching. Periarticular structures such as the infrapatellar fat pad and pes anserine bursa/tendons can become inflamed secondary to knee joint pathology,[109–111] and thus may potentially contribute to knee pain.

Practical Considerations

In clinical practice, choice of taping technique is usually determined from physiotherapy examination findings and is individualized to the patient by the therapist. There are several practical aspects to knee taping that must be considered. It is known that taping is associated with very few adverse effects, the most common of which is skin irritation.

Skin care is important to minimize the risk of adverse effects especially when tape is applied to older skin. Patients should initially be screened to ensure they are appropriate for taping and caution should be exercised with individuals with a history of skin conditions or allergies to adhesive tapes or bandages. Hypoallergenic undertape should always be used in all patients to protect skin from direct contact by the rigid strapping tape that is used to realign the patellar and unload soft tissues. The majority of skin damage is caused by frequent removal of tape. Thus in older patients with knee OA, tape should be removed and reapplied less frequently than in younger people. Patients should be instructed to carefully remove the tape in a slow and controlled manner so as to minimize risk of skin damage. In the case of skin irritation, tape should be removed and the skin rested from taping until the damage has healed. Ongoing taping may not be appropriate for some patients. For those in whom there is excessive skin irritation or who are unable to apply the tape by themselves, patellar bracing may accomplish some of the same effects (see next section).

In clinical practice, patients are usually taught by the physiotherapist how to tape their knee themselves, thus allowing taping to be used at home as a self-management strategy for relief of knee pain. However, it is not known whether self-taping is as effective as therapist-applied tape as this has not been researched specifically to date.

KNEE BRACING

A variety of commercial braces are available for knee OA and these differ in terms of construction and design, whether they are custom-made or off-the-shelf, whether they target TFJ or PFJ OA, and their price.

While a brace may be beneficial for reducing symptoms in knee OA, it should not be used as a stand-alone treatment but should complement other treatments. Given that there is limited research about the effectiveness of braces in knee OA, the decision to use a brace should be based on whether the patient demonstrates improvement on subjective and objective outcomes, particularly as individual responses vary.

Neoprene or Elastic Sleeves

Neoprene or elastic sleeves are the simplest and cheapest type of knee braces. These single piece sleeves provide compression and warmth but little support. Although only a limited number of studies have evaluated their effectiveness, some have found small short-term benefits.[112–114] In the only clinical trial, a neoprene sleeve worn for 6 months by persons with medial knee OA resulted in a significant improvement in quality of life and in function compared with a control group receiving medical treatment only.[113] However, not all people respond to this therapy. Forty-four percent of people in the neoprene sleeve group were deemed to have achieved "clinical success" based on the authors' unstated definition compared with 18% in the control group.

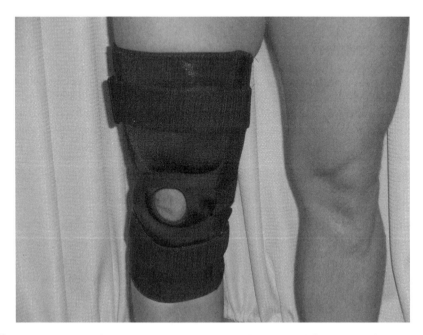

Figure 16.2. Patellofemoral joint brace. A medially directed force is applied to the patella via an adjustable strap on the anterior aspect of the brace. Proper loading of the patella minimizes lateral displacement of the patella during movement.

Patellofemoral Braces

For patients whose predominant symptoms appear to be arising from the PFJ, a patellofemoral brace (Fig. 16.2) may be considered. Similar to the rationale for patellar tape, these braces aim to correct abnormal tracking of the patella by applying a force to the patella generally in a medial direction.

Unfortunately, there are no published studies that have evaluated the effectiveness of a patellofemoral brace in patients with patellofemoral OA.

Unloader Braces

Unloader braces (Fig. 16.3) are semirigid knee braces generally made from molded plastic and foam with a hinge mechanism and straps. They can be obtained off-the-shelf or custom made, with prices varying accordingly. These braces are designed for people with predominant medial or lateral TFJ OA and tibiofemoral (varus or valgus) malalignment, with the aim of providing stability, support, and pain relief. The braces attempt to apply an external

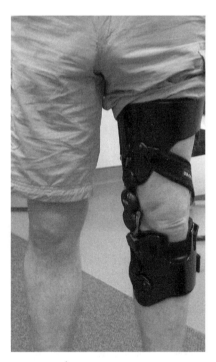

Figure 16.3. Unloader knee brace. This semirigid knee brace applies an external three-point corrective force about the knee, which reduces the load on the affected tibiofemoral compartment.

three-point corrective force that reduces the biomechanical load on the affected compartment. For example, in those with medial compartment knee OA and varus malalignment, the brace applies a valgus directed force, while in those with lateral compartment knee OA and valgus malalignment, the brace applies a varus directed force. Given the predominance of medial compartment knee OA, valgus unloader braces are most commonly used and have received the most research attention.

Effects on Unloader Braces on Gait Biomechanics and Sensorimotor Function

Studies have shown that valgus unloader braces can favorably affect knee biomechanics and sensorimotor function. Valgus unloader braces can acutely reduce varus angulation and medial compartment loads at the knee. Lindenfeld et al.[115] reported a mean 10% decrease in the KAM with an unloader brace in a group of middle-aged people with medial tibiofemoral OA. Individual responses varied and were as high as 32% in one individual. In an industry sponsored study, Pollo et al.[116] demonstrated an acute mean reduction in KAM of 13% with valgus bracing, and a reduction in medial compartment load by an average of 11%. It is believed that a direct alteration in mechanical alignment of the lower limb underlies the changes in the KAM observed with bracing. Given that a reduction in the KAM of about 10% corresponds to a 3.3-fold decrease in the risk of disease progression,[15] valgus bracing offers great potential for knee OA if the load reduction is sustained. Long-term studies are required to evaluate the effects of bracing on joint structure.

Knee bracing may also impart sensorimotor benefits to the patient with knee OA. Birmingham et al.[117] demonstrated a significant improvement in knee joint proprioception (knee joint angle replication) in patients with knee OA while wearing a knee brace. However, the mean difference between the braced and unbraced conditions was only 0.7°, which renders the clinical significance of these findings questionable. Enhanced sensory input at the knee and/or reduced pain with a brace may favorably influence muscle activation patterns. In people with medial compartment knee OA who have frontal plane knee laxity and mediolateral instability, there is increased muscle activity and coactivation of antagonistic muscles.[55,56,118] A recent small crossover study in 16 people with medial compartment knee OA and varus malalignment found that a brace either set at neutral alignment or at 4° valgus both reduced pain and muscle cocontraction.[119]

The biomechanical effects of braces may vary depending on patient and brace characteristics. Using video fluoroscopy to measure the ability of the brace to reverse joint space loss and create condylar separation in the OA affected compartment during weight-bearing conditions, Dennis et al.[120] found a brace to be less effective in obese patients. They also found that certain braces consistently improved condylar separation in most patients, whereas other braces resulted in little to no condylar separation. It may be that those with greater initial varus malalignment derive the most improvement in the KAM with a brace.[121] Finally, a comparison of a custom-made and an off-the-shelf unloader brace showed the custom-made brace to be superior in improving varus angulation and reducing the KAM.[122]

Effects of Unloader Braces on Pain and Function

Clinically, the most important parameter for braces to affect is patient symptoms. However, to our knowledge, there are only three randomized trials that have investigated the effectiveness of unloader braces for reducing pain and improving function in people with knee OA.[113,123,124] Using a double crossover design with four 6 week periods of follow-up, Horlick and Loomar[123] found that the use of a valgus unloader brace provided modest relief of pain in 40 relatively young people with medial knee OA. A significant improvement in pain or function could not be detected from a neutral brace position but this may have been due to the small sample size.

Kirkley et al.[113] conducted a 6 month comparison of a custom-made valgus unloader brace, a neoprene elastic sleeve, and medical treatment only (control) in 119 patients with varus malalignment and knee OA. They found a significant improvement in disease-specific quality of life and in function in both the brace groups compared with the control group. The unloader brace group showed greater benefits in some measures (pain during 6 minute walk test and during a timed stair climb) compared with the neoprene sleeve group. In brace and sleeve groups, the benefits were evident during the initial 6 weeks with maintenance of improvement thereafter.

In the study with the longest follow-up (12 months), the additive effect of a brace intended to reduce load in either the medial or lateral compartment was evaluated in 117 patients with unicompartmental medial or lateral knee OA.[124] Although the primary outcome measures of pain severity and knee function were improved in the intervention group in comparison with the controls at each assessment point, the differences reached only borderline significance. The reported walking distances were significantly longer in the brace group. Effect sizes ranged from 0.3 to 0.4, indicating modest benefits with bracing.

It is apparent that not all patients respond favorably to bracing therapy. In the study by Kirkley et al.,[113] 61% of patients in the unloader brace group achieved clinical "success" based on the authors' unstated definition, meaning that 39% did not respond. Exploratory subgroup analyses revealed that those who were more symptomatic gained the most benefit from bracing. No relationships were noted between age, gender, radiographic disease severity, degree of varus deformity, and status of the anterior cruciate ligament. Different results were found by Brouwer et al.[124] They showed a better bracing effect in those with varus malalignment, in patients with severe OA, in patients with secondary OA and in patients younger than 60 years.

From the few clinical trials available, it appears that an unloader brace may provide small benefits in terms of pain and function in patients with medial unicompartmental OA, although additional trial evidence confirming this is needed. Braces may not work as well in those with lateral OA.

Practical Considerations

One of the major barriers limiting the benefits of a brace for knee OA is likely to be compliance. Giori[125] found that, within 6 months, 20% of people wearing braces had discontinued their use while a further 29% ceased using them after 6 months. Those who continued to use the brace did so intermittently. Younger patients had a greater likelihood of longer brace use than did older patients. In the 12 month clinical trial by Brouwer et al.,[124] 42% of patients in the brace group changed their initial treatment. While the reasons underlying poor compliance with brace use are unknown, factors such as bulkiness, style, ease of application, fit, comfort, and lack of perceived benefit are likely to contribute. An elasticized sleeve may need to be worn under the brace to improve comfort and it is important that the brace fits snugly with no slippage during wear to maintain the biomechanical benefits. However, the brace should not be too tight, as skin irritation may be a problem, and there has been a report of a deep venous thrombosis and thromboembolism associated with use of a knee brace.[125] Persons with obese legs may experience slippage of the brace and correct positioning may be especially challenging for them. Behavioral strategies similar to those employed for exercise interventions can also be beneficial for the wearing of braces.

CONCLUSION

Although the research is not equivocal, there is sufficient evidence to indicate that physiotherapy interventions can reduce knee pain and improve function in those with knee OA. A variety of mechanisms exist, including dissipation of knee joint load, alteration of lower limb alignment (taping and bracing), and restoration of normal neuromuscular functioning. Patient responses vary, however, and therapeutic programs highlighting individual patient needs appear to be more beneficial and costeffective. No single physiotherapy intervention has been shown to provide superior results over the others, and it is likely that a combination of exercise, taping, and bracing (when appropriate) optimizes outcome as summarized below. Further research is needed to understand fully the role of physiotherapy in the overall treatment of knee OA.

Exercise

- Significant improvements in pain, physical function, and quality of life
- Physiological effects are method specific (resistance vs. aerobic training)
- No differences in overall outcome between resistance and aerobic training
- Combination therapy appears to have superior outcomes compared to resistance or aerobic training in isolation
- Long-term outcomes are dosage dependent and compliance dependent
- Methods to increase exercise compliance are necessary

Taping

- Aim is to control patellar tracking and minimize contact stress
- Most common method is medially directed taping to offload lateral compartment of PFJ
- Significant improvements in pain and physical function
- Direct effect on pain not attributable to placebo or cutaneous stimulation
- No research on long-term effects of taping or role in disease pathogenesis

Bracing

- Type of brace is dependent on affected compartment and intended outcome
- Should not be used as a stand-alone treatment
- Significant reductions in pain and knee joint load, with concomitant increases in physical function
- Outcomes are patient specific and may be influenced by clinical characteristics
- Minimal research in this area

REFERENCES

1. Zhang W, Moskowitz R, Nuki G, Abramson S, Altman R, Arden N, Bierma-Zeinstra S, Brandt K, Croft P, Doherty M, Dougados M, Hochberg M, Hunter D, Kwoh K, Lohmander L, Tugwell P. (2007). OARSI recommendations for the management of hip and knee osteoarthritis. Part I: Critical appraisal of existing

treatment guidelines and systematic review of current research evidence. Osteoarthritis Cartilage 15:981–1000.

2. Jordan K, Arden N, Doherty M, Bannwarth B, Bijlsma J, Dieppe P, Gunther K, Hauselmann H, Herrero-Beaumont G, Kaklamanis P, Lohmander S, Leeb B, Lequesne M, Mazieres B, Martin-Mola E, Pavelka K, Pendleton A, Punzi L, Serni U, Swoboda B, Verbruggen G, Zimmerman-Gorska I, Dougados M. (2003). Eular recommendations 2003: an evidence based approach to the management of knee osteoarthritis. Report of a task force of the standing committee for international clinical studies including therapeutic trials (ESCISIT). Ann Rheum Dis 62: 1145–1155.

3. Cooper C, Snow S, McAlindon TE, Kellingray S, Stuart B, Coggon D, Dieppe PA. (2000). Risk factors for the incidence and progression of radiographic knee osteoarthritis. Arthritis Rheum 43:995–1000.

4. Cooper C. (1995). Occupational activity and the risk of osteoarthritis. J Rheumatol 22(Suppl 43):1012.

5. Buckwalter JMH. (1997). Articular cartilage. Part II: Degeneration and osteoarthritis, repair, regeneration, and transplantation. J Bone Joint Surg 79A:612–632.

6. Schipplein OD, Andriacchi TP. (1991). Interaction between active and passive knee stabilizers during level walking. J Orthop Res 9:113–119.

7. Bailunas A, Hurwitz D, Ryals A, Karrar A, Case J, Block J, Andriacchi T. (2002). Increased knee joint loads during walking are present in subjects with knee osteoarthritis. Osteoarthritis Cartilage 10:573–579.

8. Wada M, Maezawa Y, Baba H, Shimada S, Sasaki S, Nose Y. (2001). Relationships among bone mineral densities, static alignment and dynamic load in patients with medial compartment knee osteoarthritis. Rheumatology 40:499–505.

9. Sharma L, Hurwitz DE, Thonar E, Sum JA, Lenz ME, Dunlop DD, Schnitzer TJ, Kirwanmellis G, Andriacchi TP. (1998). Knee adduction moment, serum hyaluronan level, and disease severity in medial tibiofemoral osteoarthritis. Arthritis Rheum 41:1233–1240.

10. Hurwitz D, Ryals A, Case J, Block J, Andriacchi T. (2002). The knee adduction moment during gait in subjects with knee osteoarthritis is more closely correlated with static alignment than radiographic disease severity, toe out angle and pain. J Orthop Res 20:101–108.

11. Shrader M, Draganich L, Pottenger L, Piotrowski G. (2004). Effects of knee pain relief in osteoarthritis on gait and stair-stepping. Clin Orthop Relat Res 421:188–193.

12. Schnitzer TJ, Popovich JM, Andersson GB, Andriacchi TP. (1993). Effect of piroxicam on gait in patients with osteoarthritis of the knee. Arthritis Rheum 36:1207–1213.

13. Henriksen M, Simonsen E, Alkjaer T, Lund H, Graven-Nielsen T, Danneskiold-Samsoe B, Bliddal H. (2006). Increased knee joint loads during walking—a consequence of pain relief in knee osteoarthritis. The Knee 13:445–450.

14. Amin S, Luepongsak N, McGibbon C, LaValley M, Krebs D, Felson D. (2004). Knee adduction moment and development of chronic knee pain in elders. Arthritis Care Res 51:371–376.

15. Miyazaki T, Wada M, Kawahara H, Sato M, Baba H, Shimada S. (2002). Dynamic load at baseline can predict radiographic disease progression in medial compartment knee osteoarthritis. Ann Rheum Dis 61:617–622.

16. Goh J, Bose K, Khoo B. (1993). Gait analysis study on patients with varus osteoarthritis of the knee. Clin Orthop Relat Res 294:223–231.

17. Maly M, Culham E, Costigan P. (2002). Static and dynamic biomechanics of foot orthoses in people with medial compartment knee osteoarthritis. Clin Biomech 17:603–610.

18. Chan G, Smith A, Kirtley C, Tsang W. (2005). Changes in knee moments with contralateral versus ipsilateral cane usage in females with knee osteoarthritis. Clin Biomech 20:396–404.

19. Thorstensson C, Henriksson M, von Porat A, Sjodahl C, Roos E. (2007). The effect of eight weeks of exercise on knee adduction moment in early knee osteoarthritis—a pilot study. Osteoarthritis Cartilage 15:1163–1170.

20. Roddy E, Zhang W, Doherty M, Arden N, Barlow J, Birrell F, Carr A, Chakravarty K, Dickson J, Hay E, Hosie G, Hurley M, Jordan K, McCarthy C, McMurdo M, Mockett S, O'Reilly S, Peat G, Pendleton A, Richards S. (2005). Evidence-based recommendations for the role of exercise in the management of osteoarthritis of the hip or knee—the move consensus. Rheumatology 44:67–73.

21. Slemenda C, Brandt KD, Heilman DK, Mazzuca S, Braunstein EM, Katz BP, Wolinsky FD. (1997). Quadriceps weakness and osteoarthritis of the knee. Ann Intern Med 127:97–104.

22. Hassan B, Mockett S, Doherty M. (2001). Static postural sway, proprioception, and maximal voluntary quadriceps contraction in patients with knee osteoarthritis and normal control subjects. Ann Rheum Dis 60:612–618.

23. Hall K, Hayes K, Falconer J. (1993). Differential strength decline in patients with osteoarthritis of the knee: revision of a hypothesis. Arthritis Care Res 6:89–96.

24. Messier SP, Loeser RF, Hoover JL, Semble EL, Wise CM. (1992). Osteoarthritis of the knee: effects on gait, strength, and flexibility. Arch Physical Med Rehabil 73:29–36.

25. Mikesky AE, Meyer A, Thompson KL. (2000). Relationship between quadriceps strength and rate of loading during gait in women. J Orthop Res 18:171–175.

26. Slemenda C, Heilman D, Brandt K, Katz B, Mazzuca SA, Braunstein E, Byrd D. (1998). Reduced quadriceps strength relative to body weight: a risk factor for knee osteoarthritis in women? Arthritis Rheum 41:1951–1959.

27. Taylor W, Heller MB, G, Duda G. (2004). Tibio-femoral loading during human gait and stair climbing. J Orthop Res 22:625–632.

28. Shelburne K, Torry M, Pandy M. (2006). Contributions of muscles, ligaments, and the ground-reaction force to tibiofemoral joint loading during normal gait. J Orthop Res 24:1983–1990.

29. Fransen M, Crosbie J, Edmonds J. (2001). Physical therapy is effective for patients with osteoarthritis of the knee: a randomized controlled trial. J Rheumatol 28: 156–164.

30. Marks R. (1993). The effect of isometric quadriceps strength training in mid-range for osteo-arthritis of the knee. N Z J Physiotherapy 21:16–19.

31. Ettinger WH, Burns R, Messier SP, Applegate W, Rejeski J, Morgan T, Shumaker S, Berry MJ, O'Toole M, Monu J, Craven T. (1997). A randomized trial comparing aerobic exercise and resistance exercise with a health education program in older adults with knee osteoarthritis. JAMA 277:25–31.

32. Rogind H, Bibow-Nielsen B, Jensen B, Moller HC, Frimodt-Moller H, Bliddal H. (1998). The effects of a physical training program on patients with osteoarthritis of the knees. Arch Physical Med Rehabil 79:1421–1427.

33. Huang M-H, Lin Y-S, Yang R-C, Lee C-L. (2003). A comparison of various therapeutic exercises on the functional status of patients with knee osteoarthritis. Semin Arthritis Rheum 32:398–406.

34. Schilke JM, Johnson GO, Housh TJ, Odell JR. (1996). Effects of muscle strength training on the functional status of patients with osteoarthritis of the knee joint. Nursing Res 45:68–72.

35. Pelland L, Brosseau L, Wells G, MacLeay L, Lambert J, Lamothe C, Robinson V, Tugwell P. (2004). Efficacy of strengthening exercises for osteoarthritis (Part I): a meta-analysis. Physical Ther Rev 9:77–108.

36. Perry J. (1992). *Gait Analysis: Normal and Pathologic Function*. Thorofare, NJ: Slack, Inc.

37. Yamada H, Koshino T, Sakai N. (2001). Hip adductor muscle strength in patients with varus deformed knee. Clin Orthop Relat Res 386:179–185.

38. Messier SP, Thompson CD, Ettinger WH. (1997). Effects of long-term aerobic or weight training regimens on gait in an older, osteoarthritic population. J Appl Biomech 13:205–225.

39. Evcik D, Sonel B. (2002). Effectiveness of a home-based exercise therapy and walking program on osteoarthritis of the knee. Rheumatol Int 22:103–106.

40. Rejeski WJ, Lawrence RB, Ettinger W, Morgan T, Thompson C. (1997). Compliance to exercise therapy in older participants with knee osteoarthritis: implication for treating disability. Med Sci Sports Exerc 29:977–985.

41. Minor MA, Hewett JE, Webel RR, Anderson SK, Kay DR. (1989). Efficacy of physical conditioning exercise in patients with rheumatoid arthritis and osteoarthritis. Arthritis Rheum 32:1396–1405.

42. Kovar PA, Allegrante JP, MacKenzie CR, Peterson MG, Gutin B, Charlson ME. (1992). Supervised fitness walking in patients with osteoarthritis of the knee. A randomized, controlled trial. Ann Intern Med 116:529–534.

43. Peterson MGE, Kovar-Toledano PA, Otis JG, Allegrante JP, MacKenzie CR, Gutin B, Kroll MA. (1993). Effect of a walking program on gait characteristics in patients with osteoarthritis. Arthritis Care Res 6:11–16.

44. Sharma L, Cahue S, Song J, Hayes K, Pai Y, Dunlop D. (2003). Physical functioning over three years in knee osteoarthritis. Role of psychosocial, local mechanical, and neuromusculsr factors. Arthritis Rheum 48:3359–3370.

45. Anderson J, Felson DT. (1988). Factors associated with osteoarthritis of the knee in the first national health and nutrition examination survey (nhanes I): evidence for an association with overweight, race and physical demands of work. Am J Epidemiol 128:179–189.

46. Spector T, Hart D, Doyle D. (1994). Incidence and progression of osteoarthritis in women with unilateral knee disease in the general poulation: the effect of obesity. Ann Rheum Dis 53:565–568.

47. Cicuttini F, Baker J, Spector T. (1996). The association of obesity with osteoarthritis of the hand and knee in women—a twin study. J Rheumatol 23:1221–1226.

48. Callaghan MJ, Oldham J, Hunt J. (1995). An evaluation of exercise regimes for patients with osteoarthritis of the knee: a single-blind randomized controlled trial. Clin Rehabil 9:213–218.

49. van Baar ME, Assendelft WJ, Dekker J, Oostendorp RA, Bijlsma JW. (1999). Effectiveness of exercise therapy in patients with osteoarthritis of the hip or knee: a systematic review of randomised controlled trials. Arthritis Rheum 42:1361–1369.

50. Suomi R, Collier D. (2003). Effects of arthritis exercise programs on functional fitness and perceived activities of daily living measures in older adults with arthritis. Arch Physical Med Rehabil 84:1589–1594.

51. Bennell K, Hinman R, Metcalf B, Buchbinder R, McConnell J, McColl G, Green S, Crossley K. (2005). Efficacy of physiotherapy management of knee joint osteoarthritis: a randomised double-blind placebo-controlled trial. Ann Rheum Dis 64:906–912.

52. Fitzgerald G, Oatis C. (2004). Role of physical therapy in management of knee osteoarthritis. Curr Opin Rheumatol 16:143–147.

53. Hurley M. (2003). Muscle dysfunction and effective rehabilitation of knee osteoarthritis: What we know and what we need to find out. Arthritis Care Res 49:444–452.

54. Hortobagyi T, Garry J, Holbert D, Devita P. (2004). Aberrations in the control of quadriceps muscle force in patients with knee osteoarthritis. Arthritis Care Res 51:562–569.

55. Childs J, Sparto P, Fitzgerald G, Bizzini M, Irrgang J. (2004). Alterations in lower extremity movement and muscle activation patterns in individuals with knee osteoarthritis. Clin Biomech 19:44–49.

56. Lewek M, Rudolph K, Snyder-Mackler L. (2004). Control of frontal plane laxity during gait in patients with medial compartment knee osteoarthritis. Osteoarthritis Cartilage 12:745–751.

57. Messier S, Loeser R, Miller G, Morgan T, Rejeski W, Sevick M, Ettinger W, Pahor M, Williamson J. (2004). Exercise and dietary weight loss in overweight and obese older adults with knee osteoarthritis. Arthritis Rheum 50:1501–1510.

58. Foley A, Halbert J, Hewitt T, Crotty M. (2003). Does hydrotherapy improve strength and physical function in patients with osteoarthritis: a randomised controlled trial comparing a gym based and a hydrotherapy based strengthening program. Ann Rhueum Dis 62:1162–1167.

59. Hinman R, Heywood S, Day A. (2007). Aquatic physical therapy for hip and knee osteoarthritis: results of a single-blind randomized controlled trial. Physical Ther 87:32–43.

60. Baker K, Nelson M, Felson D, Layne J, Sarno R, Roubenoff R. (2001). The efficacy of home based progressive strength training in older adults with knee osteoarthritis: a randomized controlled trial. J Rheumatol 28:1655–1665.

61. McCarthy C, Mills P, Pullen R, Roberts C, Silman A, Oldham J. (2004). Supplementing a home exercise programme with a class-based exercise programme is more effective than home exercise alone in the treatment of knee osteoarthritis. Rheumatology 43:880–886.

62. O'Reilly SC, Muir KR, Doherty M. (1999). Effectiveness of home exercise on pain and disability from osteoarthritis of the knee: a randomised controlled trial. Ann Rheum Dis 58:15–19.

63. Thomas K, Muir K, Doherty M, Jones A, O'Reilly S, Bassey E. (2002). Home based exercise programme for knee pain and knee osteoarthritis: randomised controlled trial. BMJ 325:752–756.

64. Belza B, Topolski T, Kinne S, Patrick D, Ramsey S. (2002). Does adherence make a difference? Results from a community-based aquatic exercise program. Nursing Res 51:285–291.

65. van Gool C, Penninx B, Kempen G, Refeski W, Miller G, van Eijk J, Pahor M, Messier S. (2005). Effects of exercise adherance on physical function among overweight older adults with knee osteoarthritis. Arthritis Rheum Arthritis Care Res 53:24–32.

66. Fielding R, Katula J, Miller M, Abbott-Pillola K, Jordan A, Glynn N, Goodpaster B, Walkup M, King A, Rejeski W. (2007). Activity adherence and physical function in older adults with functional limitations. Med Sci Sports Exerc 39:1997–2004.

67. Perri M, Anton S, Durning P, Ketterson T, Sydeman S, Berlant N, Kanasky W, Newton R, Limacher M, Martin A. (2002). Adherence to exercise prescriptions: effects of prescribing moderate versus higher levels of intensity and frequency. Health Psychol 21:452–458.

68. McCarthy C, Mills P, Pullen R, Richardson G, Hawkins N, Roberts C, Silman A, Oldham J. (2004). Supplementation of a home-based exercise programme with a class-based programme for people with osteoarthritis of the knees: a randomised controlled trial and health economic analysis. Health Technol Assessment 8:1–61.

69. Campbell R, Evans M, Tucker M, Quilty B, Dieppe P, Donovan J. (2001). Why don't patients do their exercises? Understanding non-compliance with physiotherapy in patients with osteoarthritis of the knee. J Epidemiol Community Health 55:132–138.

70. Marks R, Allegrante J. (2005). Chronic osteoarthritis and adherence to exercise: a review of the literature. J Aging Physical Activity 13:434–460.

71. Maly M, Costigan P, Olney S. (2006). Determinants of self-report outcome measures in people with knee osteoarthritis. Arch Physical Med Rehabil 87: 96–104.

72. Castro C, King A, Brassington G. (2001). Telephone versus mail interventions for maintenance of physical activity in older adults. Health Psychol 20:438–444.

73. Roddy E, Doherty M. (2006). Changing life-styles and osteoarthritis: What is the evidence? Best Pract Res Clin Rheumatol 20:81–97.

74. King A, Taylor C, Haskell W, Debusk R. (1988). Strategies for increasing early adherence to and long-term maintenance of home-based exercise training in healthy middle-aged men and women. Am J Cardiol 61:628–632.

75. Noland M. (1989). The effects of self-monitoring and reinforcement on exercise adherence. Res Q Exerc Sport 60:612–224.

76. Duncan K, Pozehl B. (2003). Effects of an exercise adherence intervention on outcomes in patients with heart failure. Rehabil Nursing 28:117–122.

77. Litt M, Kleppinger A, Judge J. (2002). Initiation and maintenance of exercise behaviour in older women: predictors from the social learning model. J Behav Med 25:83–97.

78. Oka R, King A, Rohm Young D. (1995). Sources of social support as predictors of exercise adherence in women and men ages 50 to 65 years. Women's Health 1:161–175.

79. OA ASo. (2000). Recommendations for the medical management of osteoarthritis of the hip and knee. 2000 update. Arthritis Rheum 43:1905–1915.

80. Pendleton A, Arden N, Dougados M, Doherty M, Bannwarth B, Bijlsma JWJ, Cluzeau F, Cooper C, Dieppe PA, Gunther K-P, Hauselmann HJ, Herrero-Beaumont G, Kaklamanis PM, Leeb B, Lequesne M, Lohmander S, Mazieres B, Mola E-M, Pavelka K, Serni U, Swoboda B, Verbruggen AA, Weseloh G, Zimmermann-Gorska I. (2000). Eular recommendations for the management of knee osteoarthritis: report of a task force of the standing committee for international clinical studies including therapeutic trials (ESCISIT). Ann Rheum Dis 59:936–944.

81. Szebenyi B, Hollander A, Dieppe P, Quilty B, Duddy J, Clarke S, Kirwan J. (2006). Associations between pain, function, and radiographic features in osteoarthritis of the knee. Arthritis Rheum 54:230–235.

82. Duncan R, Hay E, Saklatvala J, Croft P. (2006). Prevalence of radiographic osteoarthritis: it all depends on your point of view. Rheumatology 45:757–760.

83. Kornaat P, Bloem J, Ceulemans R, Riyazi N, Rosendaal F, Nelissen R, Carter W, Le Graverand M, Kloppenburg M. (2006). Osteoarthritis of the knee: association between clinical features and MR imaging findings. Radiology 239: 811–817.

84. Cicuttini F, Baker J, Hart D, Spector T. (1996). Choosing the best method for radiological assessment of patellofemoral osteoarthritis. Ann Rheum Dis 55:134–136.

85. Hunter D, March L, Sambrook P. (2003). The association of cartilage volume with knee pain. Osteoarthritis Cartilage 11:725–729.

86. Englund M, Lohmander L. (2005). Patellofemoral osteoarthritis coexistant with tibiofemoral osteoarthritis in a meniscectomy population. Ann Rheum Dis 64:1721–1726.

87. Boegard T, Rudling O, Petersson IF, Jonsson K. (1998). Correlation between radiographically diagnosed osteophytes and magnetic resonance detected cartilage defects in the patellofemoral joint. Ann Rheum Dis 57:395–400.

88. Lanyon P, O'Reilly S, Jones A, Doherty M. (1998). Radiographic assessment of symptomatic knee osteoarthritis in the community: definitions and normal joint space. Ann Rheum Dis 57:595–601.

89. Powers C. (2000). Patellar kinematics. Part II: The influence of the depth of the trochlear groove in subjects with and without patellofemoral pain. Physical Ther 80:965–978.

90. Ward S, Terk M, Powers C. (2007). Patella alta: association with patellofemoral alignment and changes in contact area during weight-bearing. J Bone Joint Surg 89A:1749–1755.

91. Farahmand F, Tahmasbi M, Amis A. (1998). Lateral force-displacement behaviour of the human patella and its variation with knee flexion—a biomechanical study in vitro. J Biomech 31:1147–1152.

92. Grabiner M, Koh T, Draganich L. (1994). Neuromechanics of the patellofemoral joint. Med Sci Sports Exerc 26:10–21.

93. Kalichman L, Zhang Y, Niu J, Goggins J, Gale D, Zhu Y, Felson D, Hunter D. (2007). The association between patellar alignment on magnetic resonance imaging and radiographic manifestations of knee osteoarthritis. Arthritis Res Ther 9:R26.

94. Kalichman L, Zhang Y, Niu J, Goggins J, Gale D, Felson D, Hunter D. (2007). The association between patellar alignment and patellofemoral joint osteoarthritis features—an MRI study. Rheumatology 46:1303–1308.

95. Hunter D, Zhang Y, Niu J, Felson D, Kwoh K, Newman A, Kritchevsky S, Harris T, Carbone L, Nevitt M. (2007). Patella malalignment, pain and patellofemoral progression: the health ABC study. Osteoarthritis Cartilage 15:1120–1127.

96. Harrison MM, Cooke TDV, Fisher SB, Griffin MP. (1994). Patterns of knee arthrosis and patellar subluxation. Clin Orthop Relat Res 309:56–63.

97. Hinterwimmer S, Gotthard M, von Eisenhart-Rothe R, Sauerland S, Siebert A, Vogl T, Eckstein F, Graichen H. (2005). In vivo contact areas of the knee in patients with patellar subluxation. J Biomech 38:2095–2101.

98. Cushnaghan J, McCarthy C, Dieppe P. (1994). Taping the patella medially: a new treatment for osteoarthritis of the knee joint? Br Med J 308:753–755.

99. McConnell JS. (1986). The management of chondromalacia patellae: a long term solution. Aust J Physiotherapy 32:215–223.

100. Hinman R, Bennell K, Crossley K, McConnell J. (2003). Immediate effects of adhesive tape on pain and disability in individuals with knee osteoarthritis. Rheumatology 42:865–869.

101. Hinman R, Crossley K, McConnell J, Bennell K. (2003). Efficacy of knee tape in the management of knee osteoarthritis: a blinded randomised controlled trial. Br Med J 327:135–138.

102. Callaghan M, Selfe J, Bagley P, Oldham J. (2002). The effects of patellar taping on knee joint proprioception. J Athletic Training 37:19–24.

103. Hinman R, Crossley K, McConnell J, Bennell KL. (2004). Does the application of tape influence quadriceps sensorimotor function in knee osteoarthritis? Rheumatology 43:331–336.

104. Somes S, Worrell TW, Corey B, Ingersol CD. (1997). Effects of patellar taping on patellar position in the open and closed kinetic chain: a preliminary study. J Sport Rehabil 6:299–308.

105. Worrell T, Ingersoll CD, Bockrath-Pugliese K, Minis P. (1998). Effect of patellar taping and bracing on patellar position as determined by MRI in patients with patellofemoral pain. J Athletic Training 33:16–20.

106. Larsen B, Andreasen E, Urfer A, Mickelson MR, Newhouse KE. (1995). Patellar taping: a radiographic examination of the medial glide technique. Am J Sports Med 23:465–471.

107. Pfeiffer R, DeBeliso M, Shea K, Kelley L, Irmischer B, Harris C. (2004). Kinematic MRI assessment of McConnell taping before and after exercise. Am J Sports Med 32:621–628.

108. Cowan SM, Bennell KL, Hodges PW. (2002). Therapeutic patellar taping changes the timing of vasti muscle activation in people with patellofemoral pain syndrome. Clin J Sports Med 12:339–347.

109. Jacobson J, Lenchik L, Ruhoy M, Schweitzer M, Resnick D. (1997). MR imaging of the infrapatellar fat pad of Hoffa. Radiographics 17:675–691.

110. Duri Z, Aichroth P, Dowd G. (1996). The fat pad. Clinical observations. Am J Knee Surg 9:55–66.

111. Larsson LG, Baum J. (1985). The syndrome of anserina bursitis: an overlooked diagnosis. Arthritis Rheum 28:1062–1065.

112. Hassan B, Mockett S, Doherty M. (2002). Influence of elastic bandage on knee pain, proprioception, and postural sway in subjects with knee osteoarthritis. Ann Rheum Dis 61:24–28.

113. Kirkley A, Webster-Bogaert S, Litchfield R, Amendola A, MacDonald S, McCalden R, Fowler P. (1999). The effect of bracing on varus gonarthrosis. J Bone Joint Surg Am 4:539–548.

114. Pajareya K, Chadchavalpanichaya N, Timdang S. (2003). Effectiveness of an elastic knee sleeve for patients with knee osteoarthritis: a randomized single-blinded controlled trial. J Med Assoc Thailand 86:535–542.

115. Lindenfeld T, Hewett T, Andriacchi T. (1997). Joint loading with valgus bracing in patients with varus gonarthrosis. Clin Orthop 344:290–297.

116. Pollo F, Otis J, Backus S, Warren R, Wickiewicz T. (2002). Reduction of medial compartment loads with valgus bracing of the osteoarthritic knee. Am J Sports Med 30:414–421.

117. Birmingham T, Kramer J, Kirkley A, Inglis J, Spaulding S, Vandervoort A. (2001). Knee bracing for medial compartment osteoarthritis: effects on proprioception and postural control. Rheumatology 40:285–289.

118. Lewek M, Ramsey D, Snyder-Mackler L, Rudolph K. (2005). Knee stabilization in patients with medial compartment knee osteoarthritis. Arthritis Rheum 52:2845–2853.

119. Ramsey D, Briem K, Axe M, Snyder-Mackler L. (2007). A mechanical theory for the effectivness of bracing for medial compartment osteoarthritis of the knee. J Bone Joint Surg 89A:2398–2407.

120. Dennis D, Komistek R, Nadaud M, Mahfouz M. (2006). Evaluation of off-loading braces for treatment of unicompartmental knee arthrosis. J Arthroplasty 21:2–8.

121. Gaasbeek R, Groen B, Hampsink B, van Heerwaarden R, Duysens J. (2007). Valgus bracing in patients with medial compartment osteoarthritis of the knee. A gait analysis study of a new brace. Gait Posture 26:3–10.

122. Draganich L, Reider B, Rimington T, Piotrowski G, Mallik K, Nasson S. (2006). The effectiveness of self-adjustable custom and off-the-shelf bracing in the treatment of varus gonarthrosis. J Bone Joint Surg 88A:2645–2652.

123. Horlick S, Loomar R. (1993). Valgus knee bracing for medial gonarthrosis. Clin J Sports Med 3:251–255.

124. Brouwer R, van Raaij T, Verhaar J, Coene L, Bierma-Zeinstra S. (2006). Brace treatment for osteoarthritis of the knee: a prospective randomized multi-centre trial. Osteoarthritis Cartilage 14:777–783.

125. Giori N. (2004). Load-shifting brace treatment for osteoarthritis of the knee: a minimum 2 1/2-year follow-up study. J Rehabil Res Dev 41:187–194.

17

TREATING INFLAMMATION TO RELIEVE OSTEOARTHRITIC PAIN

David T. Felson

*Boston University School of Medicine, 650 Albany Street,
Boston, Massachusetts 02118, USA*

OSTEOARTHRITIS AS AN INFLAMMATORY DISORDER

Chronic inflammation represents the extension of acute inflammation with the transformation characterized by the presence of mononuclear inflammatory cells such as monocytes and lymphocytes instead of neutrophils. Many of the acute vascular changes, a characteristic of acute inflammatory responses, diminish with chronic inflammation. An element of both acute and chronic inflammation is the secretion and action of proinflammatory cytokines, which include interleukin-1, tumor necrosis factor-α (TNF-α), and others.

All elements of chronic inflammation can be present in osteoarthritic joints. Some knees and hips with osteoarthritis show evidence of round cell inflammation within the synovium, and a proliferation of macrophages in the synovial lining. The proinflammatory cytokines, which help define the inflammatory state, can be detected in synovial fluid in the synovium and in the cartilage matrix.[1]

Pain in Osteoarthritis, Edited by David T. Felson and Hans-Georg Schaible
Copyright © 2009 Wiley-Blackwell.

The source of inflammation in osteoarthritis and the effect of proinflammatory cytokines on the disease have not been completely worked out. Historically, it is believed that cartilage destruction results in the release of cartilage breakdown products into the synovial fluid, which undergo phagocytosis by synovial cells, which, in turn, produce inflammatory mediators, triggering the ingress of more such cells and the production of cytokines. However, there is strong evidence that chondrocytes themselves produce those cytokines, leading to cartilage degeneration.

While the presence of proinflammatory cytokines in cartilage may affect loss of matrix there, it is likely not relevant to osteoarthritic pain, as cartilage does not contain pain fibers. What may be highly relevant, however, is the development of synovial inflammation as part of the osteoarthritic process and the production by synovium of excess synovial fluid, leading to capsular swelling. Both of these, synovitis and capsular distension, can produce pain.

Synovitis is a feature of some, but not all, joints with osteoarthritis.[2] In a series of careful studies evaluating pre-end stage knees and hips, Aigner and colleagues[2] have noted that, in clinical osteoarthritis, there is usually some sort of synovial pathology, although in only a minority of joints does this take on the characteristic features of inflammatory arthritis. They report four types of pathologies: hyperplastic, inflammatory, fibrotic, and detritus-rich synovial pathology. The last form is characteristic of end-stage osteoarthritis, and bone and cartilage fragments can be seen inside the synovial membrane; foreign body giant cells and some mononuclear cells can also be found in the sub lining areas of the synovium. In the hyperplastic and fibrotic forms of synovial pathology, there is villous hyperplasia at the synovial lining with varying degrees of cellular proliferation there, but little cellular infiltration in the sublining. In the inflammatory subtype, unlike the other subtypes, there is inflammation in both the synovial lining and sublining. Although representing only a minority of patients with osteoarthritis, the inflammatory subtype looks histologically like the synovium of mild rheumatoid arthritis. The form of synovitis associated with the mildest clinical osteoarthritis is the hyperplastic subtype, in which the normally flat synovial lining cells change their shape and increase their cytoplasmic volume, suggesting they have been activated. Whereas normal synovial lining is one layer thick, hyperplastic subtypes can show up to five cell layers at the surface, and there develop synovial villi, not necessarily with sublining inflammatory cells.

Perhaps similar to Aigner's characterization of inflammatory synovitis, Haywood and colleagues[3] have described severe inflammation within the synovium in 31%, mostly in patients undergoing knee or hip replacement. What is noteworthy is that vascular endothelium and endothelial cell proliferation, along with high concentrations of vascular endothelial growth factor (VEGF), are seen characteristically in the synovium, suggesting that the vascularity of the synovium increases and promotes synovial proliferation.[3]

What other evidence is there that inflammation either systemically or locally plays a role in osteoarthritis? Increases in C-reactive protein (CRP) or other systemic measures of inflammation among those with osteoarthritis might provide evidence that osteoarthritis has systemic inflammatory relationships. The presumed mechanism by which CRP would be elevated would be that mononuclear inflammatory cells trafficking through the synovium and back into the circulation would have secondary consequences on the systemic levels of inflammation.

A variety of studies have examined whether CRP or other systemic markers of inflammation, such as serum hyaluronic acid (HA), are elevated in patients with osteoarthritis. Findings have not been consistent. For example, in the Johnson County osteoarthritis project, a population-based study, persons with osteoarthritis were not found to have serum CRP elevation[4] but were found to have higher levels of serum HA than those without disease. Serum HA was thought to reflect the presence of inflamed synovium in joints with osteoarthritis, but it could reflect the coexistence of other systemic illnesses in persons with osteoarthritis. However, in one study of persons with hip osteoarthritis, CRP was found to be elevated compared with healthy controls.[5] In other studies of both hip and knee osteoarthritis, where CRP has been found elevated, an additional adjustment for body mass index (BMI) has eliminated the increase in CRP, suggesting that obesity accounts for this high CRP level in persons with weight-bearing osteoarthritis and not necessarily the osteoarthritis itself.[6,7]

In two studies, the height of CRP elevation has been linked to the likelihood of structural disease progression,[8] and in one study[9] patients with osteoarthritis who had more severe pain were likely to have higher CRP levels than those with less severe pain.

The presence of inflammation within osteoarthritic joints has several treatment implications. First, since synovium is inflamed, and that may be a source of pain along with the production of fluid, which can distend the capsule, anti-inflammatory therapy might alleviate pain. Second, as reviewed in other chapters in this book, inflammation lowers the threshold for nociceptive afferents, transforming mildly painful or nonpainful stimuli into painful ones and also produces receptor field enlargement, so that larger regions of the leg around the knee become painful.[10]

TREATMENT OF INFLAMMATION IN THE OSTEOARTHRITIC JOINT

Increasingly, there is a diversity of options available to treat inflammation in osteoarthritis. Drugs can be administered orally, topically, or by intra-articular injection. Therapies tested include conventional nonsteroidal anti-inflammatory drugs (NSAIDs), cyclooxygenase-2 (COX-2) inhibitors, interleukin-1 (IL-1) inhibitors, and corticosteroids. We review the evidence for efficacy and the expected side effects of each of these choices.

NONSTEROIDAL ANTI-INFLAMMATORY DRUGS AND COX-2 INHIBITORS

For many years, based on small, older trials, it was felt that anti-inflammatory drugs and analgesics such as paracetamol were equipotent for osteoarthritis treatment. A series of large, multicenter trials has disproved this notion, showing unequivocally that both anti-inflammatory drugs and COX-2 inhibitors are more efficacious for the treatment of pain and functional limitation than is paracetamol. In a meta-analysis of five osteoarthritis trials, Wegman and colleagues[11] showed a standardized mean difference favoring NSAIDs over paracetamol for general pain, of 0.33 (95% CI 0.15–0.51), indicating a small effect. In fact, large individual trials all showed a similar effect. For example, a randomized trial of rofecoxib, celecoxib, and acetaminophen showed that all COX-2 inhibitor groups worked better for the treatment of pain than did acetaminophen, although rofecoxib tended to show more efficacy than celecoxib. Indeed, patients often seemed to notice a difference, even though that difference was only modest. Pincus and colleagues[12] reported not only that celecoxib was more effective than acetaminophen, but that 53% of patients preferred celecoxib versus only 24% acetaminophen, with the remainder not expressing a preference. Even low dose ibuprofen (400 mg/day) was found to be significantly more efficacious than high dose acetaminophen in one large-scale trial.[13] In a large crossover trial (ACTA), Pincus and colleagues showed that NSAIDs worked better than acetaminophen in both crossover periods, but that once patients had received NSAIDs, their chances of responding to acetaminophen, when switched to it later, were extremely low. That informed current guidelines for osteoarthritis treatment, which advise that acetaminophen should be used only early in treatment of osteoarthritis and that once patients have been tried on NSAIDs they are very unlikely to experience benefits should they be switched back to acetaminophen.

While anti-inflammatory therapies are clearly more efficacious than acetaminophen for osteoarthritis, their relative efficacy is not dramatically greater, and this creates difficult treatment decisions because of the relatively high toxicity rates of many NSAIDs and COX-2 inhibitors. In fact, because of the increased rates of cardiovascular events associated with COX-2 inhibitors and with some conventional NSAIDs,[14] many of these drugs are not appropriate long-term treatment choices for older persons with osteoarthritis, especially those at high risk of heart disease or stroke. The American Heart Association has identified rofecoxib and all other COX-2 inhibitors as putting patients at high risk, although low doses of celecoxib, such as 200 mg/day, may not be associated with an elevation of risk. One widely used NSAID, diclofenac, has predominant COX-2 inhibiting actions, and in randomized trials has been found to have elevated risks of cardiovascular disease, making it similar in risk to drugs classified as COX-2 inhibitors. Thus diclofenac also should be avoided for most long-term use in osteoarthritis. The only drug scoring as safe from a cardiovascular risk perspective in these various studies is naproxen, with a risk

TABLE 17.1. Strategies to Decrease NSAID Gastrointestinal Risk

1. Use NSAIDs at low dose and intermittently.
2. Avoid use if untreated *H. pylori* present.
3. Avoid combined use with corticosteroids or aspirin.
4. Use with proton pump inhibitors.
5. Choose benign NSAID/COX-2.
6. Avoid use in persons with prior GI bleeding ulcers or upper GI surgery.

not elevated compared to nonusers or to acetaminophen users. For some NSAIDs there is insufficient data to characterize their cardiovascular risk. This includes such drugs as ibuprofen, whose use may or may not be associated with an increase in risk.

NSAIDs also cause an increased risk of gastrointestinal toxicity and the switch from COX-2 inhibitors back to conventional NSAIDs may be accompanied by a temporal increase in catastrophic gastrointestinal events attributable to NSAID use without use of gastroprotective drugs. Strategies to avoid the high risk of NSAID-related gastrointestinal (GI) side effects are shown in Table 17.1 and include the use of low doses on an as-needed basis. Other tactics include the selection of NSAIDs with a lower risk of gastrointestinal side effects, the concurrent use of gastroprotective drugs, and the selection of patients who are at low risk, including those who have no coexistent *Helicobacter pylori* infection, and other high risk patients. A composite of meta-analyses of large observational studies, which have evaluated the comparative gastrointestinal side effects of NSAIDs, is shown in Table 17.2, where drugs are ranked according to their gastrointestinal risk.

For many patients with osteoarthritis, adopting a strategy of choosing a relatively safe NSAID and keeping it at a reasonably low, well-tolerated dose

TABLE 17.2. Gastrointestinal Risk of NSAIDs/
COX-2 from Safest to Riskiest[a]

Safer
Nonacetylated salicylates
(e.g., Salsalate)
Nabumetone
Celecoxib
Ibuprofen
Diclofenac
Sulindac
Naproxen
Indomethacin
Ketoprofen
Riskier

[a]Summarizes evidence from a series of studies.[15–17]

can help avoid side effects. For those at higher gastrointestinal risk, adding a proton pump inhibitor is an effective way of minimizing that risk.

TOPICAL NONSTEROIDAL ANTI-INFLAMMATORY DRUGS

With the 2007 approval by the U.S. Food and Drug Administration of topical diclofenac and the availability of these agents in Europe, clinicians have a choice of administration modality for anti-inflammatory drugs. NSAIDs are placed into a gel or topical solution with another chemical modality that enhances penetration of the skin barrier. When absorbed through the skin, plasma concentrations are an order of magnitude lower than with the same amount of drug administered orally or parenterally. However, when these drugs are administered topically in proximity to a joint (e.g., on top of the knee), the drug can be found in joint tissues such as the synovium and cartilage.[18]

Clinical trials of topical NSAIDs versus placebo have not all been positive, and there is a worrying tendency for all published trials to be industry funded and analyzed with evidence of publication bias—the failure to publish small trials that showed no effect.[19] This publication bias suggests that readers may not have access to all evidence collected on topical NSAIDs and should be skeptical of published trial information. Among published literature, the preponderance of evidence suggests efficacy of these agents versus placebo.[19,20] They have been tested in superficial joints, in which skin application is close to the joint's surface, such as hands and knees. Compared to placebo in three trials, diclofenac topical led to a 1.6 unit improvement in WOMAC pain score (which has a range of 0–20).[20] Results of trials comparing the efficacy of topical with oral NSAIDs have varied but have generally found that topical NSAIDs are slightly less efficacious than oral agents.[21,22] In a large trial based in general practices in England, for patients given topical versus oral ibuprofen, pain improvement in the ibuprofen group was superior, especially at 12 and 24 months after starting treatment, and discontinuation for inadequate pain relief occurred in 23% of patients on topical drug versus only 13% in those on oral drug.

The major advantage of topical therapy is that, when administered by this modality, NSAIDs have fewer systemic side effects, including fewer

TABLE 17.3. Comparison of Oral and Topical NSAIDs for Osteoarthritis

Parameter	Oral	Topical
Efficacy	More potent	Less potent
Tolerability	Moderate–poor	Moderate–good
Common side effects	Upper GI symptoms and bleed, ulcer; worsening renal function	Skin irritation

gastrointestinal side effects and fewer renal and blood pressure effects.[19,20,22] Unfortunately, topical NSAIDs often cause local skin irritation where the medication is applied, inducing redness, burning, or itching in up to 40% of patients (see Table 17.3).

CORTICOSTEROIDS

Corticosteroids, used systemically in animal models of osteoarthritis, have shown inconsistent effects on cytokines and inflammatory cells within the synovium and cytokine effects within cartilage.[23] While the levels of corticosteroid attained within the joint after oral administration are sufficient to knock down cytokine levels, they do not appear to affect synovial histology in contrast to intra-articular injections of steroids, which have been found to do so. There have been no comprehensive studies in humans evaluating oral or parenteral corticosteroids in the treatment of osteoarthritis.

When instilled into the joint, corticosteroids impede the ability of inflammatory cells to leave the vascular bed and migrate into the synovium. Macrophages, prominent inflammatory cells within the synovium, are inhibited in their activity by corticosteroids. Cytokine synthesis is blocked by these drugs, especially cytokines that have potent proinflammatory effects, such as TNF-α and IL-1β. The net effect of corticosteroids is to downregulate the inflammatory process.

Since corticosteroids mitigate inflammation, of which there is often a nidus in the synovium, it makes sense that intra-articular corticosteroids might be effective for the treatment of pain in osteoarthritis. Indeed, intra-articular corticosteroids have long been a mainstay of treatment for knee osteoarthritis. In a recent meta-analysis of randomized trials comparing corticosteroid to placebo saline injections for the treatment of osteoarthritis of the knee, Arrol and Goodyear-Smith[24] reported a superiority of corticosteroid injections, with improvement lasting up to 2 weeks after injection. The treatment effect was large, and the number needed to treat for one person's improvement ranged from 1.3–3.5 patients. While effective for 2 weeks, there is inconsistent evidence that the effect of steroids lasts longer. Arrol and Goodyear-Smith[24] that of the two high quality studies examining longer term effects, there was a significant residual treatment effect of steroids even at 16–24 weeks after injection. Even so, some trial investigators have noted the favorable effect of steroid treatment diminishes after 2 weeks.[24] The studies with the shortest duration of effect tend to be those where the dose of steroid used was low, 25 mg prednisone equivalent or less, and doses higher than this may cause a more durable response. In one trial of repeated intra-articular steroid injections given every 3 months over 2 years, there was a significant favorable effect of these injections on pain and stiffness compared to a placebo.[25] Few easily identifiable predictors of steroid response have been identified.[26]

While the efficacy of intra-articular steroid injection into the knee may be short term, corticosteroid injections into an osteoarthritic hip may have more durable efficacy. Lambert and colleagues, using a 20% improvement in WOMAC as the threshold for response, noted that more than 50% of patients with hip osteoarthritis had a response up to 3 months after the steroid injection, versus a far lower response rate in patients injected with placebo. Hip injections need to be done under imaging guidance to ensure the medicine is instilled into the joint cavity.

While uncontrolled studies suggest that osteoarthritis in the thumb base may respond to steroids, especially if the disease there is mild, one well-done randomized control trial has found no efficacy of intra-articular injections there compared to placebo.[27]

The mechanism by which intra-articular steroids relieve pain is not fully worked out, but longitudinal studies of patients who have undergone steroid injections suggest[28,29] that after a steroid injection there is shrinkage of synovium with an increase in the number of fibroblast-like lining cells and a decrease in the number of inflammatory cells, especially macrophages. It is not clear whether this alteration in synovium correlates with clinical response.

OTHER INTRA-ARTICULAR TREATMENT

An alternative anti-inflammatory might be one targeting a specific cytokine active in osteoarthritis. The major prodegradative cytokine, at least in osteoarthritic cartilage, is interleukin-1, and an approved drug for rheumatoid arthritis, anakinra, which consists of a receptor blocker for IL-1β, has been tried in a large multicenter trial in patients with osteoarthritis, given as an intra-articular injection. It was unfortunately not found to be effective in treating pain or disability related to osteoarthritis. A similar biological approach targeting a specific cytokine or cell migrating into the synovium may offer treatment potential.

REFERENCES

1. Pelletier JP and Abramson SB. (2001). Osteoarthritis, an inflammatory disease: potential implication for the selection of new therapeutic targets. Arthritis Rheum 44(6):1237–1247.
2. Aigner T, Van Der Kraan P, Van Der Berg W. (2007). Osteoarthritis and inflammation—inflammatory changes in osteoarthritic synoviopathy. In Buckwater FSJ (ed.). *Osteoarthritis, Inflammation and Degradation A Continuum*. Amsterdam: IOS Press, pp. 219–235.

3. Haywood L, Pearson CI, Gill SE, Ganesan A, Wilson D, Walsh DA. (2003). Inflammation and angiogenesis in osteoarthritis. Arthritis Rheum 48(8):2173–2177.

4. Elliott A, Kraus VB, Luta G, Stabler T, Renner JB, Woodard J, Dragomir AD, Helmick CG, Hochberg MC, Jordan JM. (2005). Serum hyaluronan levels and radiographic knee and hip osteoarthritis in African Americans and Caucasians in the Johnston County Osteoarthritis Project. Arthritis Rheum 52(1):105–111.

5. Conrozier TH, Mathieu P, Colson F, Debard AL, Richard S, Favret H, Bienvenu J, Vignon E. (2000). Serum levels of YKL-40 and C reactive protein in patients with hip osteoarthritis and healthy subjects: a cross sectional study. Ann Rheum Dis 59: 828–831.

6. Nevitt M, Felson D, Peterfy C, Wildy K, Ling S, Lane N, Newman A, Carbone L, Harris T. (2002). Inflammation markers (CRP, TNF-alpha, IL-6) are not associated with radiographic or MRI findings of knee OA in the elderly: the Health ABC study. Arthritis Rheum 46(Suppl):S372.

7. Jordan J, Luta G, Stabler T, et al. (2002). Serum C-reactive protein (CRP) and osteoarthritis. Arthritis Rheum 49(Suppl 9):S373.

8. Spector TD, Nandra D, Doyle DV, Mackillop N, Gallimore JR, Pepys MB. (1997). Low-level increases in serum C-reactive protein are present in early osteoarthritis of the knee and predict progressive disease. Arthritis Rheum 40(4):723–727.

9. Sturmer T, Koenig W, Gunther KP. (2004). Severity and extent of osteoarthritis and low grade systemic inflammation as assessed by high sensitivity C reactive protein. Ann Rheum Dis 63:200–205.

10. Bonnet C and Walsh DA. (2005). Osteoarthritis, angiogenesis and inflammation. Rheumatology (Oxford) 44(1):7–16.

11. Wegman A, van der Windt D, van Tulder M, Stalman W, de Vries T. (2004). Nonsteroidal antiinflammatory drugs or acetaminophen for osteoarthritis of the hip or knee? A systematic review of evidence and guidelines. J Rheumatol 31(2):344–354.

12. Pincus T, Koch G, Lei H, Mangal B, Sokka T, Moskowitz R, et al. (2004). Patient Preference for Placebo, Acetaminophen (paracetamol) or Celecoxib Efficacy Studies (PACES): two randomised, double blind, placebo controlled, crossover clinical trials in patients with knee or hip osteoarthritis. Ann Rheum Dis 63(8):931–939.

13. Boureau F, Schneid H, Zeghari N, Wall R, Bourgeois P. (2004). The IPSO study: ibuprofen, paracetamol study in osteoarthritis. A randomised comparative clinical study comparing the efficacy and safety of ibuprofen and paracetamol analgesic treatment of osteoarthritis of the knee or hip. Ann Rheum Dis 63(9):1028–1034.

14. Antman E, Bennett JS, Daugherty A, Furberg C, Roberts H, Taubert KA. (2007). Use of nonsteroidal antiinflammatory drugs: an update for clinicians: a scientific statement from the American Heart Association. Circulation 115(12):1634–1642.

15. Lanza F. (1984). Endoscopic studies of gastric and duodenal injury after the use of ibuprofen, asprin and other nonsteroidal anti-inflammatory agents. Am J Med 77(1A):19–24.

16. Fries J, Williams CA, Bloch DA. (1991). The relative toxicity of nonsteroidal antiinflammatory drugs. Arthritis Rheum 34(11):1353–1360.

17. Hernandez-Diaz S and Rodriguez A. (2000). Association between nonsteroidal anti-inflammatory drugs and upper gastrointestinal tract bleeding/perforation. Am Med Assoc 2000(160):2093–2099.

18. Mason L, et al. (2004). Topical NSAIDs for chronic musculoskeletal pain: systematic review and meta-analysis. BMC Musculoskelet Disord 5:28.

19. Lin J, Zhang W, Jones A, Doherty M. (2004). Efficacy of topical non-steroidal anti-inflammatory drugs in the treatment of osteoarthritis: meta-analysis of randomised controlled trials. BMJ 329(7461):324.

20. Towheed T. (2006). Pennsaid therapy for osteoarthritis of the knee: a systematic review and metaanalysis of randomized controlled trials. J Rheumatol 33(3): 567–573.

21. Tugwell P, Wells GA, Shainhouse JZ. (2004). Equivalence study of a topical diclofenac solution (pennsaid) compared with oral diclofenac in symptomatic treatment of osteoarthritis of the knee: a randomized controlled trial. J Rheumatol 31(10):2002–2012.

22. Underwood M, Ashby D, Cross P, Hennessy E, Letley L, Martin J, Mt-Isa S, Parsons S, Vickers M, Whyte K. (2007). Advice to use topical or oral ibuprofen for chronic knee pain in older people: randomised controlled trial and patient preference study. BMJ 336(7636):138–142.

23. Myers S, Brandt KD, O'Connor BL. (1991). Low dose prednisone treatment does not reduce the severity of osteoarthritis in dogs after anterior cruciate ligament transection. J Rheumatol 18(12):1856–1862.

24. Arroll B and Goodyear-Smith F. (2004). Corticosteroid injections for osteoarthritis of the knee: meta-analysis. BMJ 328(7444):869.

25. Raynauld J, Buckland-Wright C, Ward R, Choquette D, Haraoui B, Martel-Pelletier J, Uthman I, Khy V, Tremblay JL, Bertrand C, Pelletier JP. (2003). Safety and efficacy of long-term intraarticular steroid injections in osteoarthritis of the knee: a randomized, double-blind, placebo-controlled trial. Arthritis Rheum 48(2):370–377.

26. Jones A and Doherty M. (1996). Intra-articular corticosteroids are effective in osteoarthritis but there are no clinical predictors of response. Ann Rheum Dis 55(11):829–832.

27. Meenagh G, Patton J, Kynes C, Wright GD. (2004). A randomised controlled trial of intra-articular corticosteroid injection of the carpometacarpal joint of the thumb in osteoarthritis. Ann Rheum Dis 63(10):1260–1263.

28. Pasquali Ronchetti I, Guerra D, Taparelli F, Boraldi F, Bergamini G, Mori G, Zizzi F, Frizziero L. (2001). Morphological analysis of knee synovial membrane biopsies from a randomized controlled clinical study comparing the effects of sodium hyaluronate (Hyalgan) and methylprednisolone acetate (Depomedrol) in osteoarthritis. Rheumatology (Oxford) 40(2):158–169.

29. Ostergaard M, Ejbjerg B, Stoltenberg M, Gideon P, Volck B, Skov K, Jensen CH, Lorenzen I. (2001). Quantitative magnetic resonance imaging as marker of synovial membrane regeneration and recurrence of synovitis after arthroscopic knee joint synovectomy: a one year follow up study. Ann Rheum Dis 60(3):233–236.

INDEX

Pain in Osteoarthritis, Edited by David T. Felson and Hans-Georg Schaible
Copyright © 2009 Wiley-Blackwell.